Living Lean and Loving It

Living Lean and Loving It

Eve Lowry, R.D.

Carla Mulligan Ennis

MOSBY/FORMAN

1988

Editor: Jacqueline Ohlgart Yaiser
Project Manager: Peggy Fagen
Design: Rey Umali

Photography by Dave Brooks, Brooks Photo

For information, contact The C.V. Mosby Company, 11830 Westline Industrial Drive, St. Louis, Missouri 63146

Printed in the United States of America

International Standard Book Number 0-8016-3215-3

Table of Contents

We dedicate this book to Eve's mother,

Aniela L. Thomas

Who sustained us with her faith, love, humor, and inexhaustible capacity to . . .
cook it one more time!

And to Carla's husband, Dave, and their daughter, Kristin,
And Eve's husband, Ken, and her father, Jan,
for all the years of eating (and cheering) our experimental cooking.

Foreword

Living Lean and Loving It is an educational masterpiece—a cookbook for accomplished or beginning cooks who want to serve their families less fat and more whole ingredients. I have served these dishes at my Lake Tahoe Fit or Fat programs and for years people have asked me for the recipes. If Americans would promote family health at the dinner table—prepare delicious foods without so darned much fat—many of the so-called "modern diseases" would be a thing of the past.

It surprises me how many times I have gone back to a favorite recipe to look at its nutritional evaluation. Some things are difficult to remember—calcium or protein or calories from fat—and the information is there at a quick glance. Beyond a doubt, the recipes are good, but Eve and Carla's nutrition graphs are what makes *Living Lean and Loving* It unique.

This book will allow you to evaluate your diet scientifically without needing a degree in nutrition. The text—especially the weight control section—is worth the price of the book by itself. It contains everything you need to know to achieve permanent weight control. The material on everything from children to fiber to sodium make this book a compendium for healthy living.

Carla and Eve have worked for me over the years, and I should have known when they told me they were writing a cookbook that it would be more than a diet book or a collection of recipes. When Eve Lowry and Carla Mulligan tackle something, it may take years but the result is well researched and well written.

Living Lean and Loving It will help people of all ages lead healthier lives whether they are fit or fat.

Covert Bailey, M.S.
Author, *Fit or Fat, The Fit or Fat Target Diet*

Acknowledgments

Six years ago, we started working on this book. Since then, we've been helped by everyone we know who likes us at all. So, to all of you who gave so generously of your time, your talent, your food, and your treasured recipes—thank you.

We would also like to gratefully acknowledge:

Dan Levine, for donating his considerable editorial talent when it was most needed;

Dr. George Briggs and Dr. Susan Oace of University of California–Berkeley; Dr. Megan Hubbard and the Tahoe Family Physicians; Dr. James Anderson of the University of Kentucky, and Drs. Earl Trumble, Craig Smith, and John Agnew of the Medical Clinic of Sacramento, for assistance with medical and nutrition research information;

Anna Thomas and Gregory Nava, for telling us no one in New York would buy the book if we put Velveeta in the nachos;

Bob Pinckney, for his enthusiastic help with photography, and Mark Thomas, for running a thousand errands;

Patrick Bennett of the "Tahoe Reader," Helen Hug, and Tom Barnes, for editorial advice;

Sharon Denton and Sharon Robbins, for professional typing, straight through the weekend;

Beverly Nash and Troy Nakamoto of the South Lake Tahoe Mikasa Store, for their generous assistance with photo props and set design; and Sierra Bookshop for prop loan;

Mrs. Eleanor Killebrew, for graciously allowing us to shoot the cover photograph in her beautiful home in Tahoe;

Len and Claudia Forman, for recognizing the worth in this project and bringing it to publication;

Jackie Yaiser, for the uncompromising professionalism, tact, and good cheer with which she directed this publication;

and finally to Peggy Fagen, our Project Editor, who made it all fit, saw a thousand details through the completion, and cheerfully informed us that "it *has* been fun, but today is the last day."

Living Lean
and
Loving It

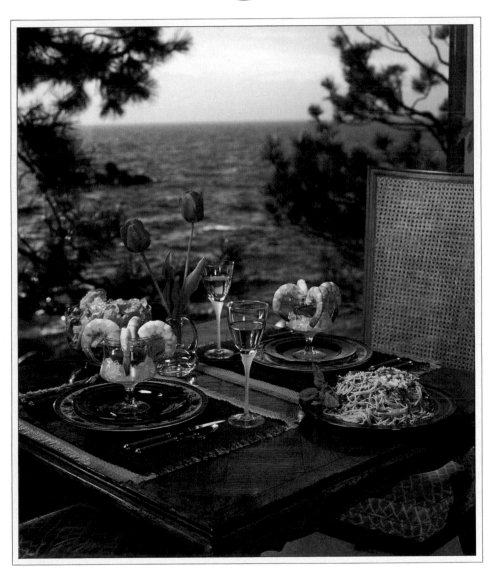

INTRODUCTION

Oliver Twist, in the musical *Oliver*, holds up a bowl of gruel and beseechingly sings, "FOOD, GLORIOUS FOOD!" Not a soul in the audience is left untouched. We all eat! But more than that, each of us has feelings, memories, even traditions, tied up with food. Try to imagine Easter without colored eggs and chocolate bunnies or Thanksgiving without turkey! While we may agree that special foods are important to holiday celebrations, many of us don't realize how much we care about everyday food choices—until our usual foods are taken away. Maybe we're in a foreign country, or maybe just on a diet. Then we notice that food is part of almost everything we do in life! Food is nachos and margaritas for TGIF, orange-frosted cupcakes for your first-grader's Halloween Carnival, and chicken noodle soup when you've got the flu. Eating isn't just vital to health, it's a joy and a comfort.

Unfortunately, some people, in fact, many people are fat. In our work as nutrition and fitness consultants, we see hundreds of patients every month, and most of them want to lose weight. They don't come to us to learn about eating the foods they love. They want to know how to stop being fat, at almost any cost. Yet, these same patients have taught us, each in their own way, that every diet plan will fail if it ignores the emotional side of eating. No two people are alike when it comes to feelings about food. One patient told us that he loved going to the movies, but if he had to cut out popcorn, he might as well stay home. Another explained to us that having a hot dog at the ballpark is just as important as yelling at the umpire.

Diets tend to tell us exactly what we don't want to hear: that we have to give up the things we most enjoy. Is it worth it, just to be slim and healthy? Maybe, maybe not. A better question is, does avoiding the foods we love even work? Americans have been obsessed with dieting for 20 years, and in that time the average adult's weight has gone up by 10 pounds!

This book is really about cooking, eating, and enjoying! It's a cookbook designed to take a difficult, painful, and often unsuccessful process and make it simple, pleasant, and satisfying. In short, instead of telling you to go on a diet, we will show you how to **put your *food* on a diet** instead.

How? In a word—less. Less fat, less sugar, less sodium, and fewer calories but not necessarily less food. The trick lies in figuring out just how much less. Take away too much, and you end up with dry and tasteless "diet food" that nobody wants to eat. Leaving in just enough to give food the good, old-fashioned flavors we love is what *Living Lean* is all about—hearty portions of favorite foods that taste the way they're supposed to taste, without the traditional fat and calories.

You can eat hamburgers, pizza, and tacos if that's what you like best, or Caesar salad and linguine with clam sauce if those are the foods that make your heart sing. The secret lies in our low-fat cooking techniques. One of the happiest discoveries you will make, as you learn to get more for less, is that there's really no need to give up your own unique style of eating. In fact, even people who resist change (like children and spouses) can be enthusiastic about leaned-down versions of foods they know and love. Quiet improvements—a bit less fat, a leaner cut of meat, a few more vegetables in the stew pot—can succeed where a whole new menu would fail.

Living Lean is not just for people who are tired of dieting. There's more to nutrition than weight control. Many highly regarded researchers now believe that 50% to 75% of modern human disease can be prevented with proper diet and exercise. In recent years, they've been giving us so much advice, sometimes we wondered if there would be anything left that was safe to eat! Diabetes doctors advised against sugar, heart specialists warned us about fats and sodium, gastroenterologists recommended more fiber, allergists debated additives, and cancer specialists questioned everything from our breakfast coffee to the burger we barbequed for supper! Happily, the muddle is beginning to clear. Instead of a different diet for each complaint, it turns out that the entire medical community has been recommending the same foods; whole grains, fruits and vegetables, beans and seeds, lean meats, and low-fat dairy products!

In preparing our recipes, we have looked for ingredients that provide the most nutrients for the fewest calories. These inevitably turn out to be whole foods; whole wheat flour instead of white, brown rice, whole grain pasta, and naturally, an abundance of fresh fruits and vegetables. When whole ingredients are used in cooking, it isn't necessary to use additives such as vitamin pills, protein powders or even raw bran. If you don't remove the nutrients from your foods to begin with, you don't have to worry about putting them back.

We know that using fresh, whole foods, prepared with a measure of art and a touch of love sounds fine for someone with a lot of time, or a kitchen staff, but the rest of us have jobs, right? The care and feeding of family, friends, and household pets is something we manage to squeeze into those few precious hours between the time clock and the alarm clock. Happily, the wonders of modern technology are on our side. With a freezer, a food processor, and a nonstick skillet, we can work epicurean wonders in record time. The following recipes will show you how to provide your family with state-of-the-art nutrition, and flavors that remind you of Grandma. In addition, our time-saving techniques are designed to let you enjoy your creations.

Finally, we included a little wickedness. Sometimes it's the small indulgences, the ones we just can't seem to do without, that sabotage a complete health program. Rather than throw in the towel on the entire effort, it makes better sense to allow for a few delightful human imperfections. That's why we include recipes for raspberry cheesecake, banana cream pudding, fried chicken, and even wine coolers.

We know that the purest of the pure will abstain from all fat, cholesterol, sugar, salt, and alcohol, now and forever. But for most of us such self-denial and food avoidance are temporary at best. Will power is a finite commodity, and even the toughest souls eventually run out.

So, it's time to stop dieting and start making food taste as wonderful as it should, without stripping it of nutrients and loading it with calories. It's time to start LIVING LEAN ... AND LOVING IT!

Weight Control

Dr. John Thomas, age 36, seemed to have it all. He was a busy family practice physician, highly regarded by patients, partners, and staff. He was happily married and had recently become a father for the second time. But he was fat. He didn't look terribly fat. The 40 extra pounds he carried were spread out pretty comfortably over his 6′2″ frame. Nevertheless, he was tired of his perennial pudge. He had been one of those cute, bright, chubby children, who had grown up to become a cute, bright, chubby adult. On the pretext of checking out our weight control clinic for patient referrals, he signed up.

It turned out that before choosing medicine as his profession, John had studied gourmet cooking in Paris. When he met Kathy, a witty, intelligent, beautiful woman, *and* a gourmet cook, it was a match. Two babies and several years later, Kathy, like John, found herself carrying extra pounds of ballast. For John and Kathy, a relaxing weekend meant inviting a few friends for a seven course feast—and spending the better part of 2 days up to their elbows in truffles, Cognac, rare meats, ripe cheeses, select wines, and, of course, the purest, freshest, sweet cream and butter they could find. It only made sense that Kathy should sign up for our clinic along with John. After all, they loved and lived and laughed together, why not grit their teeth, square their shoulders, and plunge into acute sensory deprivation (read: diet) together.

By the end of our 10-week weight control class, Kathy was 13 pounds lighter, while John had lost 27 pounds. Now the real test began. Without the support of our clinic staff, would the pounds creep back? We waited 4 months, then called them in for a checkup. Kathy had shed an additional 12 pounds, and John

had dropped another 5. Now, a year later, both maintain their weights within 5 pounds of ideal, without living under the long dark shadow of a diet.

Has their social life—cooking, eating, and sharing gourmet foods—gone by the wayside? To the contrary, since they discovered that a platter of Monterey Bay prawns can be sauteed with a tablespoon of fresh sweet butter rather than a half pound, their culinary creativity has simply taken a new direction. At the last class meeting, Kathy admitted that she had been pretty skeptical about our philosophy that the most successful pathway to permanent weight control lies in not depriving yourself of the foods you love. Nevertheless, what Kathy and John learned for themselves was that food can, in fact, be flavorful, delicious, even elegant, without being smothered in fat.

The couple made another, equally important, discovery. They learned that even very busy people can give 20 minutes each day to exercise, once they experience the benefits derived for that small price.

Recent reports have it that on Saturdays John can be seen, in sweats and sneakers, pulling two little boys in a red wagon 20 city blocks to his favorite gourmet market. Kathy, meanwhile, uses her time off from the kids to unwind at the health club. Either one will tell you that they never imagined losing weight could be so pleasurable, so permanent, and so unlike a "diet."

THE DIET SCAM

Americans are fat—and sad about it. Being fat and sad makes us susceptible to every diet scam that promises quick weight loss. At any given moment roughly 25 million American adults are on diets to lose weight, while another 25 million are between diets, rebounding from one and contemplating another. We spend an astounding 14 billion dollars per year on weight reduction books, treatments, and devices. In our pursuit of slimness we swallow just about anything, from spirulina to starch-blockers. We buy every imaginable over-the-counter drug that promises appetite suppression, be it methylcellulose (ground up trees) or phenylpropanolamine (a decongestant).

Investing all that time, money, and willpower, we would expect good results. Yet, when we count the number of people trying to lose weight and compare it with the number who succeed, the failure rate is an appalling 95%! How can it be that today, with more nutrition information available than at any other time in history, only 5% of us are getting advice that works?

We're not stupid. Rather, we fail to use our brains when we approach dieting because we are responding to two of the strongest human emotions—hope and fear. We want so badly to be thin at last (and at once) that reason itself deserts us. We become willing victims to the entrepreneurs who tell us exactly what we hope to hear. Nutrition hucksters prey on our fear of fatness to sell tonics and elixirs that promise painless and effortless weight loss.

VICTORS IN THE WAR ON FAT

It's time we looked to the 5% of dieters who do succeed. What are these people doing that's different? A person who belongs to this elite 5% is usually a veteran of the diet wars who has lost and regained the same 10 (or 30) pounds many time over. This person can count calories, carbohydrates, grams, ounces, cups, and servings—forward, backward, and standing on her head. But, more than anything else, this one person in twenty who actually achieves permanent weight control is the one who figures out that going on a diet eventually leads to going off a diet.

Will power is finite. No matter how much you have, the day you run out, the diet is over. What you won't ever lose, though, is your appetite for the foods you love, in amounts that will satisfy. If you are a habitual dieter this will mean eating more, rather than less, and eating foods you want, instead of those you think you should eat. If you have spent years cultivating the fine art of self-deprivation, this may sound a little crazy. To understand why eating well is the best way to lose fat, you just need to learn a few basic facts about nutrition—and behavior.

Fact #1: Rapid Weight Loss is not Permanent.

You didn't want to know that, did you? Why fool around losing 1 or 2 pounds a week when the world is full of people telling you how to do it faster? If you aren't quite ready to accept FACT #1, don't feel bad. Remember, that's how 95% of us react.

But, here's what the other 5% knows: Most of the weight lost on a rapid weight loss diet isn't fat. While our bathroom scales and the zippers on our jeans confirm the fact that we're losing weight fast, what they don't tell us is that it isn't fat. Metabolic balance studies done by reputable nutritionists have shown that most of the weight lost is, in fact, lean body mass. Lean body mass is everything in your body except fat, (muscles, organs, blood, bones, etc.). What you lose on a rapid weight loss diet turns out to be mostly muscle and water, along with some fat. How much fat? About the same amount you would lose on a safe weight reduction diet, about 2 pounds a week. You really can't burn fat any faster, even on the nastiest of starvation diets, so why not enjoy eating, save your muscle, and just lose fat!

But who cares what the weight we lose consists of? It's how much that counts, isn't it? Wrestlers and weight watchers have known for years that dumping water has got to be the ultimate in rapid weight loss. When they need to "make weight," they stop eating and drinking, even water, take a diuretic, and lose as much as 10 pounds overnight! Before you consider dehydration as an alternative to dieting, you should

know that the minute the rapidly reduced wrestlers are officially weighed in they head straight for the locker room and drink about a gallon of water in a desperate attempt to replace what they've lost. Water loss can be quite dangerous. Losing 10% of your body water makes you seriously sick; losing 20% generally kills you.

Diets that are very low in calories or carbohydrates cause an initial water loss of 5 to 10 pounds. This won't dehydrate you to the point of death, and it looks great on the scales, but it has nothing to do with fat. Besides, your body protects itself by replacing lost water just as soon as carbohydrate deprivation or starvation are no longer present. In other words, as soon as you go off the diet.

WHY DEPRIVATION DOESN'T WORK

So much for water. Now, how about muscle? Wouldn't it be okay to lose a little of that? It's actually a lot easier to lose a pound of muscle than a pound of fat. Here's why: lean muscle tissue contains about 500 calories per pound. You need, on the average, about 2000 calories to get through the day. If you go on a starvation diet you can enjoy rapid weight loss by burning up four pounds of muscle every day and using it for calories. The trouble with losing muscle, though, it that muscle is the very part of your body that burns calories. Every time you burn up some muscle tissue, you damage your ability to use calories. But how do we know that all those pounds falling off your body really aren't fat?

Elementary arithmetic! Fat tissue contains 3500 calories per pound. This means that a measly little pound of body fat has enough calories in it to feed you for almost 2 days (3500 divided by 2000 equal 1.75)! So, if you stop eating and start living off your fat, you should expect to lose a pound about every other day. That means it would take a whole week to lose 4 pounds, but that's not what happens. When a person goes on a total fast, he or she loses a lot more than 4 pounds per week. In fact, some of our favorite crash diets produce weight losses greater than that. The very fact that you lose 10, sometimes 15 pounds a week on these diets, should be your first clue that you are losing a whole lot of something else. You get your second clue when you gain it all back.

What do you gain back? All of the water, most of the muscle, and, ultimately, even more fat than you lost to begin with. There's nothing quite so disheartening as watching your weight go back up when you know you aren't overeating. That's why you are going to be amazed when we tell you to be thankful that you can gain back most of what you've lost. How can we say such a thing! If our bodies weren't clever enough to replace water losses almost immediately, we'd have bigger problems on our hands—like death by dehydration. If we weren't able to replace muscle tissue, half the population in this diet-happy nation would be in wheelchairs! Rebuilding lost muscle tissue takes a bit longer than rehydration, but the minute you start eating a decent amount of food (1200 to 1500 calories per day) your body starts putting it back on. Even though you are truly careful and only eat half the amount a person should be able to eat, the weight goes back up! Why? Because your thrifty body is snatching every available calorie to replace that precious muscle mass. Unfortunately, the muscles' calorie-burning ability won't be fully restored until you begin to exercise. We'll get back to that later. For now, we hope you understand that once the water and muscle are replaced so is most of the weight that was lost. You always suspected there had to be some very good reason not to put yourself through the torture of a starvation diet, didn't you? Rapid weight loss isn't permanent.

Now to the second fact.

Fact #2: Rapid Weight Loss Means Future Fat.

You've probably heard of the Yo-yo Syndrome. Dr. Jean Mayer of Tufts University calls it "the rhythm method of girth control." We think one of our weight control students put it best: "Lose 10, gain 12."

Rapid weight loss changes your metabolism. Two things happen, and neither of them are nice to hear. First, your body's ability to burn calories diminishes. Second, it's ability to store fat increases. The way our bodies function, muscle tissue uses calories, fat tissue stores calories. The more muscle you have, the more calories you burn, whether you are sitting in a chair, walking down the street, or even sleeping in your bed at night. While the fat tissue hangs around, using as few calories as possible, the muscle tissue busily burns calories, even while you are at rest, just maintaining what we call muscle tone.*

Now, does it really make sense to lose weight by burning up your muscles? Absolutely not! You may weigh 10 pounds less, but you are still fat, and now you need fewer calories to stay fat. If you could eat 2000 calories without gaining weight before the crash diet, now you may cross the line at 1500 or 1600 calories. In fact, it's entirely possible that you will now *gain* weight on the same diet which used to result in a *loss*! Why? You now have less muscle tissue and require fewer calories to perform the same activities! Once you understand what makes your body do this to you, it will be easier to resist the temptation to suffer through another diet. Do you think naturally thin people stay that way by constantly denying themselves the foods they like? Of course not! To move toward the metabolism of easy leanness, you

need to stop fighting the "losing battle" and begin eating enough to keep your muscles happy!

There's yet another reason why you gain weight so easily after an overly strict diet. Your metabolism is actually slowed down! The overall effect has been dubbed the "Survival Syndrome." To survive, the body responds to severe calorie deprivation by conserving energy. The billions of cells where calories are used don't have any way of knowing that you are starving yourself on purpose. To them, the 300 calories of liquid protein that you call the blender diet looks about the same as the 300 calories of stale bread and cabbage fed to prisoners in POW camps. At the starvation level your cells don't care where the calories are coming from, they just know they aren't getting enough.

The system goes into survival mode. Calories are saved and none are spent unless it's absolutely unavoidable. Energy cutbacks are made wherever possible. Since there aren't any extra calories for heat production, body temperature drops a bit. The dieter feels "chilly." To prevent further heat loss, blood supply to the tiny vessels near the body surface is cut back. The dieter's skin feels rough and dry. Nonessential movements are eliminated. The dieter feels listless, fatigued. Attempts at exercise are met with dizziness and cramps. Even the heartbeat and breathing rate are slowed down to conserve energy.

Repeated bouts with very low-calorie dieting can impose the survival mode as a way of life. By gradually chipping away at your calorie-burning muscles and slowing down the metabolic rate of what's left, crash dieting turns you into a slow, tired, cold person who gets fat on a diet that would starve a gnat. Rapid weight loss means future fat.

HOPE FOR THE HABITUAL DIETER

There is hope. The damage can be repaired. What's more, the rehabilitation process can be a lot of fun. It consists of playing and eating—exercise and adequate nutrition. All you have to do is forget about losing weight and learn about losing fat. There are 5 simple rules:

1. Consume enough calories to prevent muscle loss. For most women this means at least 1200 calories per day, for most men at least 1500 while you are losing fat and a good deal more once you reach your goal.

2. Eat half or more of these calories in the form of complex carbohydrates like whole-grain breads and cereals, beans, and vegetables. (Yes, we mean pasta, potatoes, pilaf, and pancakes!) Your basic metabolic functions—things like heartbeat, breathing, brain activity—require a constant supply of carbohydrate (specifically, glucose). If you don't eat enough carbohydrate, your body simply tears down muscle protein and turns it into sugar to meet energy needs.

---

*The actual number of calories burned by a pound of muscle depends on fitness and individual metabolism.

3. Eat plenty of fiber. It increases calorie-burning activity in the digestive system and can assist with appetite control as well. How much is plenty? Just exactly the amount provided by nature to the person who eats whole foods, rather than "refined" parts of foods; for example, whole-grain breads and cereals, legumes, vegetables, and fruits (things like chili, corn muffins, and even our blackberry pie).

4. Eat a variety of foods from all four of the basic food groups to achieve a balanced diet. Select low-fat, low-sugar items to get all the nutrients you need without going over your personal calorie limit.

5. Cut calories, not portions. Eat when you're hungry, and take enough to satisfy your appetite. Simply refrain from lacing foods with quite so much sugar and fat. That way you get full-sized portions of the foods you like best for about half the usual calories.

There you have it, the prescription for good nutrition and healthy weight reduction. Optimal health and ideal body weight do not require deprivation. The answer actually lies in *better* eating. Preparing the foods you love with low-fat, low-sugar, and high-fiber ingredients allows you to cut calories while actually increasing nutrients. That's good eating, and it's exactly what this book is about.

Medical research on obesity indicates that it's absolutely essential to eat, and in fact, to eat rather well, in order to lose fat. Eating healthy portions of nutritious foods signals our bodies that all is well, that we're not in danger of starving, and that its OK to burn fat. If you follow our five rules for burning fat, you will provide the vital signals of nutritional well-being to your body, and your body will respond by burning fat! While the bulges, bumps, and rolls are disappearing, you will find yourself eating more, rather than less, and choosing your favorite foods, rather than someone else's diet prescriptions.

Fact #3: There's No Law Against Lying About Nutrition

People lie about nutrition in books and magazines, on TV and radio, all the time. Your only protection is your own good judgment, based on your knowledge of nutrition. But even when you know that fat loss takes time, even when you understand why rapid weight loss can't be fat loss; there will be days you don't care. The day your husband tells you he sold more insurance than anyone else in the office and won that trip to Hawaii. The day you pick up the mail and find an invitation to your high school reunion. The Saturday night which finds you home alone, flipping through TV *Guide*. These are the times when it is critical to remind yourself that lying about rapid weight loss is not against the law.

Freedom of speech protects the right of an author to make up any story he thinks will sell, call it nutrition, and publish it. The only place misinforma-tion becomes illegal is on the label of a product. Many charming collections of nutrition fiction have topped the bestseller list for weeks. One even received a tongue-in-cheek award for "creative physiology" from an east coast medical group with a strong sense of humor. Unfortunately, to people without a background in clinical nutrition, these diets, as well as their medically ridiculous rationales, seem perfectly plausible. In fact when people try these diets and find they do lose weight, they are ecstatic! Do you think they worry about the diarrhea, the dizziness, the occasional lightheadedness? Not for a minute. What about deficiencies in such nutrients as protein, calcium, iron, and zinc? As long as the scale shows a weight loss, most are happy enough to limit themselves to nothing but fruit, or red meat and martinis, or other nutritionally unsound selections.

The greatest irony is that when such faithful dieters regain the weight after going off one of these diets, they blame themselves. They believe they are overeating, when their bodies are simply and predictably replacing lean body mass. In this case, what they don't know really *can* hurt them. Watching the scales go back up can cause the unwary dieter to conclude that its time to go on another crash diet — to do some more damage to his body.

Now, if starvation is out and eating well is in, how do we get rid of all this fat? Does losing weight have to take forever? Not at all. You can burn off between 1 and 3 pounds of actual body fat each week, while eating foods you like, in quantities that keep you satisfied. Your own individual rate of fat loss will depend on the state of your metabolism. If your metabolism could be called "sluggish," while your appetite would do justice to a lumberjack, don't despair. Stepping up your metabolism, while satisfying even the healthiest appetite is exactly what this book is about.

Switching back to whole foods and balanced nutrition is not quite all it takes to restore your body's ability to burn fat. When it comes to weight control, the bottom line is still calculated in calories. Half the adults in America are fat by the time they reach midlife simply because they have eaten too many calories. But just when did so many of us start eating so much? And why didn't we notice?

A lot of people think we eat more than our grandparents did, and that's why we're fatter. Not true. If you compare our average caloric intake to that of our grandparents, it's about the same, or even a bit less. The difference is that two generations ago people exercised more. Grandma and Grandpa didn't have jogging shoes, but they worked out every day. Remember those stories about children walking 5 miles to get to school? They weren't doing it because their parents wouldn't give them the car keys. Just getting through the day involved exercise for all.

For example, preparing breakfast started with cutting and carrying wood to build a fire in the cookstove, hauling water from the well to cook the oatmeal, gathering eggs in the henyard, perhaps milking the cows, and possibly feeding the pigs to make future hams and bacon. Somewhere along the line there was a trip into town to get flour and salt for the biscuits. Horses and buggies didn't have shock absorbers, heaters, or air conditioners, so calories were used while holding onto one's seat and maintaining one's body temperature. And, if you wanted the "high-priced spread" on those biscuits, you were looking at 20 to 30 minutes of active duty on the butter churn. . . .

In a nutshell: we don't eat more than our grandparents did, we just aren't as active. Unfortunately, our food habits hearken back to a time when we burned up a "grand slam" breakfast halfway through the morning chores. Today the same heap of bacon, eggs, and hash browns will fuel the average technocrat for a day and a half. We're caught in the middle of an unbalanced equation; more calories coming in than going out.

Exercise is the other half of the solution to the problem of fat. Exercise allows you to balance that energy equation and start Living Lean.

EXERCISE IS CHILD'S PLAY

Excuse the pun, but the answer to adult obesity is child's play. Think about it. We come into this world hellbent on energy expenditure. First we run our mothers ragged by climbing the furniture, doing chin-ups on the drapes, bouncing on our beds instead of sleeping in them, and performing somersaults in our best clothes when we visit relatives. We're sent to school where we squirm in our seats, tap our fingers, toes, and pencils, run down crowded hallways, and generally drive our teachers crazy. Finally, about the time that puberty intrudes, we begin to internalize the sedentary maxims of adulthood. It takes a few years, but eventually no one has to tell us to "sit still!", "stop running!", "slow down!", and "for goodness sake, stop fidgeting!"

Have you ever tried to keep up with a baby? You know that a crawling or toddling youngster can cover a lot of ground; but what about tiny babies who can't even stand up yet? Researchers studying the muscular development of infants invited professional athletes to lie on the floor and mimic the movements of an infant. After a mere 4 or 5 hours of "floor exercises" the athletes were exhausted, while the infants, whether awake or asleep, seemed to require these continual calisthenics to keep their bodies happy.

So do you, and so does every other human body. Never before in our history have so many of us survived with so little physical exercise. Given automatic garage-door openers, elevators, and office jobs, we manage to work longer, harder, and faster without ever flexing a muscle. Many of us are so unaccustomed to exercise we view it as a form of torture. Yet, there was a time in your life that exercise was the reward you got at recess, and sitting down in a quiet corner was called punishment. To retrieve the easy leanness of childhood we need to find ways to allow some movement back into our lives.

The fastest route to fat loss is the slow, sustained, and systemic exercise called aerobics. Aerobic exercise not only burns off "old" fat, it prevents future fat! If you want to be lean, you need to indulge in some form of regular aerobic exercise. Indulge? Yes, that's the word we wanted. Aerobic exercise is addictive. The first few weeks you hate it, but you do it because you know it's good for you. The next few weeks you keep going because you think it has to get better. At least, you're sure it couldn't get worse. Pretty soon you are running strictly on stubbornness. Then, one perfectly usual day, as you are jogging or biking or dancing along, you are astonished to notice that you are really having a very good time.

Aerobics: A High-Yield Investment

The only way to find out how good it can feel to exercise is to sweat past those first few weeks when it really doesn't. Here's a sneak preview of some of the things you are going to love about aerobic exercise:

- It curbs your appetite.
- It gives you energy.
- It makes your body look great.
- It burns a lot of calories while you do it.
- It burns more calories by stepping up your metabolic rate for hours after you do it.
- It makes you sleep better.
- It gives you a natural high!

Even skinny and naturally cheerful people can benefit from aerobics. Each day evidence mounts that aerobic exercise is a preventive factor in cardiovascular diseases, such as heart attack, stroke, hypertension, and atherosclerosis. Try it. First you'll hate it, then you'll like it, and eventually, you'll crave it!

Many people equate aerobics with jogging, but it really can be almost anything from dancing to hiking. Whether or not an exercise is aerobic just depends on the pace. It has to be fast enough to increase your heart rate, but not so fast that you're gasping for air. Aerobic exercise burns fat just as long as there is plenty of oxygen around to "fan the fire." That's why its called aerobics; it only works when you are getting enough air. Here's the "working man's" definition of aerobic exercise: . . . anything that makes you breath deeply and sweat for 15 or 20 uninterrupted minutes, but doesn't interfere with carrying on a conversation.

Men, in particular, seem to have trouble exercising without trying to break records. When it comes to losing fat, harder and faster isn't necessarily better.

Getting out of breath is a signal from Mother Nature to slow down. If you don't want to listen to Mother, ask your doctor. He or she will tell you that feeling out of breath means your body has reached its maximum ability to supply oxygen, but the supply is still not enough to keep up with the demand. At this point your body stops burning fat and starts burning blood sugar. For the person trying to lose weight, this is bad news in more ways than one. Dipping into your limited supply of blood sugar by doing too much, too fast leaves you tired, hungry, and grouchy. Not a strong position for a person trying to make wise food choices.

We started out telling you not to overdiet, and now we're telling you not to overexercise. Losing fat may not be so bad after all. But if you don't deprive yourself of the foods you love or run yourself into the ground with exercise, isn't it going to take forever to get that fat off? Well, that's the best part of all. You can actually lose fat faster with a moderate restriction of calories and a reasonable amount of exercise than you can by overdoing either one. Most people can burn from 1 to 3 pounds of fat per week by following a practically painless program of a little bit of both — cutting calories and exercising.

MAKE YOUR OWN RULES

How much is "a little bit of both"? If you're waiting for "the diet," complete with allowed foods, menu plans, and portion sizes, you haven't been paying attention. Instead of telling you what to eat, we're going to show you how to put together your very own personal diet plan.

The first step is deciding how many calories you need. You guessed it; everyone is different. (Nobody said life was going to be fair.) A typical complaint heard from less-than-lissome young housewives goes something like this: "My husband eats three times as much as I do, sits at a desk all day, watches football in the evening, and stays thin while I get fat!" The hardworking housewife isn't dreaming this up. She does eat less food and do more physical work than her husband. But he burns more calories. Here's why:

Calorie need depends on activity and on lean body mass — the amount of muscle you have. The amount of muscle you have depends on your sex (men have more muscle than women), your frame size (big people have more muscle than little people), and your fitness (fit people have more muscle than fat people).

As you can see, the typical young husband will win the calorie-burning contest hands down when competing against his wife. He's a male, he's usually bigger, and, at least for the first few years, he's generally more fit. He's reaping the benefits of high school and perhaps college athletics, which built up that calorie-burning machinery called lean body mass! But he's sliding; he's on borrowed time. About the age of 40,

he's apt to find himself in the same predicament as his wife; eating less and getting fatter.

Every individual is unique. Two people of the same sex, same age, same height, and even same weight can have very different calorie requirements. It all depends on lean body mass! (Almost!) The other thing that counts a lot is what you do all day with your lean body mass. If you let it sit in an easy chair, it just won't burn as many calories as it can if you run it around the neighborhood for 20 or 30 minutes. Calorie needs increase as you become more fit.* How would it feel to be one of those aggravatingly thin people who go about eating as they please, neither getting fat, nor worrying about it? Exercise regularly, and you will know. It feels even more terrific than it sounds.

But what about your calorie requirements right now? How many calories do you need, given your present condition, to get through your normal day? Well, there are lots of complicated regression equations devised by nutrition scientists to estimate how many calories a body needs. We're not going to give you any of them. The most accurate way to determine your individual calorie requirements is simply to keep track.

Keep a Food Record

- Carry a small notepad in your pocket for 7 days, and write down every morsel of food that you put in your mouth.
- Include both work days and weekend days in this tally. Many of us eat quite differently during the work week than we do on our days off.
- Enter each food in your record at the time that you eat it. Remembering what you've eaten from hour to hour is tricky; writing it down in the evening is a joke.
- Pay close attention to amounts. A "serving" depends on the server, the servee, and what's being served. A cryptic note about a ton of spaghetti may not evoke any memories at all by the end of the week. Better to write down "2 cups spaghetti/tomato sauce, 3 tiny meatballs." That should at least put you in the ballpark when the time comes to guess at the calorie content.
- Leave some room in the margin. At the end of the week we are going to ask you to look up the calories.

If you've never kept a food record, but you suspect it could be a bit intimidating, consider yourself astute. Behavioral scientists tell us that writing down everything you put in your mouth is one of the most powerful tools for controlling food intake. You might use this principle later on, but for now, try to eat in

---

*For an accurate, yet understandable explanation of the relationship of weight control to fitness, we refer you to *Fit or Fat* by Covert Bailey.

your usual fashion. If you are accustomed to having three beers and a large order of nachos after work on Friday, then do so but write it down ("30 corn chips, 3 oz. cheese, 2 T. chiles," etc.).

Remember, the purpose here is to find out how many calories you, personally, need to maintain the body you have right now. You will get the best information by doing the usual. This is neither the week to binge nor to diet, unless that *is* the usual. To help you do this right the first time, we've put together some food records to demonstrate the method and to point out some potential pitfalls. Here is a day in the life of a typical (overweight) American couple:

	WIFE		HUSBAND
7am	1 egg, poached 2 sl. w.w. toast 2 coffee, 2 T. skim milk	7am	coffee
10am	1 lg. orange tea, 1 t. honey	10am	2 jelly donuts coffee
12:00	tuna sandwich (½ can w.p. tuna 2 sl. w.w. bread 1 T. diet mayo. lettuce, tomato, pickle) Diet Coke sm. apple	12:00	French dip sandwich potato salad dill pickle Coke
3:30pm	diet cocoa (40 cal.)	3:30pm	coffee, Snickers bar
6pm	2 ozs. wine, club soda carrot, celery sticks	6pm	2 highballs
7pm	3 c. salad (lettuce, tomato, onion, pepper, sprouts, mushrooms) 3 T. diet dressing (60 cal.) 1 broiled chicken brst., skinned 1 lg. (10 oz.) baked pot. 2 T. LF yogurt, chives 1 c. green beans, lemon 1 coffee/½ pack cocoa (20 cal.)	7pm	sm. tossed salad Roquefort, Bacos Broiled chicken, 4pcs. baked potato, bu. green beans, bu. 2 glasses wine

Two people who live together and share meals can have very different food intakes. You already know who had the most calories, but you might be surprised at the magnitude of the difference. The wife had about 1200 calories while the husband guesses he had about 2800! He can't really be sure; he didn't write down the amounts. At any rate, if this couple wants to lose fat by cutting down on calories, we can see that the wife is in trouble already. If she only eats 1200 calories per day she's at the minimum level; she can't cut back any further. These sample food records were compiled on a Monday (the most virtuous eating day of the week). As you will see, when she gets to the next step, the wife is going to be very glad she kept her food record for a full week. Don't be a deadbeat about recording! It's not that keeping accurate food records for a week is fun. In fact, it's a pain; but the

time you invest in doing this right, can save you from ever having to go on, or off, another diet.

Calculate Your Average Daily Calories

At the end of the week look up the calories for each food, and write the numbers where you left that space in the margin. Add up each day's total. Now, list the 7 days with their total calories alongside. Add the totals for the week, then divide by seven to get your daily average. Let's go back to our samples to see how this works out:

WIFE		HUSBAND	
Monday	1200	Monday	2800
Tuesday	1400	Tuesday	2500
Wednesday	1300	Wednesday	2400
Thursday	1500	Thursday	2700
Friday	2400	Friday	2900
Saturday	2800	Saturday	3200
Sunday	2400	Sunday	3100
Total	14000	Total	19600
Average (14,000 divided by 7 equals 2000)	2000	Average (19,600 divided by 7 equals 2800)	2800

Things are definitely looking better for the wife. Based on her daily average intake of 2000 calories, she can safely eliminate up to 800 calories per day, for a predicted fat loss of a pound and a half per week. Basically, she could just eat the same way she does on Mondays. The husband has a lot of running room. Since the minimum calorie allowance for a male is 1500, he could conceivably eliminate 1300 calories per day, but we wouldn't recommend it. True, he could burn almost 3 pounds of fat per week with caloric restriction alone, but the chances are strong that he would be uncomfortable with such a drastic change in his diet.

Once you've calculated your daily average, you can use this number to decide how many calories you should eat for optimal fat loss. The number will probably surprise you. Most of our patients swear they'll never lose weight if they eat that much! They all do.

Find Your Optimal Calorie Level

In other words, decide how many calories you would like to eliminate.

The rule of thumb is:

Eliminate 500 calories per day, burn 1 pound of fat
   per week
Eliminate 1000 calories per day, burn 2 pounds of fat
   per week
Eliminate 1500 calories per day, burn 3 pounds of fat
   per week

But—remember the minimums:

Women: Eat at least 1200 calories per day!
Men: Eat at least 1500 calories per day!

more to reduce blood cholesterol than cutting down on cholesterol itself. Naturally, doing both is what works best.

Before we go on, you should know that cholesterol is strictly an animal product. You won't find cholesterol in any food from the vegetable kingdom; not in a bean, a seed, a nut, a grain, or any part or kind of fruit or vegetable! Even fatty foods like peanut butter, avocados, and olives don't contain a drop of cholesterol. That's why peanut butter labels can brag about "no cholesterol"—peanut butter is vegetable, not animal.

SATURATED, POLYUNSATURATED, MONOUNSATURATED

The terms saturated, polyunsaturated, and monounsaturated refer to the fatty acids, or building blocks, that fats are made of. All the fats we eat can be divided into these three kinds of fatty acids. The names mean just what they imply. When something is *saturated*, it is filled up. In the case of fats, these names come from their chemical structures. When all the little chemical bonds are filled up, a fat is called saturated. (It's saturated with hydrogen.) An *unsaturated* fat, on the other hand, has some unfilled chemical bonds, and a fat with many unfilled bonds is *polyunsaturated*. If it has only one unfilled bond, it's called (you guessed it!) *monounsaturated*. There is a direct correlation between how saturated a fat is and how hard it is. So you can tell how saturated a fat is just by looking at it.

Think about the fats in your own kitchen. Have you ever made a beef stew or soup? When it sits in the refrigerator, the layer of fat on top gets so hard you can lift it off and break it! Bacon grease gets hard in the refrigerator too, but not as hard as beef fat. You can scoop it out of the grease can with a spoon. The fat layer on top of chicken soup gets semi-solid in the refrigerator, but not really hard. These three fats tell the whole story about the degree of saturation of fats. Food fats are mixtures. They contain several different kinds of fat components (fatty acids). Beef fat is harder (has more saturated fatty acids) than pork fat, which is harder (has more saturated fatty acids) than chicken fat.

Vegetable oils like corn, safflower, and cottonseed oils, are high in polyunsaturated fatty acids which stay liquid, even when they are cold. Have you ever put olive oil in the refrigerator? It turns hazy and gets thick, sometimes so thick you can't pour it out of the bottle until it warms up a bit. Olive oil contains mostly monounsaturated fatty acids. Peanut oil falls somewhere between olive and safflower; it has both mono- and polyunsaturated fatty acids. The harder a fat is, the more saturated it is.

Why do we care how saturated a fat is anyway? Medical research has shown that saturated fats are the culprits when it comes to high blood cholesterol, while polyunsaturated fats actually tend to bring it down. Monounsaturated fats (olive, avocado, and peanut oils) were for many years thought to have no effect, good or bad, on blood cholesterol, but new research indicates they may be better for lowering cholesterol than polyunsaturates. That's great news for Italians, Greeks, Orientals, and all the rest of us who like to cook with these flavorful fats.

But even the good fats add up. They may be unsaturated, they may be free of cholesterol and animal fat, but oils have just as many calories as any other kind of fat. The bottom line here is that the total *amount* of fat in the diet is just as important as the *kind* of fat. So, those old "low-fat" cookbooks that substituted a cup of oil for a cup of butter missed half the boat—and in most waters, half a boat is about as good as none.

ANIMAL vs. VEGETABLE FAT

Most people equate "vegetable" with healthy polyunsaturated liquid oils and "animal" with nasty, solid, greasy stuff that makes your cholesterol go up. However, there are notable exceptions on both sides. Palm and coconut "oils" are two naturally solid (saturated) vegetable fats, while fish fats are naturally liquid (polyunsaturated) oils.

Surprisingly, palm oil and coconut oil are actually harder and more saturated than butter. Then again, when is the last time you ran to the store to get palm or coconut oil? Actually, it's likely that you bought one or both of these fats the last time you purchased groceries. Its equally likely that you didn't know it. Americans don't buy these naturally saturated vegetable fats in jars or bottles; they buy them in cookies, pastries, baking mixes, powdered coffee creamers, margarine, "natural" potato chips, ice cream, candy bars, canned pina coladas, and hundreds of other even less likely food products. These fats are used by food manufacturers because they have the flavor and texture consumers prefer. Better yet, the label can proudly proclaim "no animal fats"! The bad news is that these saturated fats have the same effect on blood cholesterol as the saturated fat from butter or lard.

There's more. The confusion about animal versus vegetable fat goes well beyond coconut and palm oils to include the issue of hydrogenation. Have you ever read a food label that listed "hydrogenated vegetable fat" or "partially hydrogenated vegetable oil" and wondered what hydrogenated means?

Hydrogenation is a wonder of modern food technology. It's a processing technique that transforms pure liquid vegetable oil into rock-hard solid white grease. Great stuff. A completely saturated fat that can be labeled "100% pure vegetable shortening—no cholesterol—no animal fats." Better yet, you can sell it to people who wouldn't eat bacon fat on a bet.

When we were talking about saturated fats, we mentioned that what they're saturated with happens to be hydrogen. Polyunsaturated fats, on the other hand, have a few chemical bonds that aren't completely filled up with hydrogen. It almost sounds like the only difference between a saturated fat and one that's not is a few hydrogen atoms, which happens to be exactly right! That's all there is to it. The food chemists figured it out years ago. You pour liquid oil into a processing vat, bombard it with hydrogen atoms and presto, whizzo—you've got shortening!

Why would anyone want to do such a thing to a perfectly good polyunsaturated oil? For a number of reasons, all of which boil down to money. Saturated fats, whether naturally solid or unnaturally solidified by hydrogenation, are stable. They don't deteriorate or go rancid. That turns out to be a significant advantage.

Have you ever taken a bite out of an old cookie . . . or potato chip? Maybe something out of an opened package that was pushed to the back of a cupboard for more months than you care to count? It tasted truly terrible; no, not just stale, but so nasty you wouldn't feed it to a rat. . . . If so, you have savored the flavor of a rancid fat. Now, just suppose you bought a package of cookies at the grocery store, opened it up on the way home in the car, and bit into one that tasted like that. The grocer knows that you wouldn't shop in his store again, and the cookie company knows you would change brands. Do you know what keeps this from happening? Saturated fat. Which is why hydrogenation caught on!

Polyunsaturated fats are vulnerable to deterioration because of those pesky unfilled bonds. A cookie made with liquid oil will go rancid a lot faster than one made with solid shortening. Oxygen (from the air) moves in, splits the double bonds, and forms a new pairing with the leftovers of the former fatty acid. At any rate, the result is oxidized free radicals—rancidity.

Saturated fats, on the other hand, can sit complacently on the grocer's shelf—for weeks, months, sometimes years—without moving a single bond, like cement. The only glitch in the system is that when you eat them, they are equally complacent about slugging around in your system and clogging up your arteries. So much for the beauty of extended shelf life.

Another advantage of saturated fats to the food industry is that these solid fats have a higher smoking point, which means foods don't scorch as easily at the high temperatures used for frying. This translates into a great savings for fast food restaurants; they don't have to change the grease as often in their deep fat fryers.

Unfortunately, recent research indicates that hydrogenated fats may not only be just as bad as naturally occurring saturated fats, they may, in fact, be

worse. While this area of investigation is too new to be conclusive, in our opinion, it is important enough to introduce, even before all the data is in.

Fats which are saturated by nature (meat and dairy fats, coconut and palm oil) are composed of fatty acids that have a very symmetrical structure. On the other hand, fats which have been artificially hardened by hydrogenation frequently contain assymetrically shaped fatty acids. (A result of the random bonding that occurs when polyunsaturated oil is bombarded with hydrogen atoms in the process of hydrogenation.) These unnatural fatty acids may or may not turn out to be a problem, but we find them worrisome for the same reason certain research scientists believe they are worth investigating.

When you eat a fat, any fat, some of the fatty acids it contains are used to build tissue in your body. We're not just talking about adipose tissue, where you store excess calories as fat, but about the actual structure of muscle and bone tissue, nerve and blood cells. All cell membranes contain fatty acids as structural components. Some of those fatty acids get built into your body tissue in *exactly* the same molecular form they had when you ate them. Aha! That's where these unnaturally shaped fatty acids become a bit questionable. You see, asymmetrical fatty acids are atypical in nature. You rarely find them in *any* natural fat, animal, or vegetable. You *only* get them in quantity in fats that have been hydrogenated.

Hydrogenation isn't just limited to shortening. This artificial hardening process is used in the production of margarine, nondairy creamer, packaged soups, gravies, dessert mixes, and hundreds of other prepared foods, including our friend from childhood—peanut butter. What Madison Avenue does not tell you in their homey, wholesome, gee-whiz-kids commercials is that those creamy delicious brands owe their delightful texture to the process of hydrogenation. Mom and the kids love the way they spread, but old-fashioned peanut butter, the messy kind with the oil at the top, is healthier. For our part, we'll stick to the liquid oils produced by Mother Nature, and when those just won't do the trick, we prefer naturally saturated fats like butter or lard to artificially hardened margarine or shortening.

A LESSON FROM THE ESKIMOS!

Fish oils are the notable exception to the rule that animal fats tend to be solid, or saturated. Fish fats have been getting a lot of press in recent years; you may have heard of them by some other names—marine oils; Omega-3 fatty acids; EPA (eicosapentaenoic acid), and DHA (docosahexaenoic acid).

Greenland Eskimos, who live on things like whale blubber and oily salmon, have an incidence of heart attack that is about 100 times lower than that in the United States! How can that be when the traditional

Eskimo diet is very high in animal fat and protein, with hardly any carbohydrate. (Fruits and vegetables don't do well in the subzero climate, nor do rice paddies or grain fields.) Since this dietary pattern flies in the face of all our best advice, Eskimos have been a bit of an embarassment to nutrition scientists. As population studies accumulated, correlating high animal fat diets with incidence of heart disease, these paradoxical Greenlanders became more than Danish investigators could bear. Denmark has a very high rate of coronary artery disease, as well as a very high (saturated) fat diet. (You've heard of Danish pastry, Danish ham, Danish bacon, etc.) The epidemiological statistics also showed that those Greenland Eskimos who moved to Denmark soon had the same incidence of heart disease as native Danes. So Danish nutritionists went off to Greenland to see what they could learn from the Eskimo life-style.

Their suspicion was that the high fish diet of the Eskimos provided large quantities of polyunsaturated fats, which might be the protective factor. Much to their surprise, when they analyzed the fats, they discovered that the Eskimo diet actually contained *less* polyunsaturated fat—and more cholesterol—than did the Danish diet. Besides that, while Eskimos have relatively low blood cholesterol levels, they are not low enough to explain the minimal heart attack rate. Yet, the unique factor about the Eskimo diet remained their high intake of fish. Eventually, the Danish research led to the current theory that it is the *kind* of polyunsaturated fat in fish oils, rather than the quantity, which makes the difference. Omega-3 fatty acids are distinguished by the location of their unsaturated bonds, specifically, the bonds that occur after the third carbon in the chain, when you start counting from the terminal or omega end. Thus the name Omega-3.

Further studies with fish oils have confirmed that these Omega-3 fatty acids do appear to be uniquely protective against heart disease for a number of possible reasons. To understand these reasons, though, you need to know a few basics about heart disease. Beginning with high blood cholesterol as a risk factor, here's a capsulized version of how it works:

1. Cholesterol is a kind of fat, and fats aren't soluble in water. In order to navigate in our bloodstreams, which are watery systems, fats need to be wrapped in a water-soluble substance; in this case, protein. These protein-coated packages of fat are called lipoproteins (*lipo*, from lipid, which means fat). Lipoproteins come in several varieties.

2. HDLs, LDLs, and VLDLs are high-density lipoproteins, low-density lipoproteins, and very low-density lipoproteins. HDLs are the good guys. People who keep their cholesterol in these kinds of packages have a lower risk of heart disease. LDLs are just the opposite. The more LDL cholesterol you have in your blood, the higher your risk of heart disease. The best evidence so far indicates that while the HDLs "pick up" cholesterol and carry it off to places in the body where it gets used up or eliminated, the LDLs are responsible for carrying cholesterol to the walls of your arteries ... and leaving it there. These cholesterol deposits become fatty plaques.

3. Fatty plaques are basically a buildup of cholesterol-containing layers of tissue on the inside of your artery walls. When you get enough of these to notice, it's called atherosclerosis.

4. Atherosclerosis means hardening of the arteries. (It's also called arteriosclerosis, just to keep you on your toes.) When fatty plaque builds up in your arteries, the normally smooth and elastic artery walls become thick, rough, and "hardened." This condition is in itself a cardiovascular disease, which impairs circulation and increases the workload of the heart. You can't feel your arteries hardening, but this process dramatically increases your risk of heart attack and stroke. The cholesterol buildup takes up space inside the artery, which becomes narrowed, making it harder for the blood to flow through. The heart is now trying to pump the same amount of blood through smaller holes in stiff, rather than resilient, tubes. The lining of these tubes is rough and bumpy, rather than smooth. Under pressure, this lining is apt to tear or crack, rather than stretch, which can result in bleeding and clot formation.

5. Heart attack occurs when a blood vessel in the heart muscle gets closed off; stroke occurs when this happens in the brain. The blockage is usually the result of a blood clot which gets caught in a narrowed portion of an artery, cutting off the blood supply.

Fish oils appear to interfere with this nasty chain of events in a number of possible ways. First, like other polyunsaturated fatty acids, they reduce total serum cholesterol and, specifically, the undesirable LDL cholesterol. Second, Omega-3 fatty acids tend to increase the beneficial HDL cholesterol fraction; and third, they reduce serum triglycerides (another kind of blood fat). But perhaps the most exciting discovery about Omega-3 fatty acids comes from an observation the Scandinavian scientists made about the Greenland Eskimos: they bruise easily. To the casual observer, that might seem to be an unrelated factor, but to a research team studying blood cholesterol, a person who bruises easily is clearly one whose blood-clotting mechanism should be studied! The Eskimo's blood proved to have fewer, as well as less easily ruptured, platelets: the blood components that help to initiate the clotting process. This means Eskimo blood takes longer to coagulate, so they bleed longer when they get cut, and they get bigger bruises (bleeding beneath the skin) when they're bumped. The significance of all this is that with fewer platelets they are also less likely to form a blood clot. Since most heart attacks and strokes are the result of blood clots getting stuck in arteries narrowed by buildup of cholesterol, blood that is less likely to clot could certainly reduce the risk that a blood vessel will suddenly get blocked. Again, the research is far from complete; and while the actual mechanism hasn't been entirely clarified, it is now generally accepted that there is a protective factor against heart disease enjoyed by people who eat more fish.

EAT MORE FISH

Meanwhile, what are we doing about these exciting discoveries in the good old U.S.A.? One would think we'd be eating more fish—and we are! The average American ate 14.5 pounds of fish last year. That was a new record high, taking American fish consumption from "practically never" to "almost once a week." It calculates out to about half an ounce per day, compared to the Greenlanders average of one *pound* per day. The logical next question is how much Omega-3 fatty acid is enough to get the beneficial effects? Right now, it appears that 3 to 6 grams per day will do the trick. That translates to a half pound of fatty fish such as salmon or mackerel, or 2 to 4 times as much other fish, or . . . more fish than most of us will eat.

American entrepreneurs have not overlooked this nutrition marketing opportunity. As quick as you can say "Omega-3," supplements appeared in the marketplace. While these fish oil extracts could present some problems if overused, that may not be much of a factor, since it takes about 20 capsules to provide 6 grams of Omega-3s. This adds up to a considerable financial commitment, as well as 180 calories. As we see it, you're certainly better off investing the money, as well as the calories, in salmon steaks or your favorite cold water fish. (See chart for Omega-3 fatty acid content of various fish and seafoods.)

If you can't imagine eating even half a pound of fish each day, you'll be pleased to know there are some studies which indicate that only two or three fish meals a week, or 1 to 2 ounces of fish per day (a tuna sandwich, a shrimp salad, or a bowl of clam chowder) may be enough to reduce your risk of heart disease. Omega-3 fatty acids also occur in some vegetable foods but in much smaller amounts. How often you include seafood in your diet may turn out to be more important than the serving size, as the protective effects appear to come from the incorporation of Omega-3 fatty acids in various blood components that are continually being used up, or torn down, refurbished and replaced. In other words, your Fourth of July clambake is a terrific idea, but the next day, consider catching a trout!

If you're thinking we've probably covered everything there is to know about fats—guess what—we've just hit the high spots! To learn more about your own lipid profile see your doctor and your registered dietitian.

Heart Friendly Fish Oils

SOURCE	Omega-3 oil content of 5 oz., raw*	CALORIES
Bass (fresh water)	.4 g	140
Calamari	.2 g	120
Catfish	.1 g	148
Clams (cherrystone)	.6 g	115
Cod (Atlantic)	.2 g	110
Crab (king and snow, 1 lb.)	.7 to .8 g	160
Flounder	.3 g	96
Haddock	.5 g	110
Halibut	.3 g	142
Herring	1.2 to 2.7 g	140-250
Langostino	.2 g	120
Lobster (Maine, 1¼ lb.)	1.4 g	240
Lobster (rock, 1 tail)	.3 g	230
Mackerel	1.8 to 2.6 g	225-270
Monkfish	.3 g	110
Mussels	1.3 g	99
Oysters (6 raw on half shell)	1.0 g	66
Perch (Atlantic) (redfish)	.4 g	125
Pollock	.5 g	120
Rockfish	.2 g	90
Salmon (pink)	1.4 g	169
Salmon (sockeye)	.6 g	205
Scallops	.4 g	115
Shark	.1 to .2 g	150
Shrimp (Atlantic brown)	.4 g	130
Sole	.1 g	120
Swordfish	.4 g	168
Trout (lake)	2.8 g	207
Trout (rainbow)	1.0 g	170
Tuna (albacore)	2.1 g	127
Tuna (yellowfin)	1.7 g	189

Other Omega-3 Sources

SOURCE	Omega-3 content in 5 oz. raw*	CALORIES
Beans (common dry, ¾ cup cooked)	.3 g	165
Beef (ground)	.3 g	280
Broccoli (1 cup cooked)	.1 g	45
Butter (1 tablespoon)	.2 g	100
Butternuts (dried, 1 tablespoon, chopped)	.7 g	51
Chicken	.1 g	145
Lamb (leg)	.4 g	192
Soybeans (green, 1 cup cooked)	4.0 g	167
Soybean oil (1 tablespoon)	1.0 g	125
Walnuts (black, 1 tablespoon, chopped)	.3 g	50
Walnut oil (1 tablespoon)	1.5 g	125

*Serving size is based on 5 oz. raw weight except where otherwise noted. Nutrient content for seafood based on analysis of cooked seafood conducted by Medallion Laboratory, MN. Current research indicates that the Omega-3 fatty acids of fish oils are beneficial in the prevention of coronary heart disease. An optimal level of intake has not been established. Studies show benefits over a range of .3 to 6.0 g.

In the meantime, keep in mind that the biggest problem with the American diet is too much fat. Heart disease has the distinction of being the number one killer, so it gets the most attention, but our high-fat diet has now also been correlated with certain kinds of cancer (colorectal, prostate, and breast), as well as diabetes, gallbladder disease, and many of the other degenerative diseases of Western society. Americans get 42% of their total calories from fat. Historically, as the fat in our diet has increased, so has the incidence of obesity. Recent research indicates fat calories are more apt to be stored than calories from carbohydrates or protein. Fat makes you fat. For all these reasons, we think it makes sense to limit dietary fat to the absolute minimum.

We have used a variety of fats in our recipes on the premise that if you get the total amount low enough, the distinction between butter, olive oil, or even bacon grease, becomes fairly academic. We have tried to choose the fats best suited to each recipe, but we suggest you use the fat you like best. Our justification for this kind of heresy comes from our work with thousands of weight control patients, who have taught us the importance of personal preference. If you're Jewish, you may have some favorite recipes that fall flat without chicken fat. If you're Italian, you obviously can't cook without olive oil. For the more clinically oriented, here's the mathematical side of this philosophy: a teaspoon of butter contains fewer saturated fats than a tablespoon of margarine, simply due to the lower total amount of fat consumed.

Diets don't work. Long-term habit change does. Food is such an integral part of life, it needs to be wonderful, in addition to being healthy. If it isn't, dietary changes won't last. So, don't eat a single fat calorie unless it's seriously delicious!

Fiber

> "Current evidence suggests diets high in carbohydrate and fiber and low in fat aid treatment or prevention of diabetes, cardiovascular disease, obesity, certain gastro-intestinal diseases, and, perhaps, cancer."

This statement was the lead sentence of a major review article by Dr. James W. Anderson on the role of fiber in health. Published in a conservative nutrition journal written for health professionals, this is a very strong statement. The article goes on to summarize 20 years of research studies on dietary fiber, from all over the world, which indicate that a high fiber diet can help with conditions ranging from constipation and hemorrhoids to high blood cholesterol and obesity.

So what is this magic stuff? Grandma called it roughage, Americans equate it with bran, but it's really a whole group of compounds that have one thing in common. Dietary fiber is, by definition, what's left over after you digest your food. Not a pretty topic. Scientists put it a bit more properly by defining fiber as "the portion of plant foods—including cellulose, hemicellulose, lignin, pectins, and gums—not digested in the human intestine." It all comes down to bowel function, which, in most circles, isn't the subject of polite conversation. Nevertheless, since fiber basically performs its magic in the confines of the intestinal tract, that is where we shall turn our attention.

The reason fiber is important is precisely because it is not a nutrient! In a sense, it never gets *inside* the body. The intestinal tract, all 26 feet of it, is really just one continuous tube, from mouth to anus, which, functionally, is outside the body. The best analogy we've heard is the donut hole concept. If you drop small objects, lets say pebbles, through the hole of the donut, they never really enter the body of the donut, do they? In the same way, objects can move through our intestinal tracts, from one end to the other, without ever entering the body proper.

DIETARY FIBER: MORE IS BETTER

Since dietary fiber can't be digested, it can't be absorbed through the wall of the intestine. What isn't absorbed, doesn't enter the bloodstream, nor does it travel to the liver, heart, brain, or any other organ. This is one of the reasons why, for many years, fiber was ignored by nutrition scientists. The general feeling was, "If it can't get into the body, it can't be a nutrient, so it probably doesn't matter."[*] That was the situation until the early 1970s, when Dr. Denis Burkitt, a British epidemiologist, brought fiber to the world's attention. He pointed out that the low intake of fiber in Western societies correlated directly with the high incidence of bowel problems such as constipation, diverticulosis, colitis, and cancer of the colon. People who live in less mechanized societies, in rural communities where the typical diet is high in natural fiber, are rarely bothered with these conditions.

Dr. Burkitt's epidemiological studies, comparing the incidence of disease in various societies, were not revolutionary. But he did capture the attention of the medical community. He provided indisputable evidence that the amount of fiber in our diets has a direct and immediate effect on bowel function. Dedicated scientist that he is, Dr. Burkitt gathered his data by monitoring the bowel movements of hundreds of individuals from both primitive and mechanized societies. He spent the better part of 20 years meticulously charting frequency and ease of evacua-

---

[*]Technically, the soluble fraction of plant fibers, while resistant to digestion by the secretions of the human small intestine, is metabolized by bacteria in the colon. The products of this bacterial fermentation include short-chain fatty acids, primarily acetate, butyrate, and propionate, which we now know are absorbed through the wall of the colon and may, in fact, be responsible for the improvement in glucose and lipid metabolism observed with diets high in soluble fibers.

tion, as well as actual weight and consistency of the end result. You have to give the good doctor credit. Some scientists walk on the moon—with TV cameras recording each small step for mankind—others do work of equal significance in settings less adaptable to media coverage.

Dr. Burkitt's findings? The average resident of the rural African region he studied moves his bowels once or twice each day and passes nearly a pound of soft stool with no discomfort. The average urban American moves his bowels once a day if things are going well and passes only 3 to 4 ounces of hard stool, often with difficulty. His conclusion: people who eat more fiber have larger, softer, and more frequent bowel movements.

This is big news to millions of successful, sophisticated Americans. Did you know that in the good old U.S.A., more money is spent, per capita, on laxatives, cathartics, suppositories, and enema preparations than on any other class of over-the-counter medications except simple pain relievers, like aspirin? The bottom line is that America is constipated—and has a headache.

People who live in primitive societies don't need to add bulking agents—be they food or drug—to their diets because they don't take them out to begin with. Their usual diet provides at least four times as much natural fiber as ours because their meals are based on beans, whole grains, and vegetables, rather than meat, eggs, and cheese.

Even though Dr. Burkitt proved only that a high-fiber diet eliminates constipation, his statistics on incidence of related medical problems were quite convincing. Doctors know from experience that people who develop other bowel problems frequently have constipation as part of their medical history. The next question for the research scientists was, did it make sense that eating a bulky diet could reduce your risk of diverticulosis, hemorrhoids, or bowel cancer? In fact, it did.

One of the simplest ways to understand how this works is by considering a tube of toothpaste. When the tube of toothpaste is full, the very slightest pressure will cause the toothpaste to squeeze out. When the tube is nearly empty, even though the toothpaste is still just as soft as it was the first day, considerable pressure is required to force the last little bit to come out. The same principles of physics apply to the digestive tract, which, if you recall, is just one long tube. The tube is made of smooth muscle. Contraction of this muscle causes segments of the tube to squeeze, while other segments relax. This rhythmic muscular action is called peristalsis, and its job is to move intestinal contents down the 26-foot line. In the stomach and small intestine, all the foods we eat provide plenty of mass to push on. In the large intestine (colon), all that is left is what didn't get

digested, which is fiber. Everything else has been absorbed. When there is a lot of this undigested residue, the muscles in the wall of the tube don't have to squeeze very hard to move the contents down the line and finally out. When there's hardly anything there, all the extra force has to come from the muscles in the wall of the tube itself.

Such straining of the bowel is believed to be what causes diverticulosis. This condition gets its name from the tiny finger-like outpocketings in the wall of the colon. These diverticuli are like miniscule hernias, weak spots where the bowel lining has ballooned out. The condition is not constantly bothersome, which is a good thing since 10% of Americans over 40 and 50% of those over 60 years of age have it. It becomes a problem when bits of waste become trapped in the little pockets, which then become inflamed, swollen, and acutely painful. At this point its called diverticulitis—and you definitely notice it.

A diet high in fiber, particularly insoluble fiber, is believed to help prevent the formation of diverticuli. The thinking goes like this: chronic constipation creates pressure from stagnating food and gas in the intestinal tract. Straining at stool increases this pressure tremendously and may cause weak portions of the bowel muscle to give way. Laxatives and cathartics, used to treat the constipation, place a sudden demand on the bowel muscles, which are "out of shape" from insufficient stimulation. Any or all of these factors may contribute to formation of diverticuli. The high-fiber diet increases stool volume, but insoluble fibers do more than just take up space. They also act like sponges, absorbing several times their weight in water, so not only is there a larger mass for the muscle to push against, it is also softer and more easily moved along. Once you have the condition of diverticulosis, it doesn't go away, but you can prevent particles from becoming trapped by consistently including foods high in cellulose (whole grain products, vegetables, and fruits) in your diet. The greater stool volume apparently stretches the bowel lining, opening up constricted diverticuli and cleaning out trapped wastes.

A high fiber intake is correlated with a lower incidence of varicose veins as well as hemorrhoids, which are swollen, distended veins in the rectal area. Again, straining at stool is implicated. Irritable bowel syndrome (IBS)—an obnoxious collection of symptoms including intermittent diarrhea and constipation, cramping, bloating, and gas—is often relieved by increasing dietary fiber, especially bran. Even the painful spasmodic bowel contractions of colitis appear to be related to our low-fiber diet.

The effects of fiber we've covered so far all relate to the insoluble fibers cellulose, hemicellulose, and lignin. Together, these make up what most of us recognize as "fiber," the tough, woody, structural material of plants; for instance, the stringy fibers in vegetables like celery stalks and broccoli stems, the hard outer coating of seeds and cereal grains (bran), and the grainy particles in fruits such as pears and berries.

Another whole group of dietary fibers, which don't contribute much to stool volume or consistency, are important for entirely different reasons. These are the water-soluble pectins and gums. Home-canners know that it's the pectin in fruit that makes jellies jell. Other similarly soluble fibers are responsible for the gumminess of cooked oatmeal and the gelling effect of cooked beans. What these fibers do in your intestine is perhaps even more amazing than what we've already covered.

Recent studies have suggested an effect called "sequestering." Certain soluble fibers, especially pectin, form irreversible bonds with food molecules, particularly fats and cholesterol, in the small intestine. Since fiber, by definition, can't be digested or absorbed, whatever it binds on the way through, can't be digested or absorbed either. Just picture it: a huge sticky pectin molecule gloms onto a fat molecule and drags it, kicking and screaming, right past every available absorption site in the small intestine. The frustrated fat molecule, laden with efficiently concentrated calories, wants nothing more than to get out of the noisy, messy intestinal tract and seek respite in a nice tidy pink fat cell. Instead of a happy home somewhere along the back of your left thigh, the fat molecule is unceremoniously ushered out of the intestinal tract, enmeshed in an unsavory tangle of crude fiber. The more fiber in your diet, the more fat and cholesterol molecules you can eliminate. While it has been shown that diets which include good sources of soluble fiber (especially oatmeal, oat bran, beans, and fruit) will result in a measurable reduction of serum cholesterol and triglycerides, the actual mechanism is not well understood.

As far as cancer of the bowel is concerned, the strongest evidence is still epidemiological. Populations with high-fiber diets have lower incidences of cancer. Just exactly why this is so has not been adequately established. There are some strong theories currently under study. One of them is that fiber, by increasing the bulk of the stools, dilutes potential cancer-causing agents; and by speeding the transit of wastes, including carcinogens, through the bowel, reduces the time these substances remain in contact with the intestinal lining. Another is that the fibers bind or detoxify some of these compounds, or that the action of intestinal bacteria alters the chemical nature of the bowel contents in more beneficial ways when there's a lot of vegetable residue around. A third theory says a high fruit and vegetable diet reduces cancer risk because these foods provide abundant natural vitamins C and A, especially beta-carotene, and that these will actually turn out to be the cancer-preventing substances, while the fiber is just a bonus. A variation on this theory holds that diets high in natural fiber tend to be low in fat, and that may be the factor that accounts for the lower incidence of cancer. Whichever of these turns out to be correct doesn't really matter, since in every case the advice will be to eat more fruits, vegetables, beans, and whole grains.

Last, but for many of us, certainly not least, is a little help from fiber in battling obesity. High-carbohydrate, high-fiber diets increase weight loss at any calorie level. Intestinal contents are propelled by the contraction of intestinal wall muscles, and the nice thing about muscular contraction is that it burns calories. If you contract your leg muscles in an appropriate sequence, it results in walking, and that burns calories. Contracting arm muscles to lift weights is another way to burn calories, and contracting your bowel muscles to move indigestible fiber 26 feet down the line also burns calories. Isn't it nice to know that eating high-fiber foods is just another name for exercising your intestines? But that's not all! Many high-fiber foods, particularly fruits and vegetables, are also low in calories. Plus, they require a lot of chewing. OK, that doesn't burn a lot of calories, but it does take a lot of time. The longer it takes you to eat something, the fewer calories you will consume before your body has time to register satiety (fullness). We used to think people felt full when they ate high-fiber foods because the insoluble fibers took up space in the stomach. Well, they do, and that helps; but now we know that the soluble fibers actually delay stomach emptying time, slow down absorption of sugar into the bloodstream, and even effect serum insulin levels, all of which increase satiety, delay the return of hunger feelings, and, basically, help you to control your eating.

Where do you get the most fiber, and how much is enough? While every major health agency in the country, from the USDA to the National Academy of Sciences has recommended that Americans increase their intake of dietary fiber, there is no agreement as to the optimal amount! In fact, even the estimates of our current (inadequate) intake, range from 5 to 20 grams of fiber per day. The sentiment against designating a number is so strong that when the National Cancer Institute stuck out its bureaucratic neck and recommended a range of 25 to 35 grams of fiber per day, it was soundly criticized by the scientific community for doing so without specifying which types of fiber or citing any controlled studies.

Believe it or not, the reasons for not making a recommendation at this point are sound. Unfortunately, explaining them opens the proverbial can of worms. The problem goes back to assessing how much fiber is in food to begin with. In a nutshell, traditional human nutrition "intake and output" studies just won't work for fiber. If you recall, dietary fiber is "what's left over after the process of human digestion." That might seem simple enough to measure. However, when our own digestive systems are through working on food, the billions of bacteria living in the colon take up where we left off. Their metabolism profoundly alters the composition of our leftovers! Not only do the bacteria break down most of the soluble fibers, they also make other fibers as they grow and multiply. To put it bluntly, bacterial bodies constitute one third of the dry weight of human fecal matter, and the fiber content of the bacterial cell walls cannot be distinguished from the fiber of food origin. So, how does one determine which part of, say, an apple was digested and absorbed, versus what remains to be called, by definition, fiber?

To get a feeling for the "confusion potential" of quantifying fiber, take a look at the labels of the cereal boxes in your cupboard. Some labels list crude fiber, others list dietary fiber (sometimes called plant fiber). Most people assume these are alternate names for the same thing. Not so.

Crude fiber is an antiquated, inadequate, and somewhat misleading measure of fiber in food. It is derived by:

1. Throwing a food sample into a test tube
2. Firing in some strong acid to duplicate what happens in the stomach when the food is exposed to the hydrochloric acid of gastric juices
3. Adding a solvent to wash out what's been "digested"
4. Dousing it with sodium hydroxide to mimic the action of the alkaline digestive juices of the pancreas and small intestine
5. Rinsing it again with solvent

What remains is called crude fiber. Unfortunately, it's a far cry from what is really left over when food moves through the intestinal tract. In fact, only a small fraction, sometimes as little as one seventh, of total dietary fiber survives this chemical gamut. Crude fiber basically includes only lignin and cellulose. Pectins, gums, and hemicelluloses are lost from the analysis.

Dietary fiber, on the other hand, is now being assessed, by several different research teams, using methods which more closely approximate what happens to food in our digestive tracts. There's just one big problem. Better methods tend to run into time and money, so, to date only a limited selection of foods have been analyzed. In addition, even the assessments that have been done, vary in method and results.

Translating crude fiber to dietary fiber is impossi-

ble. Fiber comes all mixed up in foods. We know citrus fruits, oat products, and beans are very high in the soluble fibers, while wheat bran, fruit peels, and vegetable stalks are high in cellulose, but each of these foods also contain other kinds of fibers. The mixture is so different in each food, a conversion factor can't even be approximated. Dr. James Anderson of the University of Kentucky is a leader in the very promising field of high–carbohydrate fiber (HCF) diets for the treatment of diabetes and related cardiovascular disease. His research has shown the therapeutic effects of HCF diets for diabetics to be dramatic reduction of blood sugars, blood cholesterol, and insulin requirements. While documenting the health benefits of various plant fibers, his research also underscored the lack of information on fiber content. Dr. Anderson's own research laboratory began measuring plant fiber content of commonly used foods—and yet another name for fiber was created (plant fiber is essentially the same as dietary fiber). The fiber values we have calculated for our recipes are adapted from his data. Thus, the grams of fiber per serving refer to dietary fiber. The experimental HCF diets used in Dr. Anderson's research studies provided 50 to 70 grams of plant fiber per day. These diets were also extremely low in fat (10% to 25%). To achieve such a high fiber intake, one would have to eat 4 to 6 cups of fruits and vegetables per day, including a half cup of beans or peas, plus at least six servings of whole grain bread or cereal. If this sounds like a bit much, we suggest you consider the range of possibilities between current American average of 10 grams per day and the HCF therapeutic dose of 70 grams!

While scientists continue to ferret out the details of why and how fiber does so many good things (and how many grams it takes to do them), the thing to do is eat a wide variety of high-fiber foods and enjoy the benefits. The thing *not* to do, is to use fiber supplements without a doctor's advice. Given the American fondness for the philosophy that says, "If some is good, more is better," it's not surprising that bran, guar gum, pectin, and methylcellulose compounds are available in capsules, pills, and powdered formulas. Don't kid yourself. The beneficial effects of these various types of fiber are best derived from food. Why? For purposes of this discussion, let's give Mother Nature credit for doing a good design job on the human digestive tract. Then we can turn around and blame her for being a picky mother. We're designed to get fiber from food because that's how Mother Nature provides it. From a slightly more scientific perspective, the human digestive tract processes foods in the order received. Foods from one meal are mixed by the action of the stomach, but foods eaten a half hour later will be next in line. Once food leaves the stomach, it travels through the 26 feet of tubing, pretty much without bothering what's ahead of it or following it. Therefore, fiber needs to be included in every meal. Take pectin, for example. This water-soluble fiber eaten as part of an apple will keep that apple in your stomach a bit longer, then thicken the consistency of the intestinal contents resulting from that apple and slow absorption of sugar from the apple into your bloodstream, thus moderating blood sugar levels, extending satiety, and delaying the return of hunger pangs. A dose of pure pectin, on the other hand, is so concentrated it can form a regular little plug in the intestine, causing cramping pain and nausea, sometimes to the point that medical attention is required. While that's an extreme example, it does happen. A more frequently occurring example is overuse of unprocessed bran. Folks who figure they can take their fiber in one efficient dose and get it over with, tend to push this theory to the point that it backfires. Instead of comfortable regularity, they end up with unpleasant side effects such as bloating, gas, and diarrhea. Purified fiber supplements are also apt to bind nutrients in the intestinal tract, especially trace minerals like zinc, chromium, and magnesium, rendering them unabsorbable. Fiber from food can do this too, but there are two things about food that mitigate the problem. First, foods high in fiber also provide nutrients, often in high concentrations, so a net loss of nutrients is unlikely, and, second, the fiber is mixed with and diluted by the food it came in. The point is, fiber does its job best when it enters the system as part of the food on which it will be doing that job! Doesn't that make sense?

Our recipes incorporate these recommendations for increasing dietary fiber intake:

1. Eat a wide variety of foods naturally high in fiber. These include whole grains, whole grain cereals, and whole grain baked products instead of refined white flour products, as well as larger servings and more frequent use of beans, fruits, and vegetables. This will give you the benefit of all the different types of natural food fibers.

2. The less processed the food, the better. A raw apple with its skin has more fiber than a peeled apple, which has more than applesauce, which has more than apple juice.

3. Use whole foods, rather than parts. Mother Nature likes you to get a little bran as part of your whole grain cereal for breakfast, perhaps with some fresh fruit and whole grain toast. Maybe a salad or sandwich on whole grain bread for lunch and brown rice, potatoes, or whole wheat pasta at dinnertime . . . and raspberries for dessert wouldn't hurt.

4. Drink plenty of fluids, otherwise too much fiber can actually slow down or even block digestion.

In a nutshell, don't take it out to begin with, and you won't have to worry about putting it back in! Eat and cook with good whole foods.

Sodium

Salt is an acquired taste. Newborn infants will smile when a sweet solution is dropped onto the tips of their tongues, frown when the solution is bitter, but remain entirely indifferent to varying strengths of salt solution. Babies can take salt or leave it. Not so with adults.

Salt is addictive. That's right—you get hooked on it. Have you ever noticed that some people always like their food saltier than others? Sodium abuse is not a binge and purge situation, is it? You have habitual salters, and then you have people who never think about picking up a salt shaker.

What about salt? Good stuff or bad? As usual, it's some of each. It's an essential nutrient, which means you can't survive without *some* sodium in your diet. Studies indicate people can survive on as little as 200 milligrams of sodium per day. To say we "overdo it" is putting matters politely. By most estimations, 10 to 12 grams of salt are consumed by the average American on an average day. That's 2 to 2½ teaspoons. Since salt is about 40% sodium, this means we're taking in 4 to 4½ grams of sodium (4000 to 4500 milligrams), which is about 20 times the amount of sodium our bodies require! Shocking overindulgence, to be sure, but is it a health problem?

SODIUM AND HYPERTENSION

Hypertension (high blood pressure) is one reason we're advised to use less salt. Population studies do indeed show a strong correlation between sodium intake and incidence of hypertension. For instance, in some parts of northern Japan, where the average sodium intake runs as high as 20,000 milligrams (10 teaspoons of salt) per day, an astounding 60% of the population has high blood pressure. Conversely, the Yanomamo Indians of Brazil, the Australian aborigines, and the Kalahari bushmen of Africa, along with a few other remote, isolated peoples, have remarkably low intake of sodium (500 milligrams) and virtually no hypertension. As for us, according to the American Heart Association, 60 million Americans have hypertension, or about 30% of the population. These statistics are alarming, to say the least. Yet, as is the case with any epidemiological study, other differences between populations can't be ruled out. Obesity, for instance, has been shown to quadruple risk for developing hypertension. In addition to a very low sodium intake and no hypertension, the Indians, bushmen, and aborigines are lean and well-exercised and have a different genetic pool and a very different life-style from ours. They eat a good deal less fat, protein, and cholesterol than we do, along with significantly more fiber, potassium, and vitamins A and C. Smoking, drinking, and stress, all factors which influence hypertension, are further variables.

However, when we put sodium to the test, we find that it definitely is a factor in hypertension, wherever you happen to live. Specifically, when current research is pooled, it is estimated that cutting back on salt can reduce hypertension in one third to one half of the people who have it. Whether or not reducing sodium intake can prevent hypertension, has not been established. Sodium is just like everything else in nutrition, it depends on your own individual susceptibility. If you know you have high blood pressure or a family history of heart disease, stroke, or kidney failure (all of which are related to hypertension), you'd be foolish not to cut back on salt. On the other hand, even if you don't have any of the problems that go with high blood pressure, it doesn't make a lot of sense to eat 20 times as much as your body needs, does it?

SALT IS ADDICTIVE

If you are in the habit of salting your food, you're hooked. If you've ever tried to eliminate salt, you know your palate demands it. Suddenly everything tastes like nothing. If this has been your experience, don't despair. Just stick it out for 3 weeks, and we promise you food will be food again, without all that salt. It's a fact. Some people say it's because 3 weeks is how long it takes to get new taste buds. We don't know whether letting your taste buds "grow up" in a lower salt environment really has anything to do with it. We just know that 3 weeks on a lower salt diet is usually all it takes to make foods taste right again.

Is it worth the trouble? We suggest it makes good sense to put yourself on a reduced sodium diet before someone does it for you. Imagine for a moment that you are a heart attack victim (one of 1.2 million per year in this country), regaining consciousness in the cardiac care unit of Metropolitan Hospital, U.S.A.

When the pain, the IVs, the oxygen, and the catheters are gone and the doctors are saying, "It looks like you're going to make it," the first meal arrives. You thought the worst was over, but now the low-sodium, low-fat, low-cholesterol, low-calorie diet must be faced. We've seen many patients in this predicament. A few of them have made us wonder which was going to kill them first, salt in their food or the stress generated by eating food they hate.

Jim was so hooked on salt, he would lick the top of his salt-free crackers and sprinkle them with crystalline salt substitute. The staff of the cardiac care unit learned from our friend Jim a hundred new ways to describe how truly awful food can taste without salt. When 3 weeks finally rolled by, Jim thought we had fired all the cooks and started over. Six months after his heart attack, when Jim was back in the hospital for a follow-up electrocardiogram, he dropped by the dietary department to complain again. Now he was upset over the trouble he had eating out in fast food restaurants. You guessed it, the food was too salty! If Jim can do it, we'll wager anyone can.

HOW MUCH IS HEALTHY?

There is now sufficient evidence to safely say that the average American salt intake is more than anyone needs and may, in fact, be dangerous to the health of those individuals who are sodium sensitive.

Does a fit and healthy individual need to pass up the pickles and the mustard or is it more important to skip the fat-laden hot dog he was going to put them on in the first place? How much sodium is enough? The National Research Council (the scientific body which sets the USRDAs) estimates a safe and adequate intake of sodium to be 1100 to 3300 milligrams per day.

A level teaspoon of regular salt (sodium chloride) contains 2000 milligrams (2 grams) of sodium, so the recommended 1100 to 3300 milligrams translates into ½ to 1½ teaspoons of regular salt per day. Sounds like a lot, doesn't it? Remember we said the average person in this country consumes 2 to 2½ teaspoons of salt each day. If all that salt was coming out of the salt shaker, you'd be refilling it daily.

Believing you're on a low-salt diet because you never salt food at the table is a very common mistake. The saltshaker is simply the visible tip of the iceberg. Sodium, like sugar and fat, comes to us "hidden" in foods, especially those that have been processed. And it isn't all new-fangled food technology either. One of the saltiest things you can eat is a pickle, especially the kind that tastes like it just came out of the old stone crock. Running a close second for high sodium content are the bacon, ham, and sausages hanging in the smokehouse! Salt is a preservative; it keeps foods from rotting. Salt pork, kippered herring, dried chipped beef, sauerkraut, and olives are foods which keep for a long time because they have been preserved with salt. Some foods have been so closely associated with high-sodium preservation techniques, people avoid them even when they aren't processed. Pork, for instance. Fresh pork is no higher in sodium than fresh beef, lamb, or poultry. It's the curing process that turns it into ham, bacon, and sausage that adds a lot of salt.

SALT: WHERE IS IT?

Today our sodium comes from three places. The average American gets only about 10% of it from natural sources such as fresh meat, milk, vegetables, grains, and fruits. Another 15% comes from salt added at the table or in cooking. The lion's share, 75%, comes to us in processed foods. Here's how it breaks down:

1. If you ate only whole, unprocessed natural foods—nothing from a can or box or pickle barrel—you would get about 500 to 1000 milligrams of sodium per day. This is for a balanced diet, including foods from all four food groups. Most of this sodium would come from the animal foods: meat and dairy products.

2. If you ate some processed foods, like bread, which averages 200 milligrams of sodium per slice, and natural cheese, which has 100 to 300 milligrams of sodium per ounce, you would get 2000 to 3000 milligrams of sodium per day, still well within the 1100 to 3300 milligram recommendation.

3. The average American consumes 4000 to 4500 milligrams of sodium per day, largely from processed foods. One large dill pickle has 1000 milligrams of sodium, a TV dinner has 1200, and a large fast-food burger averages 1100.

What can be done? We suggest you start in your own kitchen. Stop using the salt shaker (10%), don't add salt in cooking (15%), then address the processed foods which are common ingredients in American cooking: canned soups, bottled sauces, and prepared seasonings.

Each recipe in this book was kitchen tested with Morton's Lite Salt, which we list as "light" salt. This was calculated into the total sodium content. Light salt is half regular salt (sodium chloride) and half salt substitute (potassium chloride), which is why its sodium content (1100 milligrams per teaspoon) is about half that of regular salt. We have used this "half-salt" in all our cooking for the past 5 years. No one has noticed the difference. Light salt is an easy starting point for cutting back on total sodium.

As this is not a low-sodium cookbook, our recipes call for customary amounts of added salt. Since it is light salt, the sodium content is only half—but remember, salt is just one of many high-sodium ingredients used in normal American cooking. Books listing specific sodium content of all foods are widely available, but if you are not ready for that level of detail, we've included a dietitian's "cheat sheet" for quick sodium calculation (see chart).

To eliminate 90% of the sodium in most of our recipes, do the following:

1. Omit the light salt or use pure salt substitute instead (subtract 1100 milligrams of sodium per teaspoon light salt).

2. Substitute low-sodium broth, bouillon cubes, or powdered stock base for regular (subtract 900 milligrams of sodium per cup of broth, cube of bouillon, or teaspoon of powdered base).

3. Use low-sodium soy sauce (subtract 858 milligrams of sodium per tablespoon, but remember to add back in whatever the reduced sodium product provides).

4. Use fresh beans and other vegetables, cooked without salt, instead of canned (subtract 500 milligrams of sodium per cup).

5. Check the "cheat sheet" for ingredients which have been pickled, smoked, or cured.

Each time you make a sodium-reducing change, give it 3 weeks, and that's it!

Sodium Sources Cheat Sheet

Naturally low-sodium foods	AMOUNT OF SODIUM (in milligrams)
All fresh fruits and vegetables	Generally less
Seeds, nuts, grains (and flours)	than 10 mg
Dry beans, peas, lentils	per serving
Canned or dried fruits, jellies, syrup, sugar, honey	
Spices and herbs (no added salt)	

Foods with some natural sodium	
Milk	125/cup
Buttermilk	250/cup
Yogurt	150/cup
Cottage cheese	100/oz.
Cheese (cheddar, Jack, etc.)	100-300/oz.
Eggs	70/egg
Fresh meat, poultry, fish	25/oz.
Fresh shellfish	50-100/oz.

Condiments	
Salt (sodium chloride)	2000/teaspoon
Seasoned salt mixtures	1200/teaspoon
Baking powder	300/teaspoon
Baking soda	800/teaspoon
Soy sauce	900/tablespoon
Catsup, worcestershire, BBQ sauce	150/tablespoon
Steak sauce, chili sauce	250/tablespoon
Mustard, horseradish	200/tablespoon
Bouillon, broth, powdered soup base	1000/cup

Low-sodium substitutes	
Light salt	1100/teaspoon
Salt substitute	0
Light seasoned salt	300/teaspoon
Low-sodium baking powder	0
Mild or gentle soy sauce	500/tablespoon
Low-sodium broth, soups	50/cup

High-sodium foods	
Pickles, relish, olives, sauerkraut	200-400/oz.
Canned or dry, reconstituted broth, soups or bouillon	1000/cup
Smoked ham, bacon, sausage, lunch meat	200-400/oz.
Canned tuna, salmon	100/oz. (800/cup)
Canned beans and other vegetables	50/oz. (400/cup)

Living Lean for Children

"But what about my kids? I can't expect *them* to eat like this, can I? And when I buy the stuff they like to eat—crackers, chips, lunch meats, cookies, and ice cream—I wind up eating *that* too. Isn't there some way my 'diet' foods can taste good enough for the whole family to eat?" If you've tried to eat differently from others in your household, you know it's tough going. But take heart. There's new research—and it's on your side!

While the word on low-fat, high-fiber diets has been broadcast enough for most adults, and all dieters, to be making a symbolic effort in that direction, children, for the most part are left out of it. As we watch our children scramble on jungle gyms and streak down the streets on bicycles, it's hard to imagine that low-fat fare would hold any advantage for them. In fact, maybe they *need* all that high calorie food to fuel their incessant activity, and restriction could be harmful.

In a recent nationwide survey of parents, it was found that nine out of ten parents believe their children to be models of physical fitness. Nothing could be further from the truth.

Children today are In far worse physical condition than their counterparts of the 1960s. Recent research done by the Harvard School of Public Health documents a striking increase in weight problems among grade school and high school students alike. In children aged 6 to 11 obesity has increased by 54%, and among those between the ages of 12 and 17 it's up by 39%, prompting experts to warn of a national epidemic of childhood obesity. Almost one third of all white preteen boys are overweight as are 26% of white teenage girls. While obesity is most prevalent in white children, black youngsters are quickly closing the gap. And, while statistics vary, most authorities agree that roughly 50% of school children are unable to perform well on simple fitness tests.

And that's not all. Things don't look so good on the inside either. A significant percentage of children over age 12 years have elevated levels of cholesterol and triglycerides in their blood. And, increasingly, family doctors and pediatricians find their young patients with blood pressure readings that are too high.

Children simply aren't as active as we think. Only 36% of all students take physical education, and surveys show that the average child spends 3 to 7 hours a day parked in front of the television set.

Combine all these findings, and you have a number of factors that can predispose youngsters to heart disease, cancer, diabetes, and obesity. In short, the health and fitness of our children is sliding downhill.

As you might have guessed, *Living Lean* is not just for the over-40 set. In fact, based on the rapidly accumulating evidence, many pediatricians now recommend that we start our toddlers out on a low-fat diet at about age 2. Although you can restrict sugar and salt before age 2, you shouldn't restrict fat for babies under that age because it's possible to cause an essential fatty acid deficiency. After the age of 2, though, a diet of 40% to 60% fat, loaded with salt and sugar, isn't any more healthful for them than it is for you!

While there is little doubt that we should feed our families less fat, some recent medical and nutrition journals have documented a number of cases where children exhibited "failure to thrive" when put on severe dietary restriction. Low body weight, susceptibility to infection, and deficiency in coordination and motor skills may result when well-meaning parents are overly strict about snacks and foods that contain fat. Feeding your child as though he were in cardiac rehabilitation is not only unnecessary but potentially dangerous. We are certainly not recommending that.

The recipes in this book are filled with all the whole-grain, nutrition-packed food children need to grow on. And the food—remarkably enough—is the kind they ask you for—spaghetti, pizza, macaroni and cheese, tacos, and oatmeal cookies—all with a little less fat, sugar, and salt but with all the flavor they love. Just what you need to help them (and you) grow up lean—and love it!

Decoding the Graphs and Symbols, or How to Use This Book

SAMPLE

SERVING SIZE: 1 cup

PER SERVING: Calories 123 **Fiber:** 2 grams **Sodium:** 238 mg.

CALORIES

AT A GLANCE *this graph shows*:

1. TOTAL CALORIES per serving (numbers on *left*). The total shaded area represents calories per serving. All servings are 300 calories or less.

2. CALORIES FROM FAT, PROTEIN, AND CARBOHYDRATE per serving (numbers on *right*). The three gradations of color show how many calories come from carbohydrates, how many come from protein, and how many come from fat. These numbers do not represent percentages. (All food calories come from fat, protein, and carbohydrate. The only other source of calories is alcohol.)

WITH THIS INFORMATION *you can easily determine*:

1. PERCENT FAT: Divide calories from fat by total calories per serving, then multiply by 100 to find percentage of calories from fat:

$$\left(\frac{\text{Fat calories}}{\text{Total calories}}\right) \times 100 = \% \text{ fat}$$

2. GRAMS FAT: One gram of fat is 9 calories, so divide fat calories by 9 to get grams of fat per serving:

$$\frac{\text{Fat calories}}{9} = \text{grams fat}$$

EXAMPLE: If your goal is a diet with less than 30% of the calories coming from fat:
—Keep fat calories below 300 per 2000 calories eaten.
—Keep fat grams below 33 grams per 1000 calories eaten.

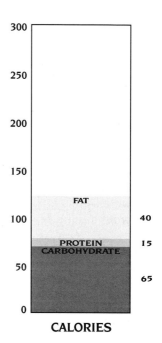

CALORIES

% U.S.R.D.A.

AT A GLANCE *this graph shows*:

1. NUTRITIONAL CONTENT per serving. The bars depict the percentage of the United States Recommended Daily Allowance U.S.R.D.A. for nine "leader" nutrients. When a single serving of a recipe provides more than 50% of the U.S.R.D.A. for any of these nutrients, a broken bar indicates that it would go off the graph.

2. NUTRIENT DENSITY. To judge how much nutrition you are getting for your calories, compare the length of the nutrient bars to the calorie bar. The calorie bar shows what percentage of 2000 calories per day is provided by one serving of the recipe. (Individual calorie needs vary; see Weight Control section.)

WITH THIS INFORMATION *you can assess*:

1. NUTRITIONAL ADEQUACY of your diet, for any given nutrient, by adding up the day's totals to see if they equal 100% of the U.S.R.D.A. for that nutrient. Keep in mind that the U.S.R.D.A.'s are not minimum requirements. (See U.S.R.D.A. CHART for further explanation.)

2. NUTRITIONAL BALANCE of your diet. Eating a wide variety of foods from the "basic four" food groups is the key to a balanced diet. The graphs demonstrate clearly that each food group is important for different nutrients. While only 9 of the 45 nutrients you need each day are graphed, if these "leader" nutrients are obtained in adequate amounts it generally means you have eaten enough nutritious food to provide all the other nutrients you need as well. (Yet another good reason to get your nutrients from foods, not pills.)

Graph: % U.S.R.D.A. based on a calorie intake of 2000 per day

Nutrient	%
CALORIES	6%
PROTEIN	4%
IRON	4%
ZINC	3%
CALCIUM	6%
VITAMIN A	35%
VITAMIN C	97%
THIAMIN	10%
RIBOFLAVIN	5%
NIACIN	2%

FIBER

Dietary (plant) fiber content of each recipe has been calculated in grams per serving (see Fiber section).

 QUICK & EASY

Recipes displaying this symbol require less than 20 minutes of "hands-on" preparation. Unattended cooking time is not included.

SODIUM

Sodium content, calculated per serving, includes sodium from all quantified ingredients. Thus, when recipe calls for "½ teaspoon light salt," the sodium content of this ingredient is calculated in, but if ingredient list includes "light salt to taste" or "optional" it is not calculated. Where alternative ingredients are listed, like "3 large tomatoes or 1 can (1 lb.) whole tomatoes," sodium is calculated for first ingredient listed.

PUTTING THE GRAPHS TO WORK FOR YOU

Each *Living Lean and Loving It* graph compares the nutrients provided in one recipe to the U.S.R.D.A. (United States Recommended Daily Allowance). The U.S.R.D.A.'s are frequently confused with the R.D.A.'s (Recommended Dietary Allowance).* While the R.D.A.'s cover individual daily requirements for people in different age categories, the U.S.R.D.A.'s are set to cover the highest expected nutritional needs of healthy adults in the U.S. (excluding pregnant and lactating women). Because the U.S.R.D.A.'s are a "blanket recommendation," the standards reflect the highest need in our population. For example, women need 18 mg of iron a day while men need only 10 mg. The U.S.R.D.A. is therefore set at 18 mg to reflect the highest need for that nutrient.

While consulting a U.S.R.D.A. chart for daily nutrient intake may be too much for even the most intrepid and inspired dieter, the four food group plan helps us achieve those very same dietary goals with a much simpler format. Eating a wide variety of low-fat, high-fiber foods in balance from all four food groups will assure you adequate intake of the nutrients that are shown on our graphs as well as the ones that are not. The following chart depicts the four food groups along with serving size and necessary daily servings. If charts aren't your cup of tea, the menu on the facing page shows how easily (and deliciously) you can meet your nutrient needs.

FOUR FOOD GROUP PLAN†

MEATS AND LEGUMES

Your Goal: **2 *Servings Per Day***

Each of the following constitutes 1 serving:

2 to 3 oz. cooked lean meat, poultry, or fish

1 cup cooked beans, lentils, or split peas

2 eggs

BREADS AND CEREALS

Your Goal: **at least 4 *Servings Per Day***

Each of the following constitutes 1 serving:

1 slice whole grain bread

½ cup cooked whole grain cereal

1 cup whole grain ready-to-eat cereal

½ cup cooked rice or pasta

DAIRY PRODUCTS

Your Goal: **2 *Servings Per Day***

Each of the following constitutes 1 serving:

1 cup (8 oz.) milk, yogurt, or cottage cheese

1 to 2 oz. cheese

FRUITS AND VEGETABLES

Your Goal: **at least 4 *Servings Per Day***

Each of the following constitutes 1 serving:

1 cup raw vegetable

½ cup cooked vegetable

½ cup fruit or juice

*Charts for U.S.R.D.A.'s and R.D.A.'s can be found in most books on general nutrition.
†Number of servings are for healthy adults. Children, pregnant and lactating women, and people with some medical conditions have different needs.

FOUR FOOD GROUP SAMPLE MENU

BREAKFAST

  2 BLUE RIBBON BRAN MUFFINS
  1 CUP FRESH BERRIES
  8 OZ. NONFAT VANILLA YOGURT

LUNCH

  1 CUP ANDERSEN'S SPLIT PEA SOUP
  1 SLICE WHOLE WHEAT BREAD
1½ CUPS SPINACH MUSHROOM SALAD
  1 CUP NONFAT MILK

SNACK

  1 APPLE

DINNER

  1 SERVING SOUTHERN FRIED CHICKEN
  ½ CUP MASHED POTATOES WITH PAN GRAVY
  1 CUP BAVARIAN COLE SLAW
  1 WHOLE WHEAT BISCUIT
  1 SERVING BANANA CREAM PUDDING

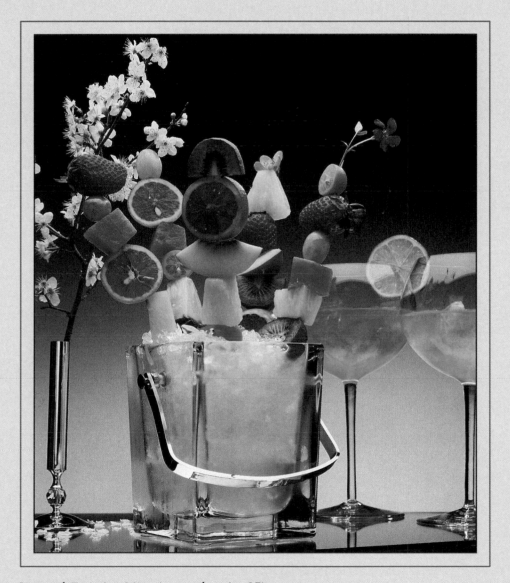

Speared Fruit (p. 36), wine coolers (p. 37)

Dips, Appetizers & Beverages

LIVER PÂTÉ

Pâté without half a pound of butter? Absolutely! This celebrated classic performs beautifully in this light variation.

INGREDIENTS

1½ LB. CHICKEN LIVERS
3 TABLESPOONS BUTTER
1 ONION, COARSELY CHOPPED
½ TEASPOON THYME
¼ TEASPOON ALLSPICE OR MACE
¼ TEASPOON BLACK PEPPER

1 TEASPOON LIGHT SALT
2 TABLESPOONS FRESH PARSLEY, MINCED
½ CUP LOW-FAT RICOTTA CHEESE
2 TABLESPOONS BRANDY OR COGNAC
ONION SLICES, FRESH PARSLEY SPRIGS,
TINY SWEET PICKLES FOR GARNISH

DIRECTIONS

Melt butter in a large nonstick skillet. Add chicken livers and onion. Sauté over medium heat until livers are brown and onions are tender, about 10 minutes.

Chop the cooked livers and onion finely. If using a food processor, do not overprocess. Stir in thyme, allspice, pepper, light salt, parsley, ricotta, and brandy. Mix well.

Grease a 3- to 4-cup mold. Pack the pâté firmly into the mold and level the top with a spatula. Chill well for at least 2 hours.

To serve, dip mold in hot water until butter melts. Unmold pâté onto platter. Garnish with sliced onions, sprigs of parsley, and tiny sweet pickles. Serve with pumpernickel or rye bread or with whole grain crackers.

SERVING SIZE: 24 Servings, 1 Oz. Each

PER SERVING: Calories 62 **Sodium:** 89 mg.

TORTA

Here's a solid little hors d'oeuvre, just right for munching while you sip wine and wait for that fashionably late Italian dinner. A tip from our very busy friend, Debbie Carniglia, who shared this treasured family recipe: torta is best made well ahead. It freezes beautifully and tastes wonderful reheated or simply thawed to room temperature.

INGREDIENTS

3 CUPS BROWN RICE, COOKED (1 CUP RAW)
3 ITALIAN SAUSAGES
1 ONION, CHOPPED
2 CLOVES GARLIC, MINCED
2 TABLESPOONS FRESH PARSLEY, CHOPPED

4 EGGS, LIGHTLY BEATEN
1 CUP GRATED PARMESAN CHEESE
1-2 TEASPOONS COARSELY GROUND BLACK PEPPER
GROUND ALLSPICE TO TASTE (1-2 TEASPOONS)
2 TEASPOONS OLIVE OIL

DIRECTIONS

Preheat oven to 350°.

Remove sausage from casings. Crumble meat into a large nonstick skillet. Cook over medium heat until well browned, about 10 to 15 minutes. Drain thoroughly on paper towels. Chop browned sausage into pea-sized pieces.

Drain grease from skillet but do not wash skillet. Add chopped onion and garlic and sauté over low heat until golden, about 10 minutes.

Combine cooked rice, cooked sausage, sautéed onion and garlic, chopped parsley, eggs, parmesan, pepper, and allspice in a large bowl.

Grease an 8-inch square pan or 6-inch by 10-inch baking dish with 1 teaspoon olive oil. Turn rice mixture into dish and pat it down evenly, with oiled hands.

Spread 1 teaspoon olive oil over top of torta.

Bake at 350° for 35 to 40 minutes, until golden-brown. Cool to room temperature and cut into 64 1-inch squares.

SERVING SIZE: 16 Servings, 4 Squares Each

PER SERVING: Calories 118 **Sodium:** 179 mg.

AL'S MARINATED MUSHROOMS 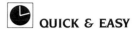 QUICK & EASY

All Italians seem to be born with discriminating palates, but our friend Al Carniglia takes this native talent one step further—he creates good food. This is his original recipe for Italian-style marinated mushrooms. They are outstanding! These are perfect for entertaining because they can be made weeks in advance, hold up beautifully at room temperature, and require only a toothpick for service.

INGREDIENTS

½ CUP VINEGAR
1 CUP WATER
1 TABLESPOON BELL PEPPER, DICED
2 TABLESPOONS PEPPERCORNS OR CRACKED
   BLACK PEPPER

1 TABLESPOON GARLIC, MINCED
2 SMALL WHOLE HOT DRIED RED CHILI PEPPERS
1 LB. SMALL WHOLE MUSHROOMS, FRESH OR
   CANNED

DIRECTIONS

Mix vinegar, water, bell pepper, peppercorns, garlic, and chiles together in a quart jar or small saucepan.

Add mushrooms to mix and microwave for 4 minutes at 70% power or heat in small saucepan, over medium heat until just below boiling.

Strain into a quart jar. Add mushrooms back to strained marinade and cool to room temperature, then refrigerate.

Marinate at least 4 to 6 hours before serving. Mushrooms are best the next day, but will keep refrigerated for up to 2 weeks.

SERVING SIZE: 8 Servings, 4 to 5 Mushrooms Each

PER SERVING: Calories 25 **Sodium:** 25 mg.

CHEDDAR-OLIVE PARTY SANDWICHES QUICK & EASY

Miniature rye bread pizzas perfect for cocktail parties and other wicked occasions. Calories for the spread alone are 18 per tablespoon; it's nice as a celery stuffing or melted on baked tomato halves.

INGREDIENTS

2 OZ. VERY SHARP CHEDDAR, (ABOUT ½C) GRATED
2 OZ. BLACK OLIVES, 4 TABLESPOONS CHOPPED
4 TABLESPOONS ONION, CHOPPED
4 TABLESPOONS LOW-FAT COTTAGE CHEESE

½ TEASPOON DIJON-STYLE MUSTARD
1 TEASPOON FRESH CILANTRO, OR PARSLEY,
   MINCED
1 LOAF (12 OZ.) PARTY RYE, 36 SLICES

DIRECTIONS

Mix all ingredients except bread in a medium bowl. You will have 1½ cups of spread, enough for 36 rye slices.

Use 2 teaspoons spread for each slice of party rye.

Heat sandwiches under broiler just until cheese melts. Serve hot.

SERVING SIZE: 12 Servings, 3 Canapes Each

PER SERVING: Calories 110 **Sodium:** 169 mg.

SPINACH SOUR CREAM DIP

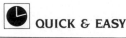 **QUICK & EASY**

Variations of this recipe turn up frequently at potluck dinners and cocktail parties involving busy people. It's quick and easy, as well as delicious, but the best part is that it can be made in advance. Originally designed for dipping chunks of sourdough bread (see Serving Suggestion), it's equally good for fresh vegetables, especially celery, zucchini, mushrooms, and broccoli.

INGREDIENTS

1 10 OZ. BOX FROZEN CHOPPED SPINACH
1 PACKAGE (2¾ OZ.) KNORR LEEK SOUP MIX
4 SMALL GREEN ONIONS, THINLY SLICED
½ CUP DIET MAYONNAISE

½ CUP SOUR CREAM
½ CUP PLAIN NONFAT YOGURT
½ CUP LOW-FAT COTTAGE CHEESE

DIRECTIONS

Heat spinach in saucepan or in microwave just until thawed and warmed through. Drain off any liquid.

Add dry soup mix to warm spinach, stir. Allow to cool. Add green onions.

Blend mayonnaise, sour cream, yogurt, and cottage cheese in blender or food processor until smooth. Add to spinach. (Do not put spinach and onions in the blender or you will have soup rather than dip!)

Chill 8 to 48 hours before serving to develop flavor.

SERVING SUGGESTION: Hollow out a large, round loaf of sourdough or sheepherder's bread by slicing off the top and tearing or carving out chunks of bread until a ½-inch thick shell remains. Eight to 24 hours before serving, put the dip in the "bread bowl," cover with bread top, then wrap in plastic or foil until ready to serve. Use the chunks of bread for dipping.

SERVING SIZE: 14 Servings, ¼ Cup Each

PER SERVING: Calories 82   **Sodium:** 373 mg.

CLAM DIP

It's hard to believe such a thick, creamy dip is only 13 calories per tablespoon.

INGREDIENTS

½ CUP LOW-FAT COTTAGE CHEESE
⅓ CUP NON FAT YOGURT
3 TABLESPOONS DIET MAYONNAISE
½ CUP COOKED POTATO (BAKED OR BOILED)
½ CUP CELERY, MINCED
2-3 TABLESPOONS ONION, MINCED
2 TABLESPOONS FRESH PARSLEY, MINCED

1 CUP CLAMS, MINCED (2 CANS, 6½ OZ. EACH)
1½ TABLESPOONS FRESH LEMON JUICE
½ TEASPOON WORCESTERSHIRE SAUCE
¼ TEASPOON WHITE OR BLACK PEPPER
FEW DROPS HOT PEPPER SAUCE
LIGHT SALT TO TASTE

DIRECTIONS

In blender or food processor, beat cottage cheese with yogurt and mayonnaise until very smooth. Add cooked potato and beat until thick, but not gummy.

Turn into medium bowl. Stir in minced celery, onion, and parsley.

Rinse clams in colander to remove any residual sand and drain thoroughly.
Add clams to dip, along with lemon juice, Worcestershire sauce, pepper, and hot pepper
sauce. Add light salt to taste.
Makes 3 Cups.

VARIATION: Add chopped fresh pimento for color or water chestnuts for crunch.

SERVING SIZE: 1 Tablespoon

PER SERVING: Calories 13   **Sodium:** 28 mg.

CRAB DIP 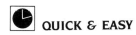 QUICK & EASY

INGREDIENTS

6 OZ. CRAB MEAT, FLAKED
½ CUP CATSUP OR CHILI SAUCE
2 TABLESPOONS FRESH LEMON JUICE
2 TEASPOONS FRESH PARSLEY, MINCED
1 TEASPOON HORSERADISH

DIRECTIONS

In a small bowl, combine all ingredients. Mix well. Cover and chill. Makes 1 cup.

SERVING SIZE: 1 Tablespoon

PER SERVING: Calories 21   **Sodium:** 118 mg.

PINTO RICOTTA DIP 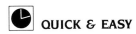 QUICK & EASY

Good hot or cold, this dip is a nice side dish with Mexican food.

INGREDIENTS

1 CAN (1 LB.) PINTO BEANS, DRAINED
8 OZ. LOW-FAT RICOTTA CHEESE
1 TABLESPOON CUMIN
1-2 TABLESPOONS SALSA

DIRECTIONS

Blend half of beans with cheese, cumin, and salsa in processor or blender until thick and
creamy. Add remaining beans and blend only slightly to retain some whole bean texture.
Use as a dip for chips or crackers.

VARIATION: Hot Bean Dip. Prepare dip. Place in a small, shallow baking dish. Sprinkle with
grated sharp cheddar. Heat in oven or microwave until bubbly.

SERVING SIZE: 10 Servings, ¼ Cup Each

PER SERVING: Calories 85   **Sodium:** 34 mg.

NOTE: To further reduce calories, substitute low-fat cottage cheese for ricotta.

BEAN DIP

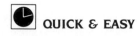 QUICK & EASY

A good dip for tortilla chips or raw vegetables. We recommend red and green sweet bell pepper strips and fresh sliced jicama for a colorful arrangement.

INGREDIENTS

      1 CAN (1 LB.) KIDNEY BEANS, WELL DRAINED
      1 CAN (4 OZ.) DICED GREEN CHILES, DRAINED
  2-3 TABLESPOONS LIME OR LEMON JUICE
      1 LARGE TOMATO, COARSELY CHOPPED
   ⅛ TEASPOON CRUSHED RED CHILI OR ½ TEASPOON HOT PEPPER SAUCE
      2 TEASPOONS WORCESTERSHIRE SAUCE
      2 CLOVES GARLIC
      4 GREEN ONION TOPS, THINLY SLICED

DIRECTIONS

Drain beans thoroughly.

Put all ingredients except green onions in a blender or food processor. Blend for 1 to 2 minutes, until smooth.

Turn mixture into serving bowl and sprinkle with green onions. Serve immediately or chill. Makes 1½ Cups.

SERVING SIZE: 6 Servings, ¼ Cup Each

PER SERVING: Calories 48   **Sodium:** 104 mg.

GUACAMOLE

The world's best guacamole is made every evening in the thatch-roofed restaurant of the Las Brisas Motel in San Blas. Strictly in the interest of culinary research, we spent a week there dutifully drinking margaritas, night after night, just to observe the barmaid's guacamole technique. It turns out that the secret to good guacamole is good avocados! While each of the other ingredients is important in the final orchestration of flavors, all must harmonize with the delicate nuttiness of the avocado, yet never overpower it.

We must admit that cottage cheese was never included by Consuelo, but it turns out to be the perfect secret ingredient. Smooth, creamy, and mild enough to virtually disappear, it allows us to make this delicious guacamole for half the usual calories.

INGREDIENTS

      1 MEDIUM AVOCADO
   ¾ CUP LOW-FAT COTTAGE CHEESE
      2 TABLESPOONS CILANTRO LEAF, CHOPPED
      1 TABLESPOON ONION, CHOPPED

      1 MEDIUM TOMATO
      1 TABLESPOON FRESH LIME JUICE
        HOT PEPPER SAUCE TO TASTE
        LIGHT SALT TO TASTE

DIRECTIONS

Peel and seed avocado. Place in blender or food processor with cottage cheese. Blend until smooth.

Add onion and cilantro to avocado mixture. Blend briefly, in spurts, just to chop cilantro a bit.

Turn mixture into a small bowl.

Cut tomato in half, horizontally. Squeeze gently to remove seeds and juice. Finely chop the meat of the tomato. Stir into the guacamole. Add lime juice.

Add hot pepper sauce and light salt to taste.

SERVING SIZE: 4 Servings, ⅓ Cup Each

PER SERVING: Calories 111   **Sodium:** 234 mg.

MICROWAVE NACHO DIP

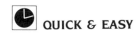 **QUICK & EASY**

We prepared a veritable mountain of nachos using this sauce recipe (multiplied by six) for a dozen friends one Labor Day weekend. Everyone said they were the best nachos they'd ever had—bar none!

INGREDIENTS

⅓ CUP ONION, FINELY CHOPPED
4 OZ. VELVEETA OR OTHER PROCESSED CHEESE*
   SLICED ¼-INCH THICK
1 CAN (4 OZ.) DICED GREEN CHILES, OR
1 SMALL BELL PEPPER, FINELY CHOPPED

1 SMALL TOMATO (ROMA TOMATO IS BEST)
TORTILLA CHIPS (FAT-FREE OR REGULAR)
PICKLED JALAPEÑO PEPPER SLICES OR FRESH
CORIANDER FOR GARNISH

DIRECTIONS

Place finely chopped onion in a small casserole dish or 2-cup glass measure. Microwave on
   high for 2 minutes, stirring once midway.
Add cheese slices. Microwave 1 minute on high.
Stir in well-drained green chiles or chopped bell pepper. Microwave 1 minute on high.
Cut tomato in half, horizontally. Squeeze each half gently to force out seeds and juice.
   Finely chop the meat of the tomato.
Stir tomato into cheese sauce. Microwave on high 1 minute more. Stir and serve immediately
   over tortilla chips or as a hot dip, with desired garnish.

SERVING SIZE: 2 Servings, ½ Cup Each

PER SERVING: Calories 198   **Sodium:** 773 mg.

*For those who harbor strong sentiments about processed cheese—rest assured this recipe turns out well with any good cheddar. So why do we recommend Velveeta? Less fat, fewer calories, and foolproof meltability.

FAT-FREE TORTILLA CHIPS

Crispy, crunchy corn chips can be yours to munch without a drop of fat! Good with guacamole, salsa, or nacho sauce. Best when freshly made but can be stored in an airtight container at room temperature.

INGREDIENTS

6 CORN TORTILLAS (6½-INCH SIZE)
   WATER
   LIGHT SALT OR CHILI POWDER (OPTIONAL)

DIRECTIONS

Preheat oven to 500°.
Line a cookie sheet with tin foil, then spray foil with nonstick cooking spray.
Working quickly, dip tortillas in water, one at a time. Shake off excess moisture, then lay tortillas
   flat on cutting board.
When all tortillas have been dipped, cut each into six pieces. Arrange pieces in a single layer
   on prepared cookie sheet.
Sprinkle with light salt or chili powder, if desired.
Bake for 4 minutes. Turn over each chip, then bake 3 to 4 minutes longer until golden brown
   and crisp. Watch carefully during the last minute because the line between "crisp" and
   "burnt" is a fine one.

SERVING SIZE: 3 Servings, 12 Chips Each

PER SERVING: Calories 134   **Sodium:** 106 mg.

SPEARED FRUIT

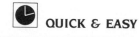 QUICK & EASY

Even if you assembled the crème de la crème of the world's cooking talent and procured the best of every food ingredient, you would still be unable to match the flavors of fresh, ripe fruit. Perfectly delicious and uncompromisingly elegant, speared fruit presents an aromatic kaleidoscope of brightness and freshness. Brilliant green kiwis, ebony grapes, golden pineapple—add a skewer and just a touch of whimsy and you have it—the ultimate showstopping hors d'ouevre! (Pictured on p. 29.)

INGREDIENTS

  2 SPANISH BLOOD ORANGES, SMALL NAVEL ORANGES, OR MANDARINS
 12 KUMQUATS OR SEEDLESS GRAPES
  2 THICK SLICES FRESH PINEAPPLE
  1 LARGE RIPE KIWIFRUIT
 12 STRAWBERRIES OR PITTED CHERRIES
    WATERMELON, HONEYDEW, OR CANTALOUPE, CUT INTO 12 (1-INCH) CUBES

DIRECTIONS

Cut fruit into bite-sized slices, cubes, or wedges.
Spear fruit on thin skewers.
Stand spears in bowl or bucket of crushed ice or use a hollowed-out pineapple or watermelon,
   filled with ice, to support the skewers.

SERVING SIZE: 12 Servings, 1 Skewer Each

PER SERVING: Calories 40   **Sodium:** 2 mg.

ORANGE JULE

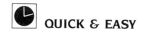 QUICK & EASY

The perfect instant breakfast for the holidays. Tis the season for a new crop of sweet navel oranges—and not a moment too soon! The kids will think this is a real treat, Mom can feel good about the extra vitamin C, but best of all, breakfast will be ready in 3 minutes.

INGREDIENTS

  2 FRESH ORANGES
 ½ CUP PLAIN NONFAT YOGURT
 ½ TEASPOON VANILLA
  2 TABLESPOONS SUGAR OR SUGAR SUBSTITUTE TO TASTE
  4 ICE CUBES

DIRECTIONS

Peel oranges, seed if necessary, and break into chunks for blending.
Place oranges and other ingredients in blender or food processor. Blend until smooth, about 2
   minutes.
Add ice cubes, blend 1 minute longer.
Strain through coarse sieve for a smoother beverage.

VARIATIONS: (1) Add a raw egg for a frothier beverage and extra protein.
(2) Freeze basic mixture halfway. Insert sticks, then freeze firm into popsicles.

SERVING SIZE: 2 Servings, About 12 Ounces Each

PER SERVING: Calories 151   **Sodium:** 45 mg.

WINE COOLERS

Stir up a tall, refreshing wine cooler and sip your way successfully through the calorie-laden cocktail hour. The original recipe for a spritzer—wine and soda with the addition of fresh citrus—lends itself to an endless variety of delicious low-calorie coolers. (Pictured on p. 29.) We've listed a few of our favorites to get you started, but here's the basic formula:

Any wine will do—white, red, rose, or blush. It need not be a fine wine, since its more subtle qualities will be covered by juice and soda.

Freshly squeezed citrus juice is essential. Try lemon, orange, lime—perhaps grapefruit or tangerine! (Bottled juices just won't do.)

Sugar-free sodas like lemon-lime, orange, grapefruit, and, of course, club soda add the fizz and the volume.

Meyer lemons (actually a crossbreed of orange and lemon) impart a subtle, freshly sweet flavor that is hard to match.

INGREDIENTS

Sunset Cooler

2 OZ. LEMON JUICE (1 LEMON, JUICED)
3 OZ. RED WINE, ⅓ CUP
6-10 OZ. DIET LEMON-LIME SODA

Citrus Cooler

1 OZ. FRESH LIME JUICE
1 OZ. FRESH ORANGE JUICE
3 OZ. WHITE WINE
4-6 OZ. DIET LEMON-LIME SODA
2-4 OZ. DIET GRAPEFRUIT SODA

Blush Cooler

3 OZ. BLUSH WINE
6 OZ. SODA
2 OZ. FRESH TANGERINE JUICE

Golden Vermouth Cooler

1 OZ. SWEET VERMOUTH
1 OZ. FRESH LEMON JUICE
2 OZ. FRESH ORANGE JUICE
6-10 OZ. DIET LEMON-LIME SODA

Orange Cooler

1 OZ. FRESH LEMON JUICE
3 OZ. WHITE WINE
6 OZ. DIET ORANGE SODA

DIRECTIONS

Fill a tall glass with ice cubes.
Pour ingredients over ice, swirl, garnish with a twist or a slice of citrus fruit and serve.

SERVING SIZE: 1 12-oz. Cooler

PER SERVING: Calories 80   Sodium content of wine and fruit juice is negligible; diet sodas vary.

NOTE: To calculate your own favorite blend:

Table wine (red, white, rose)	equals 24 calories per oz.
Lemon or lime juice	equals 8 calories per oz.
Orange, grapefruit, or tangerine juice	equals 13 calories per oz.

1 oz. equals 2 tablespoons, 8 oz. equals 1 cup

SPARKLING LEMONADE

 QUICK & EASY

A refreshing alternative to diet soda: frosty, fruity and only 15 calories. As easy to make as juicing a lemon, this old-fashioned soda provides half your daily requirement of vitamin C—naturally.

INGREDIENTS

```
    1 FRESH LEMON, JUICED (¼ CUP)
12-16 OZ. CLUB SODA
      SUGAR SUBSTITUTE OR SUGAR TO TASTE
  4-5 ICE CUBES
```

DIRECTIONS

Pour lemon juice and club soda into a tall glass.
Add sweetener and ice. Stir and serve.

SERVING SIZE: 1 Serving

PER SERVING: Calories 15   **Vitamin C:** 28 mg.

SKINNY EGGNOG

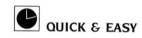 **QUICK & EASY**

The flavor of old-fashioned eggnog in a lighter medium. Cool, frothy, and creamy, this nutritious holiday drink is a children's favorite.

INGREDIENTS

```
  1 CUP NONFAT MILK
  1 EGG
  1 TEASPOON VANILLA
 ⅛ TEASPOON BRANDY EXTRACT
2-3 ICE CUBES
   ARTIFICIAL SWEETENER TO TASTE OR 4 TEASPOONS SUGAR
   NUTMEG
```

DIRECTIONS

Put all ingredients except nutmeg in blender or food processor and blend until smooth, thick, and foamy, about 1 to 2 minutes.
Pour into chilled glasses, top with a sprinkle of nutmeg, and serve immediately.

SERVING SIZE: 2 Servings, 1¼ Cup Each

PER SERVING: Calories 80   **Sodium:** 93 mg.

CITRUS BANANA SMOOTHIE 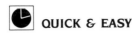 QUICK & EASY

This ready-in-a-minute breakfast drink is a lifesaver on hectic mornings. For extra protein, add an egg and blend until frothy.

INGREDIENTS

    1 FROZEN BANANA*
    ½ CUP PLAIN NONFAT YOGURT
    12 OZ. ORANGE JUICE
       SWEETENER OR SUGAR (OPTIONAL)
    1 EGG (OPTIONAL)

DIRECTIONS

Put all ingredients except sweetener in blender or processor. Blend for about 1 minute, until smooth.
Add sweetener, if desired.

SERVING SIZE: 2 Servings, 1 Cup Each

PER SERVING: Calories 172   **Sodium:** 44 mg.

*To freeze ripe bananas, simply peel, then wrap tightly in plastic wrap.

PINEAPPLE FROST 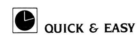 QUICK & EASY

A great thirst quencher on a hot day—one you feel good about drinking yourself or offering to your family. A nutritious alternative to the usual soft drink.

INGREDIENTS

    ½ CUP UNSWEETENED PINEAPPLE JUICE
    1 ORANGE, PEELED AND SEEDED
    1 LEMON, JUICED (¼ CUP)
    4-5 ICE CUBES
       SUGAR SUBSTITUTE TO TASTE OR 1 TABLESPOON SUGAR

DIRECTIONS

Put all ingredients in a blender and blend until smooth. Serve.

VARIATION: The fizzy version. Volume can be increased by adding 1½ cups club soda, which will also give it some fizziness.

SERVING SIZE: 2 Servings, 1 Cup Each

PER SERVING: Calories 78   **Sodium:** 2 mg.

Sauces, Gravies & Relishes

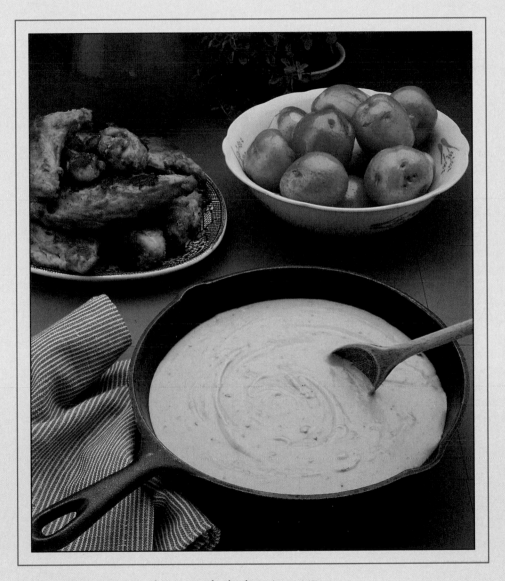

Pan Gravy (p. 48), Southern Fried Chicken (p. 144)

GREEN TOMATILLO SALSA 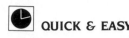 QUICK & EASY

An intensely pungent and acidic salsa. Our first taste of this bright relish arrived atop a mesquite-broiled shark steak in a trendy California dinner house. The cook cheerfully disclosed the ingredients and—after several home trials—we settled on the proportions listed below. This salsa is perfectly suited to broiled fish, but it is equally arresting over a cheese enchilada or plain bean tostada. Fresh tomatillos are available in any grocery that carries Mexican specialties. (Pictured on p. 143.)

INGREDIENTS

½ LB. FRESH TOMATILLOS*
4-6 CLOVES GARLIC
1 CUP FRESH CILANTRO LEAVES

1 TABLESPOON FRESH GREEN CHILE OR PICKLED JALAPEÑO PEPPER

DIRECTIONS

Remove brown husks from tomatillos. Wash thoroughly and cut into chunks.
Place all ingredients in a blender or food processor and chop finely but do not liquefy.
   Makes 1 cup

SERVING SIZE: 1 Tablespoon.

PER SERVING: Calories 7   **Sodium:** 3 mg.

*Tomatillo: the Mexican green tomato, or tomate verde, is a distinct species, not a red tomato that hasn't ripened. Tomatillos are bright green when ripe and are covered with a brown papery husk.

SALSA CRUDA

Salsa, the Spanish word for sauce, has become the American word for Mexican hot sauce. Cruda is the word for raw—or more politely, fresh. This ubiquitous combination of chiles and tomatoes, with herbs, onion, or perhaps garlic, ranges from pedestrian to sublime. A truly exceptional salsa can only be created from quality ingredients. Brightly flavored fresh cilantro is essential. Vine-ripened tomatoes, while equally important, sometimes simply can't be had. When tomatoes are out of season, a combination of well-drained canned tomatoes (which are always vine-ripened) with the best fresh ones you can find, actually works better than using only "fresh" tomatoes when they're not. The small green chili Serrano, with its strong, fresh flavor, is best suited to salsa, but canned green chiles plus hot pepper sauce are an acceptable substitute.

   In the summer, when you can get real tomatoes; go to the trouble of finding fresh cilantro, fresh serrano chiles and a sweet white onion. Make at least a quart of this salsa, put a shark steak or some swordfish on the barbeque—and prepare yourself for a serious gastronomic delight. Barbequed corn-on-the-cob, boiled beans, and roasted sweet peppers are recommended, but not required.

INGREDIENTS

3 CUPS FRESH RIPE TOMATOES, PEELED AND CHOPPED
1 BUNCH FRESH CILANTRO (1 CUP LEAVES) LIGHTLY CHOPPED
1 CLOVE GARLIC, MINCED

1 CUP SWEET WHITE OR RED ONION, FINELY CHOPPED OR 3 GREEN ONIONS, THINLY SLICED
JUICE OF 1 LIME
1-3 SERRANO CHILES, SEEDED AND FINELY CHOPPED
LIGHT SALT TO TASTE

DIRECTIONS

Stir together all ingredients, but do not puree.
Serve within 24 hours. Makes 1 quart.

SERVING SIZE: 1 Tablespoon

PER SERVING: Calories 4   **Sodium:** Negligible Unless Salt Is Added

AL'S HOMEMADE TOMATO SAUCE

If we asked you to taste this, on faith, you would say it's one of the best Italian sauces you have ever had. You might guess there's some wine in it, and, if you have a well-practiced palate, you might be able to identify the herbs and discern the garlic. But we are willing to lay a serious bet that you would never, in a hundred years, guess this robust, full-flavored sauce to be salt-free! We thank our ingenious friend Al Carniglio for sharing the exact blending of herbs, pepper, lemon, and sugar which magically combine to taste salty—without a grain of salt. Pay close attention to Al's technique—it is as critical to success as each ingredient. You can make a large amount of this to have on hand, for it freezes well.

INGREDIENTS

5 LB. RIPE TOMATOES (ABOUT 20 MEDIUM)— ITALIAN ROMA TOMATOES ARE BEST
2 TABLESPOONS OLIVE OIL
½ CUP ONION, FINELY CHOPPED
2 CLOVES GARLIC, MINCED
½ CUP RED WINE (BURGUNDY, CABERNET, OR PINOT NOIR)

1 TEASPOON FRESHLY GROUND BLACK PEPPER
2 TABLESPOONS SUGAR
3 TABLESPOONS LEMON JUICE
1 TEASPOON THYME
1½ TEASPOON OREGANO

DIRECTIONS

First, juice the tomatoes. This sauce requires fresh tomatoes. Substituting canned tomatoes or puree will alter the flavor substantially. Raw tomatoes can be juiced by running through a blender or food processor, then straining to remove skin and seeds. If you prefer, peel and seed tomatoes first, then puree pulp. Better yet, treat yourself to one of those wonderful Italian machines (tomato juicers) that do all of the above in a single step! You should now have 2 quarts fresh tomato juice.

Heat olive oil in a large heavy skillet. Sauté onions and garlic over low heat until golden, about 10 minutes.

Add about half the tomato juice, turn heat up to high, and "fry" the juice, stirring constantly, for about 10 minutes. It will turn deep red and develop a robust flavor.

Add remaining juice, wine, and pepper. Turn heat to low. Simmer 45 minutes, uncovered.

Add sugar, lemon juice, thyme, and oregano. Simmer 10 minutes.

Taste. Add additional wine and herbs to taste, if desired. Simmer at least 10 minutes longer to cook off alcohol and blend flavors.

VARIATIONS: Mushroom Sauce. Saute ½-1 lb. sliced mushrooms with onions and garlic.

Meat Sauce. Add cooked Italian sausage, ground round, or any lean roast meat to finished sauce. Simmer slowly in covered skillet for 30 to 60 minutes to blend flavors.

SERVING SUGGESTIONS: Serve over pasta or polenta. Use in any recipe which calls for prepared spaghetti or marinara sauce.

SERVING SIZE: 6 Servings, 1 Cup Each

PER SERVING: Calories 148   **Sodium:** 12 mg.

BASIC ITALIAN SAUCE

A basic Italian sauce to serve over pasta and use in lasagna, eggplant parmesan, spaghetti and pizza. If slow-simmering sauce is not on your agenda, make this in quantity and freeze for later use. You'll have the convenience of bottled sauce for less money, less fat, and fewer calories.

INGREDIENTS

1 TABLESPOON OLIVE OIL
1 MEDIUM ONION, MINCED
2 CLOVES GARLIC, MINCED
1 LARGE GREEN BELL PEPPER, DICED
2 BAY LEAVES
2 BOUILLON CUBES (VEGETABLE OR BEEF)
2 CANS (8 OZ. EACH) TOMATO SAUCE

1 CAN (28 OZ. EACH) TOMATOES
¼ TEASPOON ROSEMARY
½ TEASPOON THYME
½ TEASPOON BASIL
1 TEASPOON OREGANO
¼ TEASPOON BLACK PEPPER
SLICED MUSHROOMS (OPTIONAL)

DIRECTIONS

Sauté onions and garlic in oil in large cast iron skillet, over medium heat until tender.
Add remaining ingredients. Cover and simmer at least 1 hour over very low heat. Stir occasionally.

SERVING SIZE: 6 Servings, ¾ Cup Each

PER SERVING: Calories 97 **Sodium:** 913 mg.

SPAGHETTI SAUCE WITH MEAT

Spaghetti is on that list of "world's most wonderful foods that you aren't supposed to eat on a diet." We used very lean ground beef and no added fats to make this chunky spaghetti sauce. It has only 223 calories per serving, including the meat. For the die-hard dieter, serve over spaghetti squash or steamed zucchini. Having said that, remember that a cup of cooked pasta has only 200 calories.

INGREDIENTS

1 LB. EXTRA LEAN GROUND BEEF
2 LARGE ONIONS, CHOPPED
2 LARGE CLOVES GARLIC, MINCED
1 TEASPOON OREGANO
½ TEASPOON BASIL
1 LARGE BAY LEAF
1 TEASPOON LIGHT SALT

¼ TEASPOON BLACK PEPPER
¼ TEASPOON ROSEMARY
1 TEASPOON SUGAR
1 CUP SLICED FRESH MUSHROOMS OR 1 CAN (4 OZ.), DRAINED
¾ CUP DRY RED WINE
4 CUPS FRESH OR CANNED TOMATO PUREE*

DIRECTIONS

Brown meat over medium-high heat in a large cast iron skillet and drain off any fat.†
Add onions and garlic. Sauté over low heat until tender, about 15 minutes.
Add oregano, basil, bay leaf, light salt, pepper, rosemary, sugar, mushrooms, wine, and puree.
   Simmer for 1 to 1½ hours stirring occasionally.

SERVING SIZE: 6 Servings, 1 Cup Each

PER SERVING: Calories 223 **Sodium:** 276 mg.

*Fresh tomatoes, pureed in the blender, contain about 50 mg sodium per cup, while canned tomato puree contains 1000 mg sodium per cup. The sodium content of this recipe is based on fresh tomatoes plus 1 teaspoon light salt. Using canned tomato puree or sauce, skipping the 1 teaspoon salt would give you 720 mg sodium per cup.
†Using a cast iron skillet will improve iron content of food.

OKLAHOMA BARBEQUE SAUCE

This makes a lot of barbeque sauce, but it keeps for months—like catsup—at room temperature. Figuring out how to preserve it will be the least of your worries; you'll lose a jar to every friend who tastes it. In fact, poured into a fruit jar and tied with a checkered bow, it makes a perfect gift. This is a truly authentic and original secret recipe developed by W.D. Lowry of Oklahoma City. W.D. is a delightful 79-year-old butcher who gets up every morning, except Sunday, at 4:30 sharp to open the meat counter at the South Side market. On Sundays he visits his grandchildren, delighting them with raucous imitations of braying donkeys. This game has earned him the affectionate nickname of Grandpa Donkey. The handle extends to this famous sauce, known far and wide as "donkey sauce." For 20 years now, friends and family (including daughter-in-law, Eve Lowry) have encouraged W.D. to bottle and sell his secret sauce. Instead, he made a gift of it to us and now to you. (Pictured on p. 143.)

INGREDIENTS

1½ QUARTS BOILING WATER	1½ TEASPOONS CAYENNE PEPPER
1 CUP VINEGAR	2 QUARTS CATSUP
2 TABLESPOONS CHILI POWDER	1½ TEASPOONS CUMIN
¾ CUP SUGAR	1½ TEASPOONS OREGANO
1½ TEASPOONS GARLIC POWDER	2 TABLESPOONS WRIGHT'S LIQUID SMOKE
3 TABLESPOONS CAIN'S BBQ SPICE MIX	2 TABLESPOONS PAPRIKA

DIRECTIONS

Mix all ingredients in a large 5 to 6-quart pot. Simmer uncovered over lowest possible heat for 6 to 8 hours.

Stir occasionally to prevent scorching.

The sauce is ready when the consistency resembles that of catsup and the volume is reduced to about 3 quarts.

SERVING SIZE: 1 Tablespoon

PER SERVING: Calories: 15   **Sodium:** 100 mg.

SHERRIED MUSHROOM SAUCE

A golden-brown, richly flavored sauce, a bit like a Bordelaise, but softened with a touch of cream. Lovely over potatoes or almost any vegetable, but especially well suited to the cruciferous vegetables: broccoli, cauliflower, brussels sprouts, and cabbage.

INGREDIENTS

2 TABLESPOONS BUTTER	1 CUBE BEEF BOUILLON
2 MEDIUM ONIONS, FINELY MINCED	2 TEASPOONS WORCESTERSHIRE SAUCE
½ LB. MUSHROOMS, 2 CUPS, SLICED	1 TEASPOON FRESH DILL, MINCED, OR
1 CAN (10½ OZ.) CONDENSED OR DOUBLE-STRENGTH CHICKEN BROTH	¼ TEASPOON, DRIED DILL
	4 TABLESPOONS WHITE FLOUR
¼ CUP SHERRY	2 CUPS NONFAT MILK

DIRECTIONS

Melt butter in nonstick skillet and sauté onion over medium heat for 20 minutes until golden brown. Stir often to prevent scorching. Mixture will be dry but will brown nicely if stirred. Browning is important to develop the full flavor of this sauce.

Add sliced mushrooms and sauté 5 minutes more until mushrooms are limp and golden.

Add broth, sherry, bouillon, Worcestershire sauce, and dill to vegetables and heat through.

Combine flour with nonfat milk in blender or shaker jar.

Add milk mixture to sauce and stir over low heat until thick and heated through, about 5 minutes.

Continued

SERVING SIZE: 16 Servings, ½ Cup Each

PER SERVING: Calories   90   **Sodium:** 386 mg.

SAUCE BORDELAISE

Parsley root, commonly used in European kitchens to season soup stock and gravy base, is not widely available in American markets. This rich brown wine sauce uses parsley stems as a reasonable substitute. Serve this intensely flavored sauce with meats, potatoes, or rice.

INGREDIENTS

2 CLOVES GARLIC	½ TEASPOON THYME
1 LARGE CARROT	½ TEASPOON FRESHLY GROUND BLACK PEPPER
1 SMALL UNPEELED YELLOW ONION	2 CUPS DRY RED WINE
STEMS FROM ONE BUNCH PARSLEY	2 CUPS BEEF BROTH
1 TABLESPOON OLIVE OIL	2 TABLESPOONS BUTTER
1 BAY LEAF	4 TABLESPOONS WHITE FLOUR

DIRECTIONS

Wash but do not peel vegetables, since they are used to season the stock, but are then removed. Prepare as follows:
Crush garlic cloves by smashing with side of knife blade.
Scrub carrot and chop coarsely.
Rinse onion. Cut off root end, then coarsely chop the rest, including skins, which help color the sauce.
Cut stems off bunch of parsley and rinse.
Heat olive oil in a large heavy pan. Add all prepared vegetables plus bay leaf, thyme, and pepper. Sauté over medium heat until vegetables are very well browned, about 20 to 25 minutes, stirring often.
Add wine and broth. Bring to a boil, reduce heat, and simmer uncovered for 30 minutes. Strain. You should have about 2 cups.
In a heavy saucepan, over medium heat, melt butter. When it stops spattering, add flour, stirring constantly, to make a rather dry roux. Stir constantly for 1 minute, to brown flour.
Add strained broth, stirring constantly until sauce thickens and bubbles. Reduce heat, simmer 10 to 12 minutes, to blend flavors and reduce to desired consistency. Makes 2 cups, 32 tablespoons.

SERVING SIZE: 1 Tablespoon

PER SERVING: Calories   18   **Sodium:** 55 mg.

BACON CHEESE SAUCE QUICK & EASY

This is a quick and easy sauce for broccoli, cauliflower, or steamed cabbage. It's also delicious on baked potatoes.

INGREDIENTS

2 TEASPOONS BUTTER	1 TABLESPOON WHITE FLOUR
2 TABLESPOONS ONION, FINELY MINCED	⅔ CUP NONFAT MILK
1½ OZ. VELVEETA, SHARP CHEDDAR, OR SWISS	1 TEASPOON BACON BITS, CRUSHED
CHEESE, SHREDDED (ABOUT ½ CUP)	DASH WHITE PEPPER

DIRECTIONS

Melt butter and sauté minced onion in small saucepan or nonstick skillet over medium heat until golden, about 5 minutes.

Combine shredded cheese, flour, and milk in a small bowl. Add to onions. Stir until cheese
  melts and sauce thickens and bubbles.
Add crushed bacon bits and pepper to taste.
Serve over steamed vegetables.

SERVING SIZE: 4 Servings, 2 Tablespoons Each

PER SERVING: Calories 75 **Sodium:** 201 mg.

NORWEGIAN HOT MUSTARD SAUCE QUICK & EASY

This wonderful recipe came from Anne Tye, who adapted it from her grandmother's Norwegian
cookbook. The original recipe says this sauce is to be served over poached cod, but we find
it's equally delicious with many other kinds of fish and just perfect on Lentil Loaf.

INGREDIENTS

⅓ CUP DIET MAYONNAISE
3 TABLESPOONS VINEGAR
3 TABLESPOONS PREPARED GRAINY (DIJON) MUSTARD
1-1½ TABLESPOONS DRY MUSTARD (DEPENDING ON HOTNESS DESIRED)

½ TEASPOON LIGHT SALT
¼ TEASPOON WHITE PEPPER
3 TABLESPOONS SUGAR
⅛ TEASPOON CARDAMOM
1 TABLESPOON OLIVE OIL (OPTIONAL)

DIRECTIONS

Combine all ingredients in a small bowl or blender. Adjust the amount of dry mustard you use
  according to how hot you want your sauce to be. The olive oil lends a smoothness to the
  flavors but is not necessary to the success of the sauce.
Beat well to combine. Cover and chill for at least 2 hours. Makes 1 cup.

SERVING SIZE: 1 Tablespoon

PER SERVING: Calories 28 **Sodium:** 102 mg.

COCKTAIL SAUCE 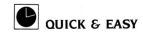 QUICK & EASY

INGREDIENTS

½ CUP CATSUP
3 TABLESPOONS LIME JUICE

2 TABLESPOONS HORSERADISH
1-2 TEASPOONS FRESH PARSLEY, VERY FINELY CHOPPED

DIRECTIONS

Combine all ingredients in a small bowl. Chill and serve.

SERVING SIZE: 12 Servings, 1 Tablespoon Each

PER SERVING: Calories 13 **Sodium:** 107 mg.

JANIS' SEAFOOD SAUCE 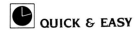 QUICK & EASY

Janis Arch, expert massage therapist and consummate cook, shared this recipe with us.

INGREDIENTS

¼ CUP DIJON MUSTARD
1 CUP PLAIN NONFAT YOGURT

2 TABLESPOONS HORSERADISH, DRAINED
1 TABLESPOON FRESH PARSLEY, MINCED

Continued

DIRECTIONS

Mix all ingredients together in a small bowl and chill. Serve with hot or cold fish. Makes
1½ Cups (24 Tablespoons).

SERVING SIZE: 1 Tablespoon

PER SERVING: Calories 8   **Sodium:** 41 mg.

PAN GRAVY

Here's a traditional "country gravy" for about half the fat and calories of standard pan gravy. (Pictured on p. 41.)
For a completely fat-free sauce method, see Kettle Gravy.

INGREDIENTS

  2 TABLESPOONS BACON FAT, CHICKEN FAT, OR OTHER MEAT FAT
  4 TABLESPOONS WHITE FLOUR
2½ CUPS NONFAT MILK
  2 BOUILLON CUBES OR 2 TEASPOONS POWDERED BOUILLON, DISSOLVED IN ¼ CUP HOT WATER
⅛ TEASPOON FRESHLY GROUND BLACK PEPPER
¼ TEASPOON THYME

DIRECTIONS

Melt fat in a heavy skillet.
Add flour. Heat, stirring constantly until flour begins to turn golden. You will have a rather
   lumpy roux.
Stir in milk all at once, then heat, stirring constantly, until thickened.
Add dissolved bouillon, pepper, and thyme.
Simmer for 2 minutes, stirring. Adjust seasonings. Serve.

SERVING SIZE: Makes 2½ Cups or 10 Servings, ¼ Cup Each

PER SERVING: Calories 58   **Sodium:** 270 mg. (from bouillon)

KETTLE GRAVY

Have you ever wondered how it is that frozen diet dinners can be swimming in sauce and still
call themselves low-calorie? Experienced cooks know there is more than one way to make
gravy. Most sauces and gravies begin with a roux: a mixture of fat and flour to which the liquid
is added. In contrast, a kettle gravy begins with broth or meat juices, which are then thickened
with flour or cornstarch to achieve the desired consistency. By this method a rich, full-bodied
gravy can be made without a drop of fat!

   The goodness of your gravy will depend directly on how good a broth you use to begin
with. Savory meat juices from a slowly simmered, well-seasoned pot roast, or broth from a
chicken stewed with vegetables and herbs will certainly produce the most elegant of fat-free
sauces; but even ordinary canned broth can be brought along nicely with the addition of
herbs and spices. Fresh herbs can work an instant transformation; dried are good too, if some
simmering time is allowed to blend flavors.

INGREDIENTS

2 CUPS GOOD STRONG BROTH OR MEAT
  DRIPPINGS, SKIMMED OF ALL FAT
⅛ TEASPOON WHITE OR FRESHLY GROUND
  BLACK PEPPER
½ TEASPOON ONION POWDER
⅛ TEASPOON THYME OR SAGE

¼ TEASPOON MARJORAM OR BASIL (OR
  ½-1 TEASPOON FRESH HERBS)
1 CUP NONFAT MILK
5 TABLESPOONS WHITE FLOUR*
  LIGHT SALT (OPTIONAL)
  FRESHLY CHOPPED PARSLEY, DILL, CHIVES,
  OR SCALLIONS FOR GARNISH

DIRECTIONS

Heat broth or meat juices in a 2-quart saucepan, with all seasonings except fresh parsley, dill, or chives. Simmer 5 minutes or longer to develop flavor.

Dissolve flour in nonfat milk in blender or shaker jar.

Bring seasoned broth to a full, rolling boil. Slowly add milk and dissolved flour, stirring constantly until mixture thickens and returns to boiling.

Turn heat very low, simmer uncovered 5 to 10 minutes more to thoroughly cook the flour and further reduce the fluid. Stir occasionally to prevent scorching. Adjust seasonings; add light salt, if desired.

Sprinkle with freshly chopped parsley, dill, chives, or scallions just before serving. Makes 2½ to 3 Cups, 6 Generous Servings.

SERVING SIZE: ⅙ of recipe

PER SERVING: Calories 50   **Sodium:** 334 mg. (with canned broth)

*For a thicker gravy, use 6 to 7 tablespoons flour. Three to four tablespoons nonfat dry milk solids can be dissolved along with the flour, if a very creamy flavor is desired.

MIDDLE EASTERN CUCUMBER RELISH 🕐 QUICK & EASY

Serve this cool, flavorful relish with shish kebab or any barbequed fish.

INGREDIENTS

1 MEDIUM CUCUMBER, PEELED, SEEDED, AND CUT IN ¼-INCH CUBES, ABOUT 1 CUP
¼ CUP RADISHES, THINLY SLICED
½ CUP SCALLIONS, THINLY SLICED

½ CUP PLAIN NONFAT YOGURT
¼ CUP DIET MAYONNAISE
BLACK PEPPER TO TASTE

DIRECTIONS

Combine all ingredients in a medium bowl. Cover and chill. Makes 2 cups.

SERVING SIZE: 8 Servings, ¼ Cup Each

PER SERVING: Calories 33   **Sodium:** 63 mg.

INSTANT CRANBERRY RELISH 🕐 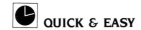QUICK & EASY

Bright, piquant, and flavorful, this relish is excellent with poultry. For a special garnish, mound this colorful relish on pear halves or in orange cups.

INGREDIENTS

1 BAG (12 OZ.) FRESH CRANBERRIES
1 WHOLE ORANGE, PEELED AND SEEDED

GRATED PEEL OF ½-1 ORANGE (TO TASTE)
SUGAR SUBSTITUTE OR ½-1 CUP SUGAR (TO TASTE)

DIRECTIONS

Place cranberries and peeled orange in food processor or blender.

Blend intermittently to desired consistency. Do not overblend. Consistency should resemble that of granola.

Add sugar substitute or sugar and orange peel to taste. Orange peel adds aroma and improves flavor. Flavor will range from very tart to much sweeter, depending on amount of sweetener used.

SERVING SIZE: 5 Servings, ½ Cup Each

PER SERVING: Calories 40   **Sodium:** 2 mg.

Soups & Stews

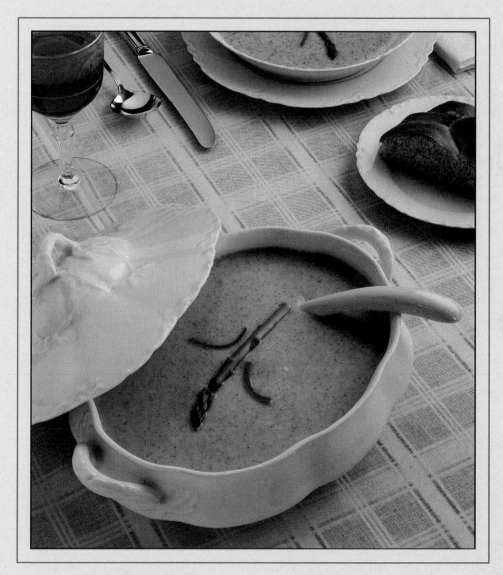

Asparagus Soup (p. 68)

LENORE FINNEY'S NAVY BEAN SOUP

QUICK & EASY

One of the very nicest things that can happen to anyone is to be invited into Judge and Mrs. Finney's kitchen at Lake Tahoe. The big butcher block is likely to be laden with an assortment of quick breads and cookies, and if you're really lucky, navy bean soup will be simmering on the stove. This simple and soul-warming recipe comes from Lenore's kitchen to yours.

INGREDIENTS

    8 CUPS WATER
    1 LB. DRY SMALL WHITE BEANS
    1 ONION, DICED
 1½ CUPS CELERY, CHOPPED
 1½ TEASPOONS LIGHT SALT
    1 BAY LEAF
  ½ TEASPOON ITALIAN SEASONING
    2 TABLESPOONS BUTTER

DIRECTIONS

Rinse and sort beans. Soak them overnight in a large covered soup pot with 5 cups of water.
Add remaining 3 cups water, onion, celery, light salt, bay leaf, Italian seasoning, and butter.
    Bring mixture to a boil. Then cover, leaving lid slightly ajar, reduce heat, and simmer for 3 to
    4 hours until beans are very tender.
Check several times during cooking. Add more water if needed to obtain desired consistency.
Adjust seasonings.

SERVING SIZE: 8 Servings, 1 Cup Each

PER SERVING: Calories 226   **Fiber:** 9 grams   **Sodium:** 273 mg.

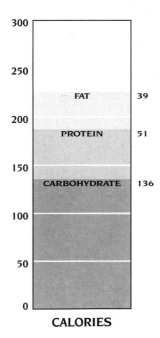

FAT	39
PROTEIN	51
CARBOHYDRATE	136

CALORIES

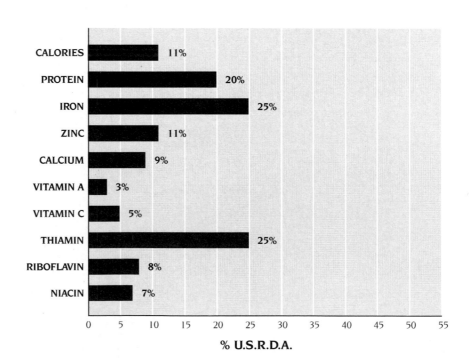

	% U.S.R.D.A.
CALORIES	11%
PROTEIN	20%
IRON	25%
ZINC	11%
CALCIUM	9%
VITAMIN A	3%
VITAMIN C	5%
THIAMIN	25%
RIBOFLAVIN	8%
NIACIN	7%

% U.S.R.D.A.

BLACK BEAN SOUP

The Columbia restaurant, a landmark of Tampa's Latin quarter, has earned its reputation by offering consistently delicious Spanish cuisine. In our opinion their black bean soup is the very best. Artfully presented in a broad-rimmed white bowl, this decidedly black soup surrounds an island of steamed rice and is garnished with a starkly contrasting sprinkle of white onion. This soup makes an elegant first course or an impressive vegetarian entree.

INGREDIENTS

1 LB. DRY BLACK BEANS
2 QUARTS WATER
2 TABLESPOONS OLIVE OIL
4 CLOVES GARLIC, MINCED
3 LARGE ONIONS, FINELY CHOPPED
2 LARGE BELL PEPPERS, CUT IN THIN STRIPS
¼ TEASPOON CUMIN

½ TEASPOON BLACK PEPPER
1 BAY LEAF
1 TEASPOON OREGANO, CRUSHED
1 TABLESPOON LIGHT SALT
COOKED BROWN RICE
CHOPPED WHITE ONION FOR GARNISH

DIRECTIONS

Wash and sort beans. Soak overnight in 2 quarts water.

Pour beans into a 4-quart soup kettle and bring to a boil in same soaking water. Simmer over lowest possible heat, partially covered.

Meanwhile, heat olive oil in a large nonstick skillet. Sauté garlic, onions, and bell pepper strips over low heat until tender, about 20 minutes. Add cumin, black pepper, bay leaf, oregano, and light salt. Add vegetable mixture to beans and stir well. Continue to cook slowly until beans are tender, about 2½ to 3 hours.

Cook brown rice. Use ½ to 1 cup cooked rice per person.

SERVING SUGGESTIONS: Place a mound of rice to one side of a broad-rimmed soup bowl, then carefully ladle soup into bowl, so that it flows around, but doesn't cover the "rice island." Sprinkle with chopped white onion. Chopped parsley, lemon slices, or hard-boiled egg slices are alternate garnishes.

SERVING SIZE: 10 Servings, 1 Cup Each

PER SERVING: Calories 202 **Fiber:** 7 grams **Sodium:** 342 mg.

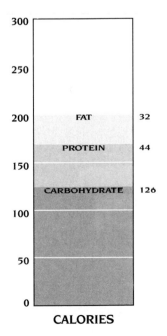

FAT	32
PROTEIN	44
CARBOHYDRATE	126

CALORIES

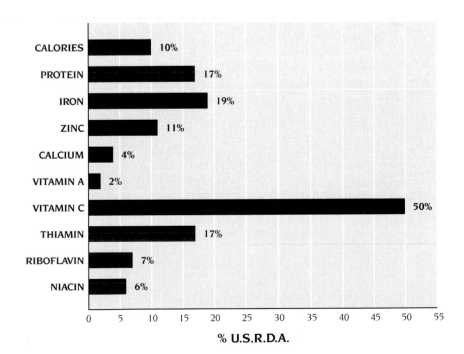

CALORIES 10%
PROTEIN 17%
IRON 19%
ZINC 11%
CALCIUM 4%
VITAMIN A 2%
VITAMIN C 50%
THIAMIN 17%
RIBOFLAVIN 7%
NIACIN 6%

% U.S.R.D.A.

SOPA DE LENTEJAS
(LENTIL SOUP)

Lentils, like beans and peas, make excellent soups. In Mexico, lentil soup appears frequently as the "soup of the day," much like our Navy Bean soup. We tasted this delicious soup at the El Presidente in Loreto, then ventured into the hotel kitchen to request the recipe from the sous-chef. While quite the gentleman, and most "simpatico," he didn't speak English. After an entertaining session of pantomime, assisted by our waiter, two cooks, and a busboy, we came away with what we believe to be the authentic formula. If it isn't, it should be, as it is superb.

INGREDIENTS

1 CUP LENTILS
3 QUARTS WATER
3 LARGE CARROTS, CHOPPED
4 LARGE TOMATOES, PEELED AND CHOPPED OR
  1 CAN (28 OZ.) TOMATOES, CHOPPED
2 SLICES (2 OZ.) LEAN BACON, DICED
1 TABLESPOON RESERVED BACON FAT
2 MEDIUM ONIONS, CHOPPED

4 CLOVES GARLIC, MINCED
1 BELL PEPPER, DICED
3 CUBES CHICKEN BOUILLON OR 3 TEASPOONS
  POWDERED SOUP BASE
¼ TEASPOON BLACK PEPPER
1-2 TABLESPOONS CHILI POWDER
2 TABLESPOONS WORCESTERSHIRE SAUCE
  CUMIN AND RED PEPPER TO TASTE (OPTIONAL)

DIRECTIONS

Rinse and sort lentils. Put in a large kettle with 3 quarts water, carrots, and tomatoes. Bring to a
  boil; then reduce heat, cover, and simmer for 30 to 60 minutes, until lentils are tender.
Meanwhile, in a nonstick skillet, sauté diced bacon until crisp. Drain bacon on a paper towel.
  Reserve 1 tablespoon bacon fat and discard the rest.
Sauté onion, garlic, and bell pepper in the fat until onion and garlic are golden brown.
Add sautéed vegetables and crisp bacon to lentils along with chicken bouillon, black pepper,
  chili powder, and Worcestershire. Simmer 30 minutes to blend flavors.
Taste and adjust seasonings. Add cumin and red pepper, if desired, and simmer 10 minutes more.

SERVING SIZE: 12 Servings, 1 Cup Each

PER SERVING: Calories 113   **Fiber:** 3 grams   **Sodium:** 299 mg.

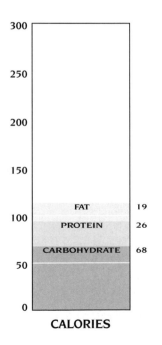

FAT	19
PROTEIN	26
CARBOHYDRATE	68

CALORIES

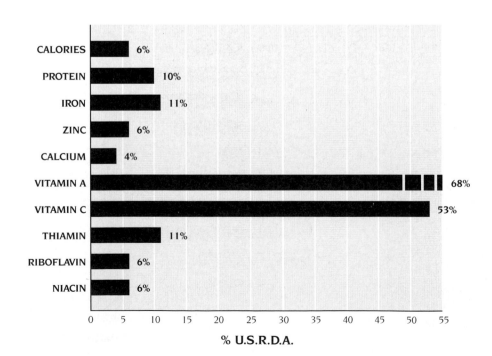

CALORIES	6%
PROTEIN	10%
IRON	11%
ZINC	6%
CALCIUM	4%
VITAMIN A	68%
VITAMIN C	53%
THIAMIN	11%
RIBOFLAVIN	6%
NIACIN	6%

% U.S.R.D.A.

PEA SOUP
ANDERSEN'S ORIGINAL RECIPE FOR SPLIT PEA SOUP

This well-loved soup dates back to June, 1924, when Anton and Juliette Andersen arrived in California's beautiful Santa Ynez Valley and opened their restaurant in Buellton. Anton was from Denmark and Juliette from France, both with years of experience in the preparation of fine foods. Juliette's recipe for split pea soup was an immediate favorite, and Anton's flair for the dramatic soon popularized the restaurant as the "Original Home of Split Pea Soup." Today Pea Soup Andersen's serves over 400,000 gallons of their delicious and nutritious soup every year at their three California locations.

INGREDIENTS

2 QUARTS OF SOFT WATER
2 CUPS OF GREEN SPLIT PEAS
1 BRANCH OF CELERY, COARSELY CHOPPED
1 LARGE CARROT, CHOPPED
1 SMALL ONION, CHOPPED

¼ TEASPOON GROUND THYME
1 PINCH CAYENNE PEPPER
1 BAY LEAF
SALT AND BLACK PEPPER

DIRECTIONS

NOTE: While directions on the limited space of a bag of split peas read simply, "Boil hard for 20 minutes, then slowly, until peas are tender. Strain through a fine sieve and reheat to boiling point," more detailed directions follow here:

Combine water, split peas, celery, carrot, onion, thyme, cayenne, and bay leaf in a large kettle. Bring to a boil and boil vigorously, uncovered, for 20 minutes.

Reduce heat, cover, and simmer until peas are tender, about 40 minutes.

Taste and season as desired with light salt and black pepper.

To achieve the exact texture and flavor of the soup served by Pea Soup Andersen's, strain through a fine sieve before serving. For a finely textured soup which retains full fiber value, simply whirl in blender or food processor.

SERVING SIZE: 8 Servings, 1 Cup Each

PER SERVING: Calories 185   **Fiber:** 9 grams   **Sodium:** 35 mg.

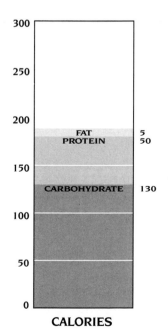

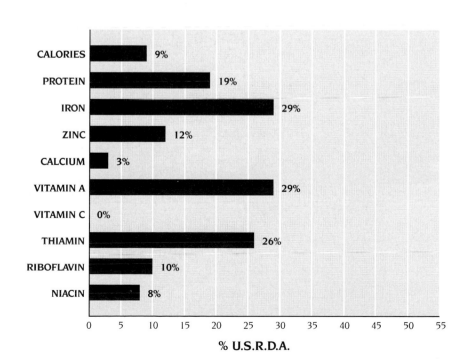

% U.S.R.D.A.

MINESTRONE SOUP

Of all the minestrone soups we tested, this was our favorite. Thick and rich, it needs only a fresh green salad and a loaf of crusty bread to complete the menu. This soup freezes well, so you might like to double the recipe.

INGREDIENTS

- 1 TABLESPOON OLIVE OIL
- 4 CLOVES GARLIC, MINCED
- ¼ TEASPOON FRESHLY GROUND BLACK PEPPER
- 1 CAN (1 LB.) KIDNEY BEANS, WITH LIQUID
- 1 CAN (1 LB.) GREEN LIMA BEANS, WITH LIQUID
- 4 CUPS WATER
- ¼ CUP CHOPPED FRESH PARSLEY
- 2 SMALL STALKS CELERY WITH TOPS, THINLY SLICED

- 1 LARGE CARROT, THINLY SLICED
- 6 SMALL GREEN ONIONS, SLICED
- 1 BUNCH SWISS CHARD (3-5 LARGE LEAVES), CUT IN 1-INCH PIECES
- 1 CAN (8 OZ.) TOMATO SAUCE
- ⅓ CUP SHERRY
- 1 CUP WHOLE WHEAT ELBOW MACARONI

DIRECTIONS

Heat the olive oil in a large, heavy soup kettle. Sauté garlic and ground pepper for 1 to 2 minutes.

Add about half the kidney beans and half the lima beans along with their liquid. Mash with a wooden spoon or potato masher. Then add remaining beans and leave them whole.

Add water, parsley, celery, carrot, green onions, Swiss chard, and tomato sauce. Bring to a boil then reduce heat, cover, and simmer for 30 to 40 minutes, until vegetables are tender.

Add sherry and macaroni. Simmer, uncovered, for 15 to 20 minutes until macaroni is tender.

VARIATIONS: Add 1 to 2 cups of one of the following: potato, zucchini, onion, leeks, green beans, or peas along with other vegetables.

Substitute 1 large head of shredded Chinese cabbage for the chard.

SERVING SIZE: 8 Servings, 1 Cup Each

PER SERVING: Calories 162 **Fiber:** 15 grams **Sodium:** 612 mg.

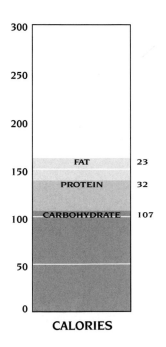

CALORIES

FAT	23
PROTEIN	32
CARBOHYDRATE	107

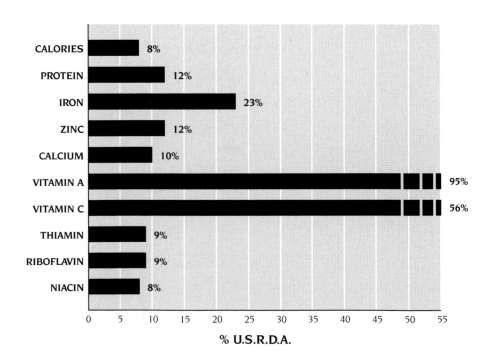

	% U.S.R.D.A.
CALORIES	8%
PROTEIN	12%
IRON	23%
ZINC	12%
CALCIUM	10%
VITAMIN A	95%
VITAMIN C	56%
THIAMIN	9%
RIBOFLAVIN	9%
NIACIN	8%

OLD-FASHIONED SPLIT PEA SOUP WITH HAM HOCKS

INGREDIENTS

1 LB. DRY GREEN SPLIT PEAS	1 BAY LEAF
1½ LB. HAM HOCKS	½ TEASPOON THYME
3½ QUARTS WATER	¼ TEASPOON ALLSPICE
1 LARGE ONION, FINELY CHOPPED	1 CLOVE GARLIC, MINCED
1 LARGE CARROT, FINELY CHOPPED	¼ TEASPOON BLACK PEPPER
1 LARGE STALK CELERY, FINELY CHOPPED	1 TEASPOON LIGHT SALT OR TO TASTE

DIRECTIONS

Rinse and sort split peas. Soak them in 6 cups water for several hours or overnight.

Simmer ham hocks in 2 quarts water until meat falls away from bones, about 1½ to 2 hours.

Remove ham hocks, cool, then separate meat from bone and fat. (You will have 5-7 oz. lean meat.)

Cool broth and skim off fat or refrigerate overnight and lift fat from gelled broth.

To the skimmed broth, add the split peas along with their soaking water. Stir in meat, vegetables, and seasonings. Bring to a boil, then reduce heat. Cover and simmer for 1½ hours over very low heat. Stir occasionally; add water if needed.

VARIATIONS: Quick Version. In place of ham hocks, use 12 oz. lean turkey ham cut in ¼-inch cubes. Reduce water to 2½ quarts. In a very large kettle, combine all ingredients plus 2 cups chicken broth. Cook over low heat for 1½ to 2 hours, stirring occasionally.

Pea Soup With Mushrooms. Add 1 lb. sliced or chopped fresh mushrooms to other vegetables.

SERVING SIZE: 12 Servings, 1 Cup Each

PER SERVING: Calories 167   **Fiber:** 17 grams   **Sodium:** 247 mg.

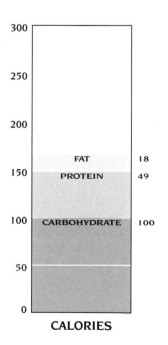

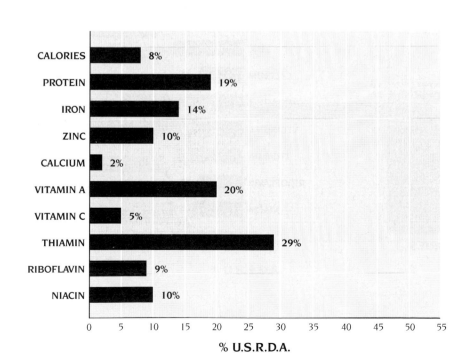

MULLIGATAWNY SOUP

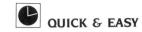 **QUICK & EASY**

Hearty, warmly spiced, richly textured, and satisfying to the soul—everything a soup should be.

INGREDIENTS

1½ TABLESPOONS BUTTER
1 MEDIUM ONION, CHOPPED
1 MEDIUM CARROT, PEELED AND DICED
1 BELL PEPPER, DICED
1 STALK CELERY, TRIMMED AND DICED
1 LARGE, TART APPLE, PEELED AND CHOPPED
2 CUPS COOKED CHICKEN, CUBED, OR 1 CAN (12 OZ.) CHICKEN CHUNKS
¼ CUP WHITE FLOUR

4 WHOLE CLOVES
2-3 TEASPOONS CURRY POWDER
¼ CUP FRESH PARSLEY, MINCED
¼ TEASPOON NUTMEG
2 CUPS CHICKEN BROTH OR 1 CAN (14½ OZ.)
2 CUPS TOMATOES, PEELED AND CHOPPED, OR
1 CAN (1 LB.) PEELED TOMATOES, CHOPPED
FRESHLY GROUND BLACK PEPPER
LIGHT SALT (OPTIONAL)

DIRECTIONS

Melt butter in a large saucepan over medium high heat. Add onion and sauté for 5 minutes.

Add carrot, pepper, celery, apple and chicken. Sauté, stirring often until vegetables are tender, about 10 to 12 minutes.

Sprinkle flour, cloves, curry, parsley, and nutmeg over vegetable mixture in pan. Sauté 1 minute, stirring constantly.

Stir in broth and tomatoes with their liquid. Season with pepper to taste and light salt, if desired.

Cover, reduce heat to low, and simmer gently for about 30 minutes.

If a thinner soup is desired, add more chicken broth. Remove whole cloves and serve.

SERVING SIZE: 10 Servings, 1 Cup Each

PER SERVING: Calories 127 **Fiber:** 2 grams **Sodium:** 249 mg.

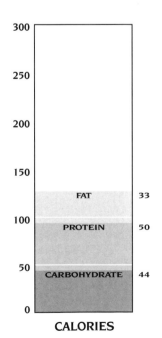

FAT 33
PROTEIN 50
CARBOHYDRATE 44

CALORIES

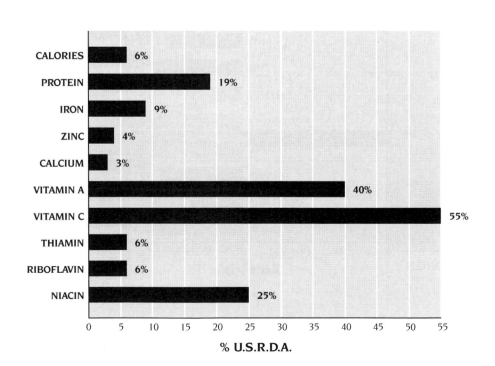

CALORIES 6%
PROTEIN 19%
IRON 9%
ZINC 4%
CALCIUM 3%
VITAMIN A 40%
VITAMIN C 55%
THIAMIN 6%
RIBOFLAVIN 6%
NIACIN 25%

% U.S.R.D.A.

FATIMA'S BEEF STEW

Fatima is Portugese, but her beef stew is an international favorite. As head cook in a California retirement home, her food is taste-tested by residents and staff of every nationality. On the day Fatima is making stew, no one leaves the premises for lunch. This stew freezes well, so make a big batch.

INGREDIENTS

- 2 TEASPOONS OIL
- 2 LB. LEAN BEEF, TRIMMED AND CUT IN 1-INCH CUBES
- 1 LARGE OR 2 SMALL ONIONS, CHOPPED
- 3 CUPS WATER
- 2 CHICKEN BOUILLON CUBES
- 1 BEEF BOUILLON CUBE
- ½ TEASPOON GARLIC POWDER
- ½ TEASPOON THYME
- 1 BAY LEAF
- 6 MEDIUM POTATOES, PEELED AND CUT IN CHUNKS
- 3 LARGE CARROTS, CUT IN ½ INCH SLICES
- 1 SMALL HEAD CABBAGE, FINELY CHOPPED
- 1 CAN (1 LB.) STEWED TOMATOES
- 2 TABLESPOONS FLOUR IN ½ CUP COLD WATER
- ¼ TEASPOON BLACK PEPPER AND LIGHT SALT TO TASTE

DIRECTIONS

Brown cubed beef in oil in a large heavy skillet or Dutch oven over medium-high heat.

Add onion and brown, stirring for 1 to 2 minutes.

Add water, chicken and beef bouillon cubes, garlic powder, thyme, and bay leaf. Bring mixture to a boil, then reduce heat, cover, and simmer for 1½ to 2 hours, until meat is tender.

Add potatoes, carrots, cabbage, and tomatoes. Cover and simmer for 30 minutes until vegetables are tender.

Add flour dissolved in cold water, stir until thickened, then simmer 2 to 3 minutes.

Add pepper and light salt to taste.

SERVING SIZE: 16 Servings, 1 Cup Each

PER SERVING: Calories 153   **Fiber:** 3 grams   **Sodium:** 293 mg.

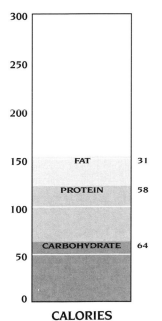

	CALORIES
FAT	31
PROTEIN	58
CARBOHYDRATE	64

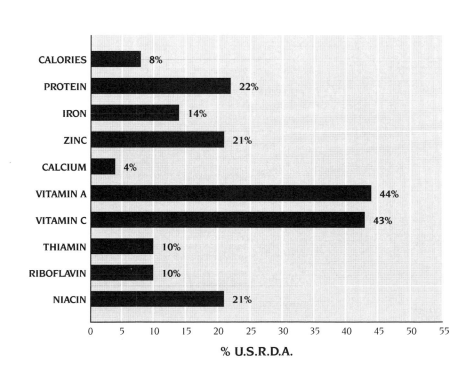

	% U.S.R.D.A.
CALORIES	8%
PROTEIN	22%
IRON	14%
ZINC	21%
CALCIUM	4%
VITAMIN A	44%
VITAMIN C	43%
THIAMIN	10%
RIBOFLAVIN	10%
NIACIN	21%

ASPARAGUS SOUP

We fell in love with Lili Kozerski's asparagus soup with the first spoonful. Assuming it would have to be filed under "sinful dishes for special occasions," we were amazed to discover that this delicacy is not only low in fat and calories, but also loaded with fiber and nutrients. What's more, it's a frugal homemaker's dream. Lili created it from the part of the asparagus we usually throw away! (Pictured on p. 52.)

INGREDIENTS

        4 CUPS ASPARAGUS STALKS, WITH OR WITHOUT TIPS*
        3 CUPS CHICKEN BROTH
        2 CUPS NONFAT MILK
        4 TABLESPOONS WHITE FLOUR
    ¼-½ TEASPOON CURRY POWDER
            LIGHT SALT (OPTIONAL)

DIRECTIONS

Simmer asparagus in the 3 cups chicken broth in a medium, covered saucepan, 30 to 50
    minutes until tender.
Puree mixture in blender or food processor in two batches.
Strain through large-mesh sieve or colander to remove coarse fibers. Return to saucepan and
    reheat. You will now have about 2 cups puree.
Dissolve flour in milk and stir into asparagus puree. Add curry powder. Continue stirring over
    low flame, until mixture returns to boiling and thickens.
Add light salt, if desired.

SERVING SIZE: 4 Servings, 1 Cup Each

PER SERVING: Calories 95   **Fiber:** 2 grams   **Sodium:** 545 mg.

*To save time, use 3 cups asparagus tips, skip the stems and
the straining.

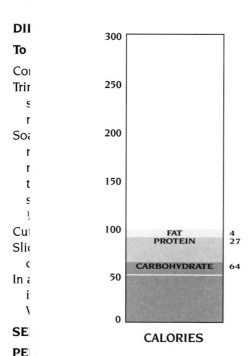

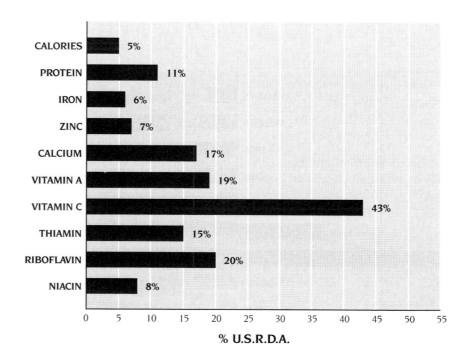

ZUCCHINI SOUP

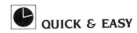 **QUICK & EASY**

This soup is smooth, creamy, and delicate, with the special flavor which comes only from garden-fresh ingredients. The fact that you spent all of 5 minutes preparing this delightful first course need never get past you and your blender.

INGREDIENTS

3 LB. ZUCCHINI, 6 CUPS DICED
½ CUP ONION, FINELY CHOPPED
6-8 GREEN ONIONS, SLICED
½ CUP FRESH PARSLEY, CHOPPED

3 CHICKEN BOUILLON CUBES*
1 TEASPOON LIGHT SEASONED SALT*
WATER TO COVER WELL
1 SMALL CAN (6 OZ.) NONFAT EVAPORATED MILK

DIRECTIONS

Put all ingredients except milk in a large saucepan. Bring to a boil. Reduce heat, cover, and simmer for about half an hour until vegetables are quite soft.

Puree soup mixture in blender or food processor. Add milk. Return mixture to pan, heat through, and serve. Soup may also be served chilled.

SERVING SIZE: 8 Servings, 1 Cup Each

PER SERVING: Calories 62   **Fiber:** 5 grams   **Sodium:** 501 mg.

*95% of the sodium content of this recipe comes from the bouillon cubes and seasoned salt. For a low-sodium soup (33 mg. per cup), substitute salt-free chicken broth and seasoned salt substitute.

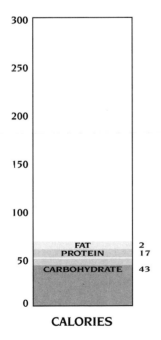

CALORIES

FAT 2
PROTEIN 17
CARBOHYDRATE 43

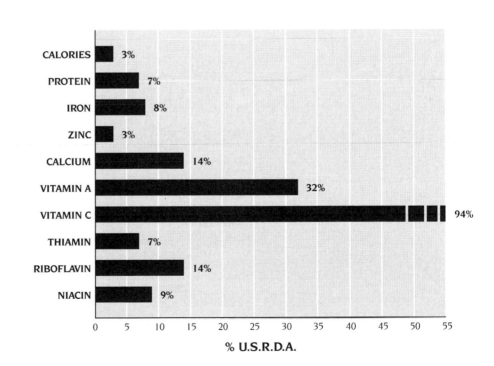

CALORIES 3%
PROTEIN 7%
IRON 8%
ZINC 3%
CALCIUM 14%
VITAMIN A 32%
VITAMIN C 94%
THIAMIN 7%
RIBOFLAVIN 14%
NIACIN 9%

% U.S.R.D.A.

POTATO LEEK SOUP

Leeks belong to the onion family but have a distinctive, delicate flavor all their own. Because leeks grow underground, they tend to collect sand, and require thorough washing. To clean, cut off the roots, then the coarse green tops, leaving 1 to 2 inches of green. Slice lengthwise to within an inch of the root end. Spread the leaves and rinse well under cold running water. Wash the green tops as well, because they will be used to add flavor to the stock even though they are too coarse to be included in the finished soup.

INGREDIENTS

- 4 TENDER YOUNG LEEKS
- 4 MEDIUM POTATOES, PEELED AND DICED
- 3 CUPS CHICKEN BROTH
- 1½ CUPS NONFAT MILK
  FRESHLY GROUND BLACK PEPPER
  LIGHT SALT (OPTIONAL)
- 1 TABLESPOON CHOPPED FRESH DILL OR 1 TEASPOON DRIED

DIRECTIONS

Thoroughly clean leeks (see above), reserving green tops. Thinly slice bottoms.

In a covered pot, simmer whole leek tops, sliced leek bottoms and diced potatoes in chicken broth until very soft, about 45 minutes.

Remove leek tops. Add milk. Heat through. Just before serving, add dill, pepper, and light salt, if desired.

If fresh dill is used, it should not be cooked as it loses some of its flavor. If dried dill is used, add it with the milk to give it time to rehydrate.

SERVING SIZE: 6 Servings, About 1 Cup Each

PER SERVING: Calories 97   **Fiber:** 2 grams   **Sodium:** 403 mg.

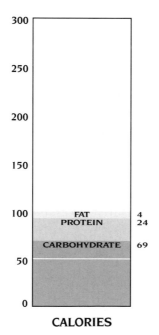

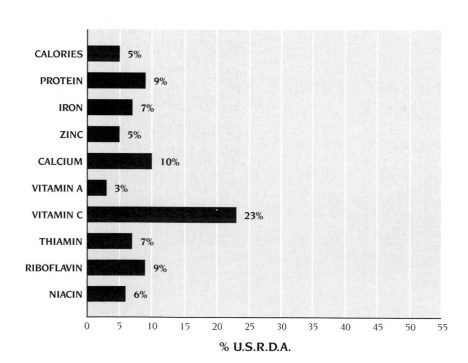

WINTER VEGETABLE SOUP 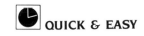 QUICK & EASY

Something special happens to vegetables when you cook them together in a flavorful stock. They are magically transformed into a food that children will eat—soup! It's an afterschool snack Mom can feel good about, and even the pickiest of little squirrels will be partial to this soup if they help chop the carrots (or push the button on the food processor).

INGREDIENTS

1 LARGE ONION, DICED
2 LARGE CARROTS, SLICED
2 LARGE STALKS CELERY, SLICED
1 SMALL TURNIP, DICED
2 LEEKS, BOTTOM HALF, THINLY SLICED
2 LARGE OR 4 SMALL POTATOES, CUBED
1 CAN (1 LB.) TOMATOES

1 PACKAGE (10 OZ.) FROZEN CORN
1 PACKAGE (10 OZ.) FROZEN CUT GREEN BEANS
½ TEASPOON MARJORAM
½ TEASPOON OREGANO
2 QUARTS BEEF BROTH OR 4 CANS (14½ OZ. EACH)
PARMESAN CHEESE, GRATED (OPTIONAL)
TO GARNISH

DIRECTIONS

Put all ingredients except Parmesan cheese in a large (6- to 8-quart) pot.
Bring to a boil, reduce heat, and simmer for approximately 1 hour or until vegetables are tender and flavors are blended. Garnish with grated Parmesan if desired.

SERVING SIZE: 10 Servings, 1 Cup Each

PER SERVING: Calories 112 **Fiber:** 5 grams **Sodium:** 308 mg.

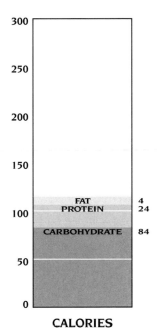

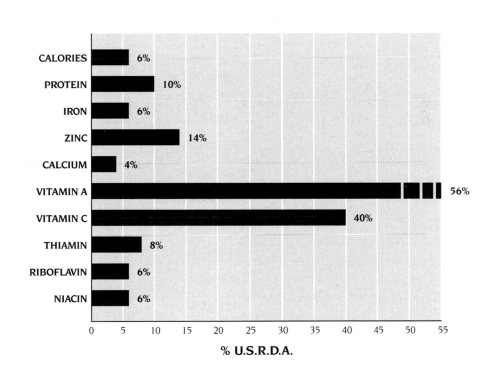

OLD-FASHIONED TOMATO SOUP

 QUICK & EASY

Old fashioned cream of tomato soup . . . it's "M m m-m m m Good." For a delicious low-sodium soup, use unsalted fresh or canned tomato juice.

INGREDIENTS

- 4 CUPS TOMATO JUICE
- 2 TABLESPOONS ONION, FINELY MINCED
- ½ BAY LEAF
- ⅛ TEASPOON BAKING SODA
- 1 TABLESPOON WHITE FLOUR
  DASH BLACK PEPPER
- 2 TEASPOONS SUGAR
- 2 CUPS HOT NONFAT MILK

DIRECTIONS

In medium saucepan (preferably nonaluminum since soup is acidic), heat tomato juice, onion, and bay leaf to boiling. Reduce heat, simmer for 10 minutes.
Remove from heat, stir in baking soda.
In large saucepan, make a thin white sauce: combine flour, pepper, and sugar. Gradually stir in milk. Heat, stirring constantly, to boiling. Simmer 1 minute.
Add tomato juice mixture to white sauce, stirring constantly. Heat through, but do not boil.
Serve immediately.

SERVING SIZE: 6 Servings, 1 Cup Each

PER SERVING: Calories 75 **Fiber:** 1 gram **Sodium:** 511 mg.

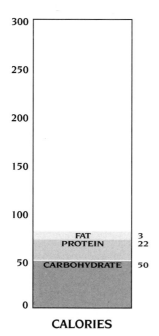

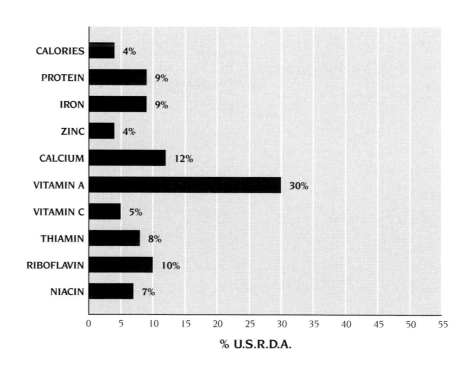

NEW ENGLAND CLAM CHOWDER

INGREDIENTS

2 POTATOES, PEELED AND CUT IN ½-INCH CUBES
(1½ CUPS)
1½ CUPS WATER
½ TEASPOON LIGHT SALT (OPTIONAL)
1 SLICE BACON (1 OZ.), CUT IN THIN SHREDS
1 SMALL ONION, 1 CUP CHOPPED
2 TABLESPOONS WHITE FLOUR
2 CUPS NONFAT MILK

DASH ALLSPICE
½ TEASPOON CHICKEN BROTH GRANULES
2 CANS (6½ OZ. EACH) CLAMS AND JUICE
1 TABLESPOON SHERRY WINE
½ TEASPOON WORCESTERSHIRE SAUCE
¼ CUP FRESH PARSLEY, CHOPPED
FRESHLY GROUND BLACK PEPPER

DIRECTIONS

Place peeled and cubed potatoes in a large saucepan with water and light salt, if used. Bring to a boil, cover, and simmer for 15 to 20 minutes until tender.

Sauté bacon shreds in a large nonstick skillet until crisp and brown. Remove to a small bowl, leaving fat in pan.

Add minced onion to bacon fat. Sauté over medium heat until golden brown, 10 to 12 minutes.

Add flour to well-browned onions in skillet. Sauté 4 to 5 minutes, stirring constantly to brown the flour.

Add milk, allspice, and broth granules to skillet. Stir until mixture begins to bubble and forms a thin cream sauce. Add this sauce to the undrained boiled potatoes.

Add clams with their juice, sherry, and Worcestershire sauce. Heat through. Add chopped parsley, season to taste with pepper, and serve immediately.

SERVING SIZE: 5 Servings, 1 Cup Each

PER SERVING: Calories 160   **Fiber:** 1 gram   **Sodium:** 493 mg.

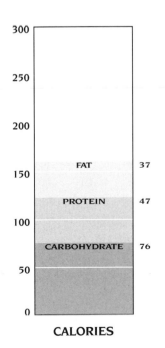

CALORIES

FAT 37
PROTEIN 47
CARBOHYDRATE 76

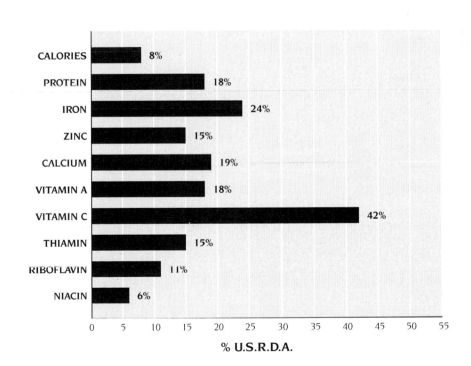

% U.S.R.D.A.

CALORIES 8%
PROTEIN 18%
IRON 24%
ZINC 15%
CALCIUM 19%
VITAMIN A 18%
VITAMIN C 42%
THIAMIN 15%
RIBOFLAVIN 11%
NIACIN 6%

Salads & Dressings

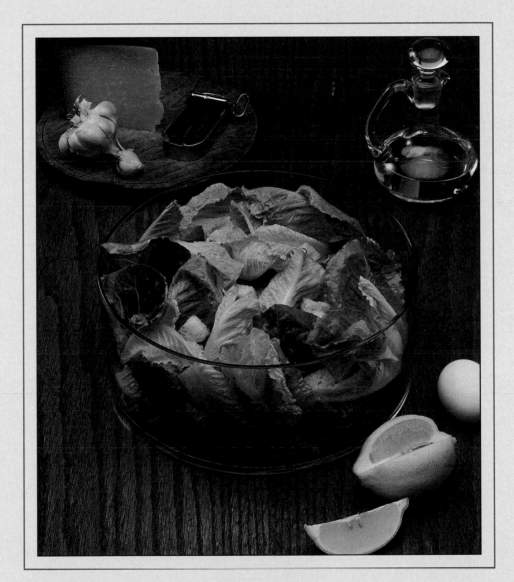

Ingredients for Traditional Caesar Salad (p. 76)

TRADITIONAL CAESAR SALAD

This Caesar Salad is traditional in every respect except the fat content. For a real show, toss the salad at tableside, the way it's done in certain pricey dining establishments—with a flourish!

INGREDIENTS

- 2 TEASPOONS AND 2 TABLESPOONS OLIVE OIL (EXTRA VIRGIN IS BEST)
- 2 CLOVES GARLIC, CRUSHED
- 2-3 CLOVES GARLIC, MINCED
- 4 SLICES (4 OZ.) SOURDOUGH FRENCH BREAD, CUT INTO ½-INCH CUBES

- 2 HEADS ROMAINE LETTUCE
- 1 CAN (2 OZ.) ANCHOVIES (FLAT FILLETS)
- 1 EGG
- 3 TABLESPOONS FRESH LEMON JUICE
- 2 TABLESPOONS PARMESAN CHEESE, GRATED FRESHLY GROUND BLACK PEPPER

DIRECTIONS

Heat 2 teaspoons olive oil in a large heavy (cast iron) skillet with the 2 cloves crushed garlic. Add bread cubes, toss lightly to coat. Reduce heat to low and allow the croutons to toast for 10 to 15 minutes until crisp. Stir them every 2 to 3 minutes to prevent scorching. (Croutons can also be "finished" under the broiler or in a toaster oven.)

Combine remaining 2 tablespoons olive oil with the 2-3 cloves minced garlic in a small bowl.

Drain anchovies, cut into ¼-inch pieces, cover, and chill.

Rinse romaine leaves, pat or shake dry, and tear

into pieces. Place in a large wooden salad bowl, cover, and chill until serving time.

Coddle the egg by immersing in boiling water for 60 seconds.

Juice the lemon; grate the parmesan; and set out the pepper grinder.

To serve, bring out the bowl of chilled romaine.

Crack the coddled egg into the prepared garlic oil, beat lightly with fork.

Pour over greens. Toss to coat.

Sprinkle on parmesan cheese, chopped anchovies, and finally, lemon juice.

Toss again, then add croutons; toss and serve.

SERVING SIZE: 8 Servings, 1½ Cups Each

PER SERVING: Calories 116 **Fiber:** 2 grams **Sodium:** 158 mg.

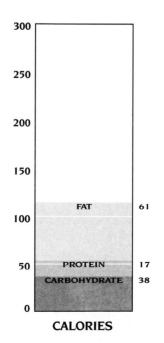

FAT 61
PROTEIN 17
CARBOHYDRATE 38

CALORIES

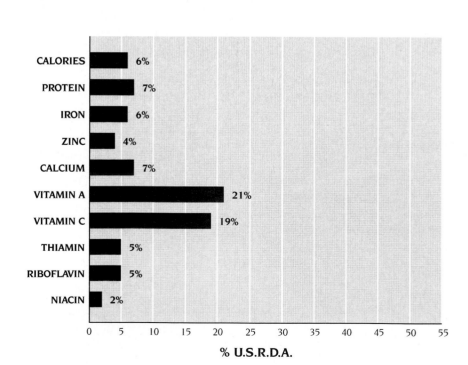

	%
CALORIES	6%
PROTEIN	7%
IRON	6%
ZINC	4%
CALCIUM	7%
VITAMIN A	21%
VITAMIN C	19%
THIAMIN	5%
RIBOFLAVIN	5%
NIACIN	2%

0 5 10 15 20 25 30 35 40 45 50 55

% U.S.R.D.A.

SWEET AND SOUR SHRIMP SALAD

QUICK & EASY

A chilled vegetable salad borrows the flavors of sweet and sour shrimp.

INGREDIENTS

4 LARGE CARROTS, PEELED AND CUT IN ¼-INCH
  SLICES
1 LARGE BELL PEPPER, CUT IN 1-INCH PIECES
1 SMALL ONION, MINCED

Sauce

½ CAN (10 OZ.) CONDENSED TOMATO SOUP
½ CUP CIDER VINEGAR
¼ CUP BROWN SUGAR
1 TEASPOON PREPARED MUSTARD
½ TEASPOON WORCESTERSHIRE SAUCE

1 CUP COOKED TINY SHRIMP OR 2 CANS
  (6½ OZ. EACH), DRAINED AND CHILLED
2 HARD-BOILED EGGS, SLICED
  FRESH PARSLEY SPRIGS FOR GARNISH

DIRECTIONS

Boil or steam sliced carrots until just tender, about 20 minutes.
Combine sauce ingredients in a small bowl.
Drain carrots and turn them into a medium bowl. Add bell pepper and onion to hot carrots.
  Add sauce and toss lightly. Chill at least 1 hour.
Just before serving, add cooked, chilled shrimp. Arrange sliced eggs and parsley sprigs on
  top and serve.

VARIATION: Use fresh or canned pineapple rings in place of egg slices.

SERVING SIZE: 6 Servings, 1 Cup Each

PER SERVING: Calories 168   **Fiber:** 4 grams   **Sodium:** 325 mg.

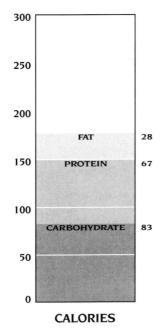

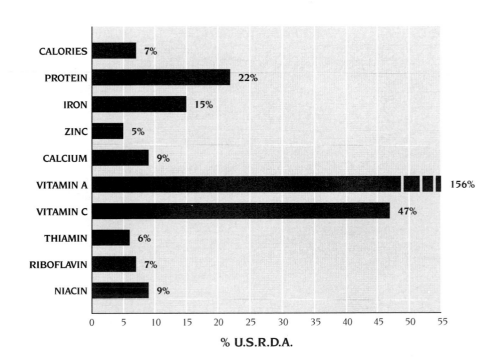

BARBEQUED FISH SALAD

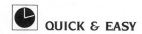 **QUICK & EASY**

The next time you barbeque more fish than you can eat, keep this delectable salad in mind. A Baja California fishing expedition and an abundance of fresh dorado (Mexican mahimahi) inspired this breezy meal-in-one salad. It borrows the bright flavor blend of Latin American *ceviche* (marinated raw seafood) and happily works just as well with fish that has been cooked! Add some soft French rolls (bolillos) and a pitcher of sangria, and you might believe your sundeck overlooks a beach in Baja.

INGREDIENTS

    2 BARBEQUED FISH STEAKS (ABOUT ½ LB. EACH) (SWORDFISH, MAHIMAHI, SALMON,
       SHARK, OR HALIBUT)
    ½ LARGE, SWEET ONION, COARSELY CHOPPED
       JUICE OF 1 LIME
       DASH OF HOT CHILI PEPPER, HOT SAUCE, OR SLICED MARINATED JALAPEÑO CHILES TO TASTE
    1 TABLESPOON FRESH CILANTRO, CHOPPED
    4 RIPE TOMATOES, EACH CUT INTO EIGHT WEDGES
    4 CUPS BABY ROMAINE OR BUTTER LETTUCE LEAVES
       LIME WEDGES AND FRESH CILANTRO FOR GARNISH

DIRECTIONS

Using your fingers, break fish into bite-sized pieces. Remove any fat or bones.
In a medium bowl, toss all ingredients *except* tomatoes and lettuce leaves.
   Chill until ready to serve.
Arrange romaine or butter lettuce leaves on four chilled salad plates. Spoon fish salad onto
   center of plate. Surround with tomato wedges and garnish with limes and cilantro.

SERVING SIZE: ¼ Recipe

PER SERVING: Calories 256   **Fiber:** 4 grams   **Sodium:** 123 mg.

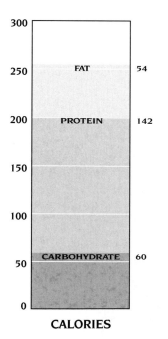

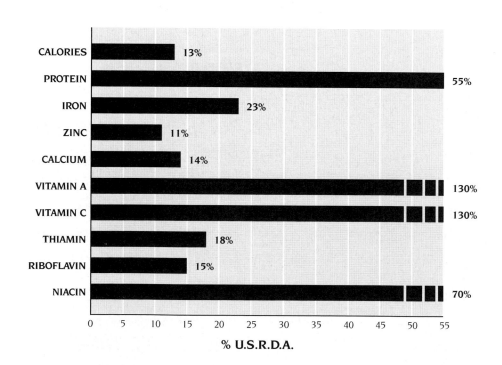

TACO SALAD

INGREDIENTS

Meat

1 LB. GROUND ROUND OR EXTRA-LEAN GROUND BEEF
3 MEDIUM TOMATOES, PEELED, OR 1 CAN (1 LB.)

2 TEASPOONS CUMIN
2 TEASPOONS CHILI POWDER
LIGHT SALT (OPTIONAL)

Salad

8 CORN TORTILLAS
1 HEAD ICEBERG LETTUCE, 8 CUPS BITE-SIZED PIECES
1 BELL PEPPER, QUARTERED AND SLICED THINLY
2 MEDIUM TOMATOES, CUT IN SMALL CHUNKS
1 LARGE RED ONION, QUARTERED AND THINLY SLICED
1 CAN (2¼ OZ.) BLACK OLIVES, SLICED

1½ CUPS COOKED KIDNEY BEANS OR 1 CAN (1 LB.), DRAINED
6 PEPPEROCINNI (ITALIAN PICKLED PEPPERS) THINLY SLICED (OPTIONAL)
4 OZ. SHARP CHEDDAR CHEESE, GRATED
½ CUP OIL-FREE ITALIAN SALAD DRESSING*
SALSA

DIRECTIONS

Brown meat and drain off any fat. Add tomatoes, cumin, chili powder, and light salt, if used. Simmer for 10 to 15 minutes to blend flavors and cook off liquid. Set aside to cool.

Preheat oven to 300°.

Cut tortillas into wedges and spread on foil or cookie sheet sprayed with nonstick cooking spray. Bake for 10 to 12 minutes, until crisp. Cool and crumble the chips.

Layer lettuce, bell pepper, tomatoes, and onion in a large salad bowl.

Sprinkle on kidney beans, olives, and pepperocinni, if used.

Spoon cooled meat mixture over salad and top with shredded cheese.

Refrigerate until serving, up to 8 hours.

To serve, pour oil-free dressing over salad. Toss lightly. Sprinkle with crushed tortilla chips. Serve with salsa and additional oil-free dressing.

VARIATION: Use avocado salad dressing in place of Italian.

SERVING SIZE: ⅛ Recipe

PER SERVING: Calories 300   **Fiber:** 8 grams   **Sodium:** 444 mg.

*110 mg. sodium per serving comes from the commercial oil-free dressing. To reduce sodium use homemade or low-sodium dressing.

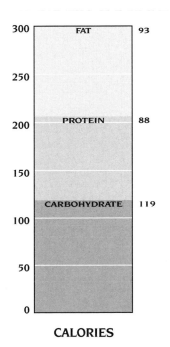

CALORIES

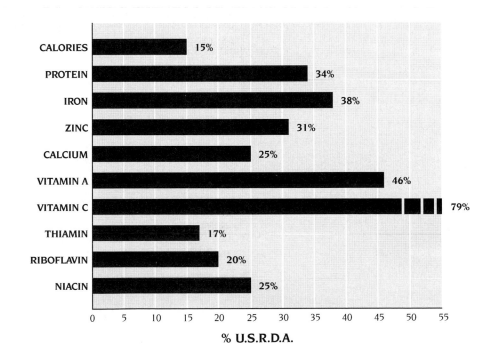

% U.S.R.D.A.

SPINACH MUSHROOM SALAD

INGREDIENTS

1 LARGE BUNCH SPINACH, (1 LB.)
½ LB. MUSHROOMS, 2 CUPS SLICED

2 OZ. FETA CHEESE
PINE NUTS FOR GARNISH (OPTIONAL)

Pecan Vinaigrette Dressing

1 CLOVE GARLIC
2 TABLESPOONS OLIVE OIL
2-3 TABLESPOONS CIDER OR WINE VINEGAR
2 TABLESPOONS LEMON JUICE
2 TABLESPOONS WATER
¼ TEASPOON DRY MUSTARD
¼ TEASPOON FRESHLY GROUND BLACK PEPPER

1 TEASPOON SUGAR
¼ TEASPOON LIGHT SALT
2 TABLESPOONS (½ OZ.) CHOPPED PECANS
OR WALNUTS
½ TEASPOON FRESH TARRAGON LEAF OR
¼ TEASPOON DRIED TARRAGON

DIRECTIONS

Wash spinach leaves thoroughly. Remove stems and discard tough and discolored leaves.
Blot leaves on paper towels.

Wash mushrooms, blot dry, and cut into thick slices.

Crumble feta cheese or slice it thinly and then cut into slivers.

Combine all dressing ingredients in blender or food processor. Begin with 2 tablespoons
vinegar. Taste and add more vinegar, if desired.

Just before serving, toss dressing with spinach, mushrooms, and cheese. Garnish with pine
nuts if desired.

VARIATION: Spinach and Pasta Salad. Prepare spinach, mushrooms, and cheese, but do not
combine them. Double the dressing recipe. Boil ½ lb. farfalle (bow-tie pasta) or fusilli
(corkscrew pasta) until barely tender (al dente). Drain and rinse with cold water. Arrange
pasta, then spinach leaves and mushrooms on four large salad plates. Sprinkle with feta
cheese, then drizzle with dressing. Garnish with pine nuts, if desired. Pasta adds 220
calories to each serving.

SERVING SIZE: ¼ Recipe

PER SERVING: Calories 138   **Fiber:** 3 grams   **Sodium:** 268 mg.

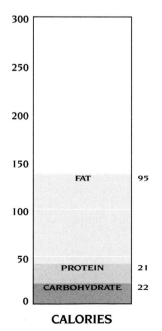

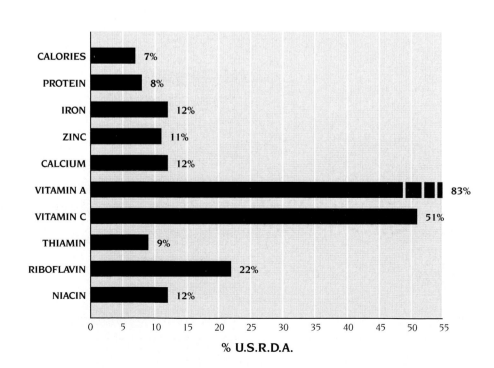

% U.S.R.D.A.

SPINACH SALAD WITH BACON DRESSING

INGREDIENTS

1 LARGE BUNCH SPINACH (10 CUPS LEAVES)
½-1 SWEET RED ONION, THINLY SLICED
1 SMALL RED OR GREEN BELL PEPPER, THINLY SLICED
2 MEDIUM TOMATOES, CUT IN SMALL WEDGES
1 SMALL, RIPE AVOCADO, PEELED AND DICED
1 HARD-BOILED EGG, CHOPPED

2 SLICES BACON, COOKED AND DICED
1 TABLESPOON BACON FAT
3 CLOVES GARLIC, MINCED
½ TEASPOON COARSELY GROUND BLACK PEPPER
2 TEASPOONS SUGAR
3 TABLESPOONS CIDER VINEGAR
2 TABLESPOONS CATSUP

DIRECTIONS

Wash spinach thoroughly in cold water to remove sand and grit. Remove stems and discard discolored or tough leaves. Shake off excess moisture, tear larger leaves into bite-sized pieces and place in a large bowl.

Slice onion as thinly as possible. Adjust amount used depending on how sweet or hot it is.

Add onion, bell pepper, tomatoes, avocado, and egg to spinach.

Cut bacon into small shreds and fry in medium skillet until very crisp. Remove meat from pan and drain on paper towel. Save 1 tablespoon of bacon fat and discard the rest.

Sauté garlic in reserved bacon fat until golden. Add black pepper and sauté 10 seconds longer. Remove from heat.

Add sugar, vinegar, and catsup to skillet. Stir quickly and pour over vegetables. Sprinkle with bacon bits, toss, and serve immediately.

VARIATION: Low-Cholesterol Spinach Salad. Substitute 1 tablespoon imitation bacon bits and 1 tablespoon olive oil for the bacon and fat. Use 2 hard-boiled egg whites instead of the whole egg.

SERVING SIZE: 6 Servings, 1½ Cups Each

PER SERVING: Calories 126   **Fiber:** 2 grams   **Sodium:** 125 mg.

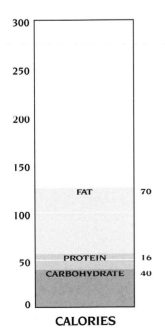

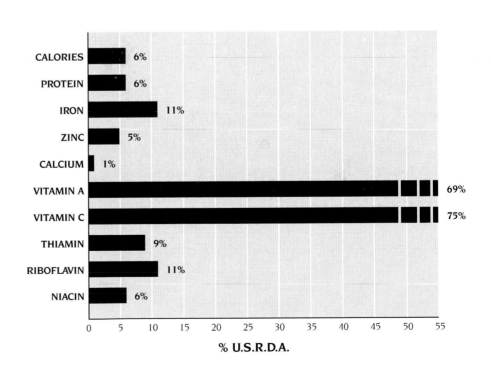

OLD-FASHIONED POTATO SALAD

A cupful of regular deli-type potato salad provides 350 calories. Ours is not only lower in fat and calories, it's also much better. In fact, this creamy potato salad is so good, when we served it at a big Fourth of July picnic, we had to *work* to convince our friends that it was really low fat.

INGREDIENTS

6 LARGE POTATOES (3 LB.)
¼ CUP OIL-FREE ITALIAN SALAD DRESSING
½-1 ONION, MINCED
3 LARGE STALKS CELERY, CHOPPED
¾ CUP SWEET PICKLE RELISH
6 HARD-BOILED EGGS, CHOPPED

Dressing

½ CUP SOUR CREAM
⅓ CUP DIET MAYONNAISE
2 TEASPOONS PREPARED MUSTARD
1 TEASPOON LIGHT SALT
2 TABLESPOONS VINEGAR OR DILL PICKLE JUICE
¼ TEASPOON FRESHLY GROUND BLACK PEPPER

DIRECTIONS

In a large kettle, boil potatoes in their skins, just until fork tender, 40 to 45 minutes.

Drain potatoes. Cool until they can be handled, then peel and cut into ½-inch cubes. Place in a large bowl and drizzle with Italian dressing.

Onion is a critical ingredient in this salad. It should be minced with a sharp knife, rather than a food processor, since the crushing and bruising of mechanical chopping tends to bring out the bitterness. Taste the onion. If it's a sweet, mild summer onion, use a large one. In the winter, when *all* varieties of onions have intensified in flavor from months of storage, use just half a small one and chop it finely.

Add onion, celery, and pickle relish to potatoes and mix well.

Chop eggs and set aside.

In a small bowl, combine sour cream, mayonnaise, mustard, light salt, vinegar or pickle juice, and pepper. Stir well and add to potato salad, along with chopped eggs. Stir thoroughly but lightly, then cover and chill several hours to develop flavor.

VARIATIONS: Dilled Cucumber Potato Salad. Omit mustard. Add 1 fresh cucumber, diced, and 1 tablespoon chopped fresh dill. **Potato Salad with Peppers.** Add chopped red and sweet, green bell peppers or pimento to taste.

SERVING SIZE: 10 Servings, 1 Cup Each

PER SERVING: Calories 224 **Fiber:** 3 grams **Sodium:** 419 mg.

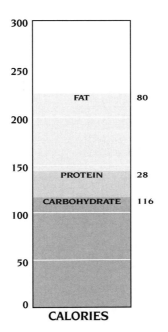

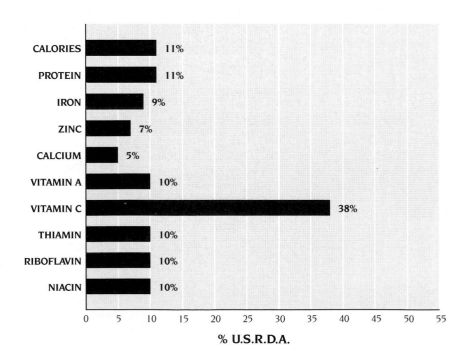

CHINESE CHICKEN SALAD 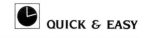 QUICK & EASY

Sesame oil is used by Oriental cooks as a seasoning, rather than a fat. Just a few drops of this nutty oil imparts a distinctly Oriental flavor. Try this simple salad as a first course or a luncheon entree.

INGREDIENTS

Salad

4	CHICKEN BREASTS, COOKED
	(12 OZ. WHITE MEAT)
4	LARGE STALKS CELERY
10-12	SMALL GREEN ONIONS
1	HEAD ICEBERG LETTUCE
	(ABOUT 4 CUPS)
	SESAME SEEDS OR STRIPS OF PIMENTO
	FOR GARNISH

Dressing

4	TABLESPOONS WHITE OR RICE VINEGAR
4	TEASPOONS SUGAR
1	TEASPOON SESAME OIL
2	CLOVES GARLIC, MINCED, OR ½ TEASPOON
	GARLIC POWDER
2	TEASPOONS SHERRY
¼	TEASPOON WHITE PEPPER OR FRESHLY
	GROUND BLACK PEPPER
	LIGHT SALT (OPTIONAL)

DIRECTIONS

Cut chicken breasts into slivers, about matchstick size.
Thinly slice celery and green onions, diagonally.
Shred iceberg lettuce.
Combine dressing ingredients in a small cruet or jar.
To serve toss lettuce, celery, and green onions in a serving bowl. Top with chicken slivers.
   Garnish with pimento or sesame seeds. Drizzle on dressing and serve immediately.

SERVING SIZE: 4 Servings, 1¾ Cups Each

PER SERVING: Calories 200   **Fiber:** 3 grams   **Sodium:** 132 mg.

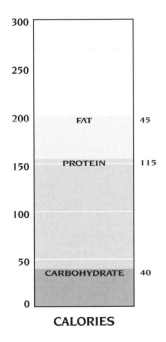

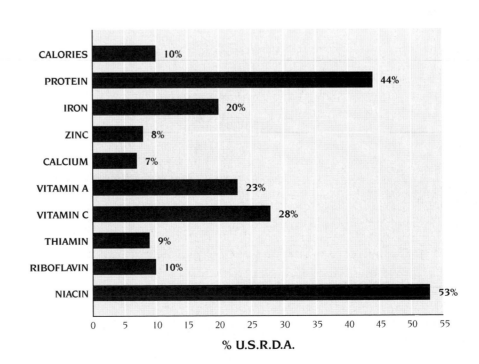

CHICKEN SALAD

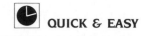 **QUICK & EASY**

Here's a basic chicken salad to mound atop mixed greens. Garnish with tomato wedges, pineapple rings, or asparagus spears for a luncheon entree. It also makes an excellent sandwich filling.

INGREDIENTS

2 CUPS COOKED CHICKEN, CUBED, OR 1 CAN
(12 OZ.) WHITE CHUNKED CHICKEN
2 STALKS CELERY, 1 CUP CHOPPED
4 TABLESPOONS PICKLE RELISH
½ CUP GREEN ONION, SLICED

Dressing

2 TABLESPOONS DIET MAYONNAISE
½ CUP PLAIN NONFAT YOGURT
SUGAR AND BLACK PEPPER TO TASTE
LIGHT SALT (OPTIONAL)

DIRECTIONS

In medium bowl toss chicken with celery, pickle relish, and green onions. In small bowl mix mayonnaise and yogurt. Add sugar and pepper to taste. Combine salad with dressing, then add salt, if desired.

SERVING SIZE: 4 Servings, ¾ Cup Each

PER SERVING: Calories 169   **Fiber:** 2 grams   **Sodium:** 248 mg.

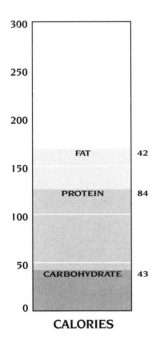

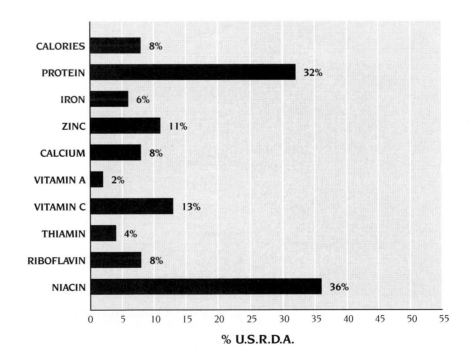

SMOKED TURKEY WALDORF 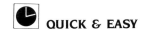 QUICK & EASY

Smoked turkey breast lends a distinctly rich and nutty flavor to this Waldorf-type salad.

INGREDIENTS

8 OZ. SMOKED TURKEY BREAST, 1½ CUPS CUBED
2 CRISP UNPEELED APPLES, CUBED
2 LARGE STALKS CELERY, THINLY SLICED
   RED LEAF LETTUCE LEAVES

Dressing

¼ CUP DIET MAYONNAISE
¼ CUP PLAIN NONFAT YOGURT
½ TEASPOON CURRY POWDER
2 PACKETS SUGAR SUBSTITUTE OR
  1 TABLESPOON SUGAR
  CHUTNEY FOR GARNISH (OPTIONAL)

DIRECTIONS

Combine turkey, apples, and celery in a large bowl.
Blend dressing ingredients.
Toss turkey mixture with dressing. Cover and chill.
Serve on bed of red leaf lettuce. Garnish with chutney, if desired.

VARIATIONS: Add ½ cup plumped raisins or 1 cup pineapple tidbits.
Garnish with slivered pecans or walnuts.

SERVING SIZE: 5 Servings, 1 Cup Each

PER SERVING: Calories 156   **Fiber:** 2 grams   **Sodium:** 290 mg.

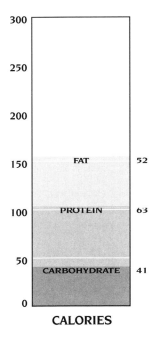

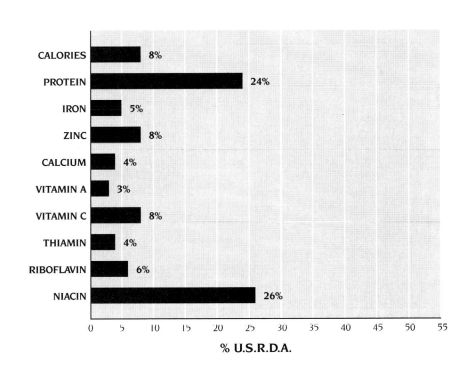

MAIN COURSE TUNA SALAD QUICK & EASY

A large and satisfying lunch for a mere 170 calories.

INGREDIENTS

½ SMALL HEAD ICEBERG LETTUCE, ABOUT 3 CUPS CUBED
½ CUP ALFALFA SPROUTS
1 BELL PEPPER, SLICED
4 GREEN ONIONS, SLICED
6 LARGE MUSHROOMS, SLICED
1 CAN (6½ OZ.) SOLID WHITE TUNA, PACKED IN WATER, DRAINED AND FLAKED
1 TABLESPOON DIET CUCUMBER DRESSING
1 TABLESPOON LEMON JUICE
  COARSELY GROUND BLACK PEPPER

DIRECTIONS

Chill prepared vegetables in a medium bowl.
Just before serving, add tuna.
Toss salad with cucumber dressing, lemon juice, and pepper.
Serve immediately.

SERVING SIZE: 2 Main Servings, 4 Side Dish Servings

PER SERVING: Calories 167   **Fiber:** 4 grams   **Sodium:** 445 mg.

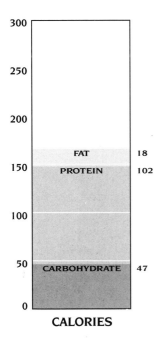

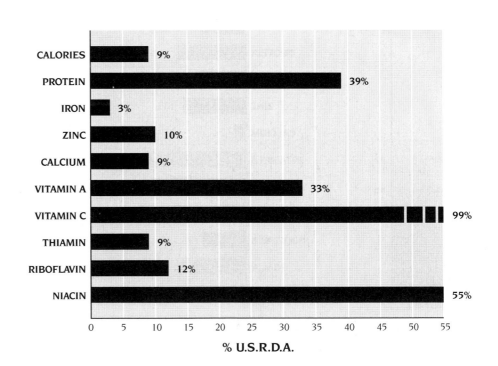

BROCCOLI RICE SALAD

Colorful and delicious . . . this is one of our favorite buffet salads. It keeps for several days in the refrigerator. Good as a side dish or as a light main dish with the addition of the optional egg or seafood.

INGREDIENTS

2 CUPS COOKED BROWN RICE, COOLED
¼ CUP DIET ITALIAN SALAD DRESSING
2 TABLESPOONS DIET CUCUMBER OR OTHER CREAMY SALAD DRESSING
1 BUNCH FRESH BROCCOLI
1 TABLESPOON FRESH PARSLEY, CHOPPED
1 TABLESPOON ONION, FINELY MINCED

2 TOMATOES, CUT IN THIN WEDGES, OR 1 RED BELL PEPPER, CUT IN THIN STRIPS
2 TABLESPOONS PARMESAN CHEESE, GRATED
⅛ TEASPOON BLACK PEPPER
LIGHT SALT TO TASTE
CHOPPED EGG, TUNA, CRAB, OR SHRIMP (OPTIONAL)

DIRECTIONS

Add Italian and creamy dressing to cooled brown rice. Stir and set aside.

Remove rough stems from broccoli and cut head into bite-sized florets. Steam broccoli until just tender, about 10 minutes, depending on size of florets. Drain and cool.

Add all vegetables to rice. Toss lightly, sprinkle with parmesan, and season to taste with salt and pepper. Chill.

Add optional ingredients, if desired.

SERVING SIZE: 8 Servings, 1 Cup Each

PER SERVING: Calories 103 **Fiber:** 4 grams **Sodium:** 236 mg.

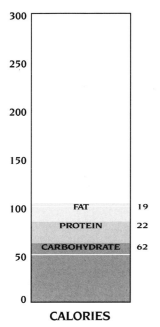

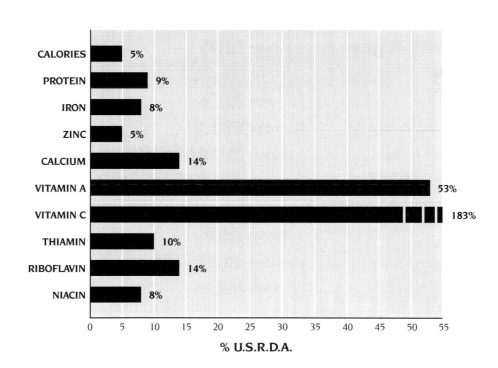

CRANBERRY JELLO MOLD

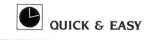 **QUICK & EASY**

Intensely flavored and deliciously piquant, this molded salad is the perfect accompaniment to a traditional turkey dinner or any unembellished roasted poultry.

INGREDIENTS

- 1 BAG (12 OZ.) FRESH CRANBERRIES
- 1 PACKET (8-SERVING) SUGAR FREE CHERRY OR STRAWBERRY GELATIN
- 2 CUPS BOILING WATER
- ¼ CUP SUGAR OR HONEY
- 1 CAN (20 OZ.) JUICE-PACKED CRUSHED PINEAPPLE

DIRECTIONS

Rinse and sort cranberries, discarding any that are soft or broken.

Dissolve gelatin in boiling water. Add sugar or honey, stirring until dissolved.

Grind cranberries in food processor or in blender, using some of the juice from the canned pineapple if needed for processing.

Add ground cranberries and pineapple with all the remaining juice to the gelatin mixture.

Pour into a 6-cup mold. Chill until firm.

To unmold, dip mold into a bowl of hot water for 3 to 4 seconds, then invert on serving plate.

SERVING SIZE: 8 Servings, ½ Cup Each

PER SERVING: Calories 95   **Fiber:** 3 grams   **Sodium:** 10 mg.

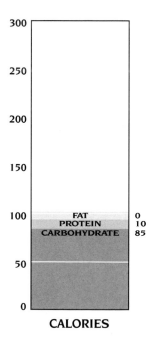

FAT 0
PROTEIN 10
CARBOHYDRATE 85

CALORIES

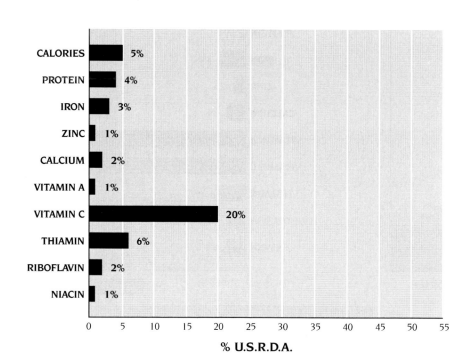

CALORIES 5%
PROTEIN 4%
IRON 3%
ZINC 1%
CALCIUM 2%
VITAMIN A 1%
VITAMIN C 20%
THIAMIN 6%
RIBOFLAVIN 2%
NIACIN 1%

% U.S.R.D.A.

GRANDMOTHER SHAPLEIGH'S FRUIT COCKTAIL

Our friend Anne, who gave us this heirloom recipe, tells us that for special holiday dinners, this elegant fruit cup should be served in decorated grapefruit shells (see holiday directions below).

INGREDIENTS

- 6 LARGE PINK GRAPEFRUITS
- 1 FRESH RIPE PINEAPPLE, CLEANED AND CRUSHED OR 1 CAN (20 OZ.) JUICE-PACKED CRUSHED PINEAPPLE
- ½ CUP BOGGS CRANBERRY LIQUEUR OR ½ CUP APRICOT BRANDY
- 12 LARGE MARASCHINO CHERRIES, DRAINED OR 12 FRESH CHERRIES

DIRECTIONS

Peel grapefruit. Remove membranes. Break grapefruit segments into bite-sized pieces and place in large bowl.

Add pineapple and mix.

Pour in Boggs or brandy. Cover and chill until serving time.

Divide among 12 bowls and top each with a cherry.

VARIATION: For a fancier presentation, cut each grapefruit in half, crosswise. With a sharp paring knife, cut around each grapefruit section, removing fruit to a large bowl. Using a sharp-edged spoon, scrape out membranes and discard. Now take sharp kitchen shears or a paring knife and cut little triangular notches around the edge of each grapefruit shell. Mix fruit filling, as above. Serve in grapefruit shells, topping each with a maraschino cherry and mint leaf.

SERVING SIZE: 12 Servings, ¾ Cup Each

PER SERVING: Calories 100   **Fiber:** 3 grams   **Sodium:** 2 mg.

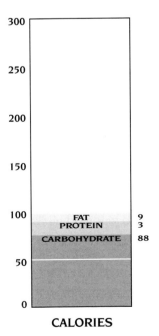

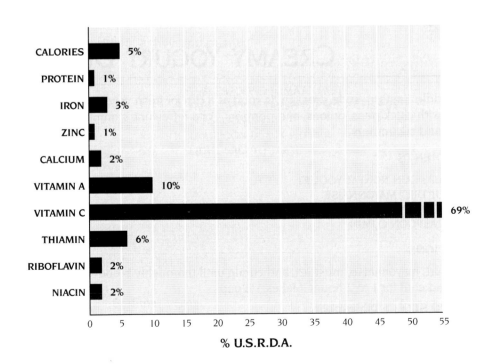

LOUISIANA RED BEANS

Deeply red, richly spiced, smoky, and hot! We had these red beans the first night we were in New Orleans—and every night after that for the rest of the week! Each restaurant had its own secret formula, but the basic ingredients were red beans (not kidney beans, but a smaller, distinct variety), something smoky, and something seriously hot. If you can get the fiery sausage links typical in Creole cooking (called boudin), they're the best; but if they aren't available in your area, a well-smoked Polish kielbasa plus some red chiles comes pretty close.

INGREDIENTS

1 LB. DRY RED BEANS
8 CUPS WATER
1 TEASPOON LIGHT SALT
1 LB. LOUISIANA HOT SMOKED SAUSAGE (BOUDIN) OR POLISH KIELBASA PLUS ¼ TO ½ TEASPOON CRUSHED RED CHILES
2 LARGE ONIONS, CHOPPED
1 BELL PEPPER, CHOPPED

2 STALKS CELERY, CHOPPED
2-3 CLOVES GARLIC, MINCED
½ CUP FRESH PARSLEY, CHOPPED
1 BAY LEAF
1-2 TEASPOONS CRUSHED RED PEPPER (CAYENNE) OR HOT PEPPER SAUCE TO TASTE
¼ TEASPOON LIQUID SMOKE (OPTIONAL)
1 TEASPOON BLACK PEPPER

DIRECTIONS

Wash and sort beans. Add 8 cups water and soak overnight in a large, nonaluminum soup pot.

Bring beans to boil in their soaking water. Skim off foam, add salt and simmer, partially covered, for 45 minutes.

Cut sausage in quarters lengthwise, then slice very thinly (⅛-inch slices).

In a large nonstick skillet, fry sausage slices over low heat to cook off fat. Tip up pan during last half of cooking to drain fat as it is released. Blot browned sausage on paper towels.

Add sausage and all remaining ingredients to beans. Bring to boil, reduce heat, and simmer, partially covered, over very low heat for about 1½ hours until beans are tender. Check water during cooking and add more if necessary to prevent scorching.

SERVING SIZE: 10 Servings, 1 Cup Each

PER SERVING: Calories 245 **Fiber:** 7 grams **Sodium:** 441 mg.

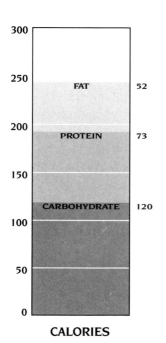

CALORIES

FAT	52
PROTEIN	73
CARBOHYDRATE	120

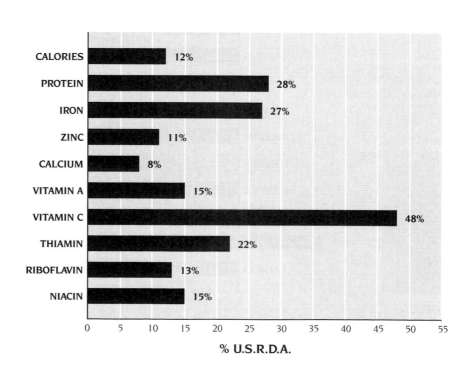

% U.S.R.D.A.

CALORIES	12%
PROTEIN	28%
IRON	27%
ZINC	11%
CALCIUM	8%
VITAMIN A	15%
VITAMIN C	48%
THIAMIN	22%
RIBOFLAVIN	13%
NIACIN	15%

DEBBIE'S BEAN AND PASTA STEW **QUICK & EASY**

Debbie Ornsdorff leads such an active life that most of us would get tired just watching her! In addition to her job as a high school coach, Debbie enters 10K runs on a regular basis, tours from state to state on her bicycle, is an avid backpacker—and an excellent cook. This recipe reflects her life-style because—like Debbie—it is quick and low in fat!

INGREDIENTS

2 TEASPOONS OLIVE OIL
1 SMALL ONION, CHOPPED
½ CUP BELL PEPPER, CHOPPED
3 CLOVES GARLIC, MINCED
1 CAN (1 LB.) TOMATOES, CHOPPED
1 CAN (1 LB.) KIDNEY BEANS, UNDRAINED
1½ CUPS SMALL WHOLE GRAIN PASTA SHELLS, 6 OZ.

1 CUP WATER
½ TEASPOON OREGANO
¼ TEASPOON BASIL
⅛ TEASPOON BLACK PEPPER
1 CAN (1 LB.) GARBANZO BEANS, UNDRAINED
PARMESAN CHEESE (OPTIONAL)

DIRECTIONS

Heat oil in a medium saucepan. Add onion, bell pepper, and garlic, and sauté over medium heat until soft, about 10 to 12 minutes.

Add tomatoes and kidney beans with their liquid. Bring to a boil.

Add shell pasta, water, oregano, basil, and pepper.

Reduce heat, cover, and simmer for 10 to 12 minutes until pasta is tender.

Add garbanzo beans with their liquid. Simmer until heated through. If a thicker stew is desired, allow to simmer, uncovered to reduce fluid.

Sprinkle with parmesan, if desired.

SERVING SIZE: 8 Servings, About 1 Cup Each

PER SERVING: Calories 203   **Fiber:** 7 grams   **Sodium:** 533 mg.

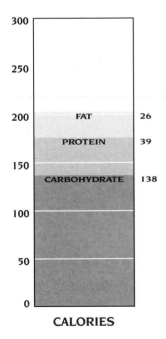

CALORIES

FAT 26
PROTEIN 39
CARBOHYDRATE 138

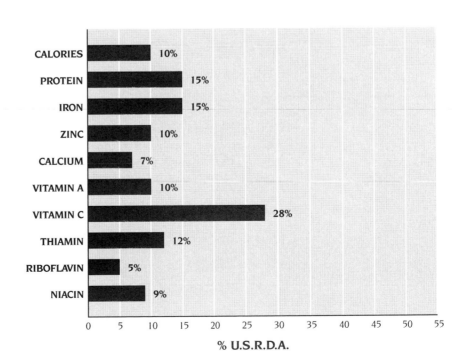

CALORIES	10%
PROTEIN	15%
IRON	15%
ZINC	10%
CALCIUM	7%
VITAMIN A	10%
VITAMIN C	28%
THIAMIN	12%
RIBOFLAVIN	5%
NIACIN	9%

% U.S.R.D.A.

SOUTHERN-STYLE LIMA BEANS AND HAM

If childhood memories of bland, mushy lima beans dim your enthusiasm for this nutritious legume, try our flavorful Southern classic. It's a natural with Country Cornbread.

INGREDIENTS

1 LB. DRY LIMA BEANS	1 TEASPOON GARLIC POWDER
10 CUPS WATER, DIVIDED	¼ TEASPOON CRUSHED CHILI
1½ LB. HAM HOCKS	½-1 TEASPOON ROSEMARY
2 ONIONS, CHOPPED	DASH DILL
3 TABLESPOONS HOT CATSUP (OR REGULAR	BLACK PEPPER TO TASTE
CATSUP PLUS DASH HOT SAUCE)	LIGHT SALT (OPTIONAL)
2 TABLESPOONS WORCESTERSHIRE SAUCE	

DIRECTIONS

Rinse and sort beans. Place in very large saucepan. Add 4 cups water. Bring to a boil. Boil 2 minutes, then remove from heat, cover, and allow to soak for 2 hours.

In second saucepan, cover ham hocks with 6 cups water. Boil, partially covered, for 2 to 3 hours until meat is falling away from bones.

Remove meat from broth. When cool enough to handle, separate lean meat from fat, skin, and bone. Skim fat from broth.

To soaked beans add lean meat, skimmed broth, plus water to make 4 cups. Add all remaining ingredients. Simmer, partially covered, for 1 to 2 hours until beans are very tender. Taste, adjust seasonings, and serve.

SERVING SIZE: 10 Servings, 1 Cup Each

PER SERVING: Calories 203   **Fiber:** 6 grams   **Sodium:** 287 mg.

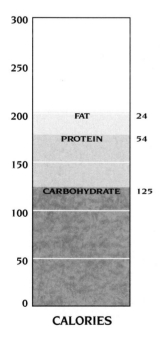

CALORIES

FAT 24
PROTEIN 54
CARBOHYDRATE 125

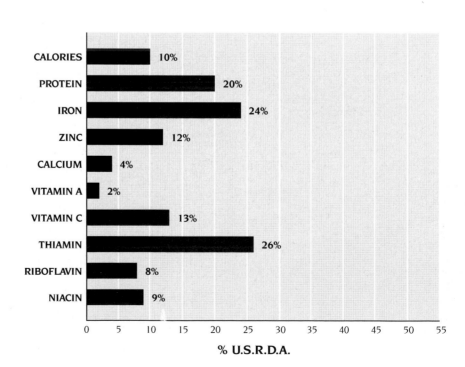

CALORIES	10%
PROTEIN	20%
IRON	24%
ZINC	12%
CALCIUM	4%
VITAMIN A	2%
VITAMIN C	13%
THIAMIN	26%
RIBOFLAVIN	8%
NIACIN	9%

% U.S.R.D.A.

BURRITOS DELEGADOS

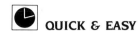 **QUICK & EASY**

These simple bean burritos received a unanimous "thumbs up" rating from the fifth graders of Meyers Elementary in South Lake Tahoe, California.

INGREDIENTS

1½ CUPS COOKED PINTO OR KIDNEY BEANS OR
  1 CAN (1 LB.) WELL DRAINED
2-3 TABLESPOONS MILD SALSA
 ½ CUP LOW-FAT COTTAGE CHEESE
    DASH CUMIN (OPTIONAL)
  5 WHOLE WHEAT FLOUR TORTILLAS

DIRECTIONS

Place well-drained beans in a small heavy saucepan. Use a potato masher to crush beans slightly. Add salsa, cottage cheese, and cumin, if desired.

Cook, stirring constantly, over medium heat until cheese begins to melt and mixture bubbles and thickens.

Heat a heavy skillet over medium heat. When it's quite hot, warm the tortillas, one at a time, for about 30 seconds on each side until softened.

Spread filling in a vertical line down the center of each tortilla. Fold up bottom edge, then roll tortilla sideways to form burrito. Serve immediately or wrap and freeze for microwave reheating. Serve with additional salsa or hot sauce.

SERVING SIZE: 5 Servings, 1 Burrito Each

PER SERVING: Calories 204   **Fiber:** 5 grams   **Sodium:** 473 mg.

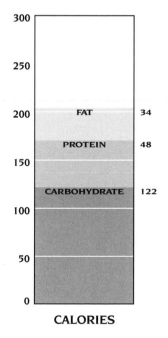

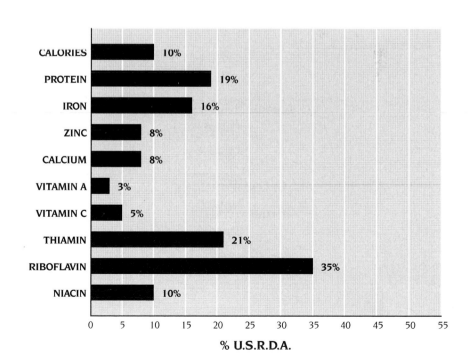

LENTIL BURGERS

Lentil burgers have been joked about for years as something only the most far-out health-food nut would eat and actually enjoy. We served this recipe at one of Covert Bailey's seminars and everyone from a football coach to a dental assistant begged for the recipe. These marvelous lentil burgers cost about 8 cents each! Try them on whole wheat buns with all the trimmings, just the way you would serve a regular burger. (Pictured on p. 103.)

INGREDIENTS

½ CUP LENTILS
2½ CUPS WATER
¼ CUP BULGAR WHEAT
1 TEASPOON LIGHT SALT
½ TEASPOON EACH GARLIC POWDER, CELERY SEED, CUMIN, AND SAGE

¼ TEASPOON NUTMEG
1 LARGE ONION, FINELY MINCED
2 EGGS, BEATEN
3 TABLESPOONS PARMESAN CHEESE
1 CUP WHOLE WHEAT FLOUR
4 TEASPOONS VEGETABLE OIL FOR FRYING

DIRECTIONS

Wash and sort lentils. Place in a large saucepan with 2½ cups water. Bring to a boil, then reduce heat and simmer uncovered, 30 to 40 minutes until just tender.

Add bulgar, light salt, and seasonings. Simmer, covered, for 5 to 10 minutes or until all water is absorbed.

Remove from heat and stir in minced onion. Cover and allow to cool to room temperature.

Add eggs and mix well. Add parmesan and flour. Stir thoroughly.

Wet hands and form into eight patties, each ½-inch thick. Over medium heat, fry in two batches in a nonstick skillet using 2 teaspoons oil per batch. Cook approximately 5 minutes per side.

SERVING SIZE: 8 Servings, 1 Patty Each

PER SERVING: Calories 170 **Fiber:** 4 grams **Sodium:** 194 mg.

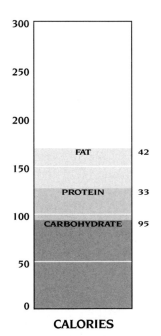

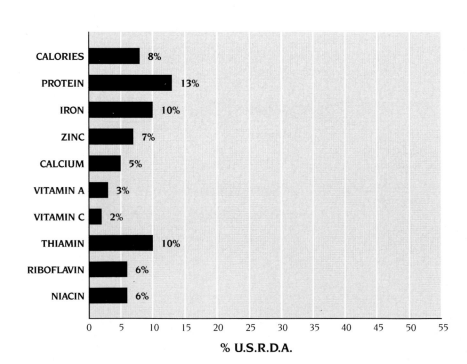

CURRIED LENTIL PATTIES

These patties can be served on whole wheat hamburger buns, but we like to break them up and put them into pocket bread along with cucumber chunks, sprouts, tomatoes, and our Creamy Cucumber Dressing. Serve with rice, curried vegetables, and a cucumber salad.

INGREDIENTS

1	CUP DRY LENTILS	1	CARROT, GRATED
5	CUPS WATER	1	ZUCCHINI, GRATED
¾	-INCH PIECE FRESH GINGER, MINCED	1	STALK CELERY, MINCED
3	CLOVES GARLIC, MINCED	1	SMALL BUNCH GREEN ONIONS, THINLY SLICED
1½	TEASPOONS LIGHT SALT	3	EGGS
1	TEASPOON CORIANDER SEED, GROUND	½	CUP WHOLE WHEAT PASTRY FLOUR
½	TEASPOON TURMERIC	¼	CUP BRAN CEREAL (PELLET SHAPED)
1	TEASPOON CUMIN	2	TEASPOONS OIL
	PINCH HOT RED CHILI		SOY SAUCE FOR SERVING (OPTIONAL)

DIRECTIONS

Wash and sort lentils.

Put lentils and water in a large saucepan and bring to a boil. Skim foam off top, reduce heat, and simmer, uncovered, for 15 minutes.

Add ginger, garlic, light salt, coriander, turmeric, cumin, and red chili. Continue to simmer until lentils are softened and mixture has thickened, about 10 minutes.

Add carrot, zucchini, celery, and green onions. Mix well. Continue cooking until lentils are com-pletely cooked, about 20 minutes more. Remove from heat and allow to cool.

Stir in eggs, flour, and cereal. Mix well.

Heat 1 teaspoon oil in a large nonstick skillet over low heat. Using half the lentil mixture, drop it by large spoonfuls into a hot skillet. Flatten into patties with a spoon. Cook about 10 minutes on first side and about 5 minutes on second side. Patties will be about ½-inch thick. Repeat with second teaspoon of oil and remaining lentil mixture.

Serve with soy sauce, if desired.

SERVING SIZE: 10 Servings, 1 Patty Each

PER SERVING: Calories 142 **Fiber:** 5 grams **Sodium:** 215 mg.

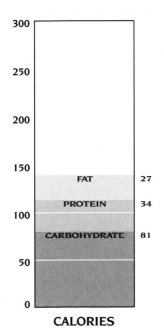

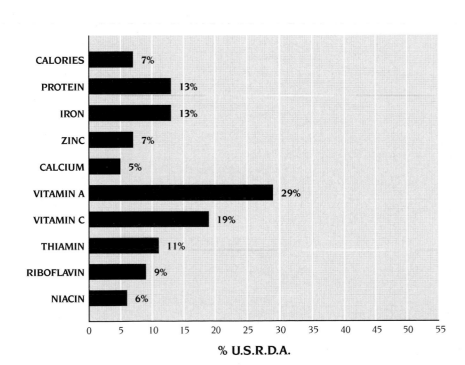

JO'S LENTIL LOAF

INGREDIENTS

- 3 CUPS WATER
- 1½ CUPS LENTILS
- ½ TEASPOON LIGHT SALT
- ½ TEASPOON BLACK PEPPER
- ½ TEASPOON CLOVES
- 1 TEASPOON BASIL
- ¼ CUP FRESH PARSLEY, CHOPPED
- 3 CLOVES GARLIC, MINCED
- 2 LARGE ONIONS, CHOPPED
- 6 OZ. EXTRA SHARP CHEDDAR CHEESE, 2 CUPS GRATED
- ½ POUND MUSHROOMS, 2 CUPS SLICED
- 2 SLICES WHOLE WHEAT BREAD, CRUMBLED
- 1 EGG, BEATEN
- ½ CUP PLAIN NONFAT YOGURT

Crust

- 1 CUP WHOLE WHEAT PASTRY FLOUR
- ½ CUP CORNMEAL
- 1 TEASPOON BAKING POWDER
- 1-1¼ CUPS BUTTERMILK OR SOUR SKIM MILK

DIRECTIONS

Put water, lentils, light salt, pepper, cloves, basil, parsley, garlic, and onions in a large saucepan. Bring mixture to a boil over high heat, then reduce heat and simmer, uncovered, until lentils are soft, about 30 minutes. Stir occasionally to prevent scorching.

When liquid has cooked off and lentils are fairly soft, remove from heat and add mushrooms, cheese, bread crumbs, egg, and yogurt. Preheat oven to 350°.

Spray a 9-inch by 5-inch by 3-inch loaf pan with nonstick cooking spray. Turn lentil mixture into loaf pan.

Mix flour, cornmeal, and baking powder in a medium bowl. Stir in enough buttermilk or sour skim milk to make a batter the consistency of pancake batter.

Smooth batter over top of lentil loaf. Bake for 45 minutes. Let cool for a few minutes before slicing.

VARIATIONS: Lentil Pie. Bake in 9-inch deep-dish pie plate, with crust.
Streamlined Loaf. Omit crust. Chill and slice for sandwiches.

SERVING SUGGESTION: Norwegian Mustard Sauce is nice with this savory loaf.

SERVING SIZE: 10 Servings, 1 Slice Each

PER SERVING: Calories 292 **Fiber:** 7 grams **Sodium:** 285 mg.

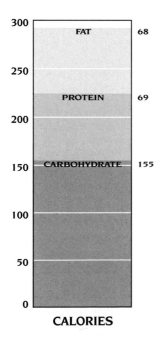

CALORIES

FAT	68
PROTEIN	69
CARBOHYDRATE	155

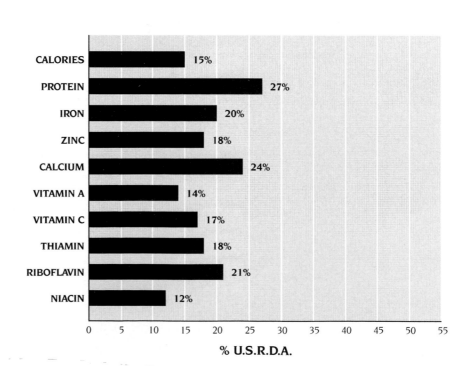

	% U.S.R.D.A.
CALORIES	15%
PROTEIN	27%
IRON	20%
ZINC	18%
CALCIUM	24%
VITAMIN A	14%
VITAMIN C	17%
THIAMIN	18%
RIBOFLAVIN	21%
NIACIN	12%

STOVE-TOP
BARLEY LENTIL CASSEROLE 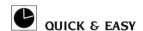 QUICK & EASY

INGREDIENTS

1 TABLESPOON OIL	4-5 CUPS HOT WATER
1 LARGE ONION, CHOPPED	1 TEASPOON LIGHT SALT
4 CLOVES GARLIC, MINCED	½ TEASPOON BLACK PEPPER
1 CUP BARLEY	1 MEDIUM LEMON, JUICED
1 CARROT, CHOPPED	1 CUP LENTILS
1 STALK CELERY, CHOPPED	1 CUP PLAIN NONFAT YOGURT
2 TEASPOONS CUMIN	FRESH CILANTRO FOR GARNISH (OPTIONAL)
½ TEASPOON CURRY POWDER	

DIRECTIONS

Heat oil in a large, heavy Dutch oven or covered saucepan over medium heat. Add onion, garlic
and barley and sauté until onion is golden, about 10 to 12 minutes. Stir frequently.

Add carrots, celery, cumin, and curry powder. Sauté 10 minutes more.

Add 4 cups water, light salt, pepper, lemon juice, and lentils. Bring mixture to a boil. Reduce
heat, cover, and simmer for about 1 hour until barley is tender and water has cooked off.
Add water only if necessary to prevent scorching. When barley is tender, remove lid and cook
off any remaining fluid.

Serve with a heaping tablespoonful of yogurt on each serving. Garnish with fresh cilantro,
if desired.

SERVING SIZE: 7 Servings, 1 Cup Each

PER SERVING: Calories 250   **Fiber:** 8 grams   **Sodium:** 209 mg.

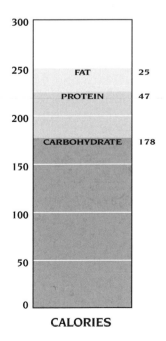

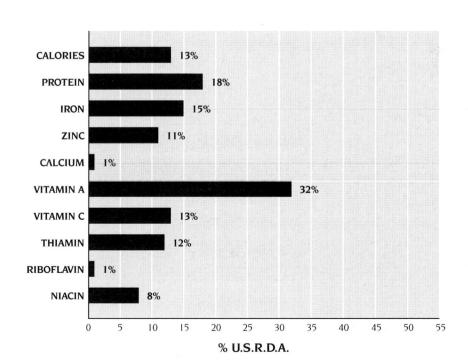

DALL

In India, dall (also dal or dhal) is an everyday dish made of lentils or yellow split peas and is served along with meat curries or as a main dish with rice. In the United States many people have never heard of lentils at all, much less the fact that they come in a variety of colors, sizes, and flavors. If you like beans, you will enjoy getting acquainted with lentils. To obtain the more colorful varieties, check an Oriental grocery. We suggest you make this dish several hours ahead of time or even the day before, since cooking time will vary with the type of lentils used.

INGREDIENTS

1 TEASPOON OIL	½-1 TEASPOON TURMERIC
4-5 THIN STRIPS OF BELL PEPPER	¾ TEASPOON LIGHT SALT
½ SMALL HOT GREEN CHILI PEPPER, SLICED IN ¼-INCH ROUNDS*	3-4 SMALL DRIED SHRIMP, MINCED (OPTIONAL)
1 CLOVE GARLIC, MINCED	1 CUP DRIED YELLOW SPLIT PEAS OR LENTILS
2 TEASPOONS CURRY POWDER	1 CUP NONFAT MILK
	1½ CUPS WATER

DIRECTIONS

Heat oil in a medium saucepan. Sauté bell pepper strips, hot chiles, garlic, curry powder, turmeric, light salt, and dried shrimp, if used. Sauté and stir over medium-low heat until peppers are tender and flavors blended, about 3 to 5 minutes. Mixture will be dry so watch for scorching.

Sort, then wash, split peas or lentils.

Add peas or lentils, milk, and water to saucepan. Cover and simmer over low heat for 1 to 2 hours until tender. Cooking time will vary according to type of split peas or lentils used. Additional fluid may be needed for longer cooking times.

SERVING SIZE: 6 Servings, ½ Cup Each

PER SERVING: Calories 141   **Fiber:** 6 grams   **Sodium:** 160 mg.

*Use more or less hot chili depending on desired degree of spiciness. One small (1½-inch long) chili makes for a very firey dish. Use care when handling chiles. Avoid touching your eyes. Wash hands thoroughly after handling. Chili slices can be removed before serving, if desired.

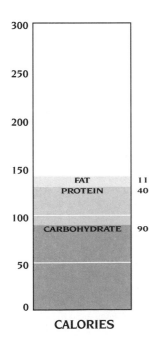

CALORIES

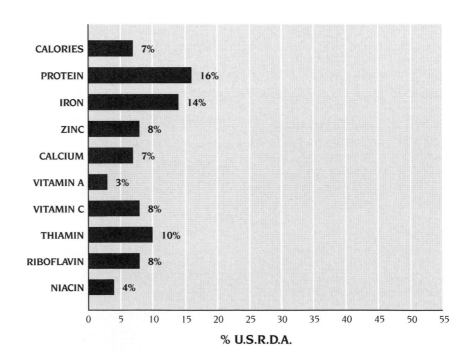

% U.S.R.D.A.

MA-PO TOFU

The correct name for this dish is "Chen Ma-Po Dou-Fu." Variations are numerous: some replace pork with beef, some call for fermented black beans or bean sauce (see Variations), but all are typically hot and spicy!

INGREDIENTS

1 LARGE PORK CHOP
1 TEASPOON PEANUT OIL
1 TABLESPOON FRESH GINGER ROOT, MINCED
3 LARGE CLOVES GARLIC, MINCED
⅛-¼ TEASPOON CRUSHED DRIED RED CHILES
½ CUP WATER
1 BEEF BOUILLON CUBE OR ½ TEASPOON BOUILLON GRANULES
10 OZ. TOFU, 1½ CUPS CUT INTO ½-INCH CUBES

1 TABLESPOON SOY SAUCE
½ CUP GREEN ONIONS, SLICED

Sauce

1 TABLESPOON SHERRY
1 TABLESPOON SOY SAUCE
2 TABLESPOONS WATER
1 TABLESPOON CORNSTARCH

DIRECTIONS

Trim all fat from pork chop. Slice meat thinly, then cut into little shreds.

Heat 1 teaspoon oil in a large nonstick skillet. Add pork shreds. Stir fry over high heat until brown, about 5 minutes.

Add minced ginger, garlic, and crushed chiles. Stir-fry 1 minute to blend flavors.

Dissolve bouillon in ½ cup water.

Add cubed tofu, dissolved bouillon, soy sauce, and green onions to skillet. Simmer until mixture is almost dry.

In a small bowl, mix sauce ingredients.

Add sauce to tofu mixture. Cook 1 minute until thickened, stirring gently.

Serve over steamed rice with a vegetable side dish.

VARIATIONS: Add 1-2 teaspoons fermented black beans or hot bean sauce with minced ginger.
Low-Sodium version. Since 97% of the sodium in this recipe comes from the 2 tablespoons soy sauce and the bouillon, using low-salt products will dramatically reduce sodium content.

SERVING SIZE: 2 Servings, Main Dish; 4 Servings, Side Dish

PER SERVING: Calories 246   **Fiber:** 6 grams   **Sodium:** 1370 mg.

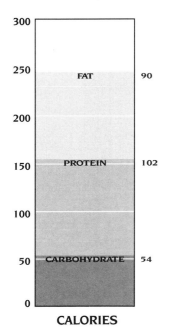

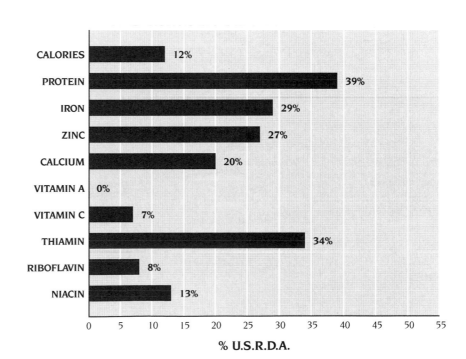

SNOW PEAS WITH TOFU

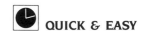 **QUICK & EASY**

A simple stir-fry of crisp green pea pods, dark earthy mushrooms, and delicate white tofu.

INGREDIENTS

1 TABLESPOON OIL
2 CLOVES GARLIC, MINCED
1 ONION, SLICED
12 LARGE MUSHROOMS (¾ LB.) SLICED*
½ LB. SNOW PEAS

1 TABLESPOON SOY SAUCE
¼ CUP SHERRY
1 CUBE CHICKEN BOUILLON DISSOLVED IN ¼ CUP WATER
1 PACKAGE (14 OZ.) TOFU, CUBED

DIRECTIONS

Heat oil in a wok or large skillet. Sauté garlic over medium heat until lightly browned, about 1 to 2 minutes.

Add sliced onion. Stir fry over medium-high heat for 3 to 5 minutes until onion begins to brown around the edges.

Add mushrooms and snow peas. Turn heat to high. Stir fry until snow peas are crisp tender, 3 to 4 minutes.

Add soy sauce, sherry, bouillon, and tofu. Simmer, uncovered, until tofu is heated through. Serve.

SERVING SIZE: 4 Servings, 1 Cup Each

PER SERVING: Calories 191 **Fiber:** 9 grams **Sodium:** 477 mg.

*Chinese black mushrooms will give this dish a more intensely Oriental flavor. To substitute these dried mushrooms for fresh, soak 6 large or 12 small black mushrooms in 1 cup hot water until soft (15 to 30 minutes). Remove tough stems, cut larger mushroom caps into halves or quarters.

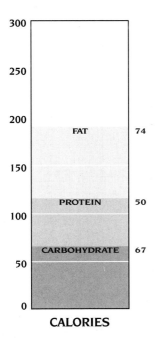

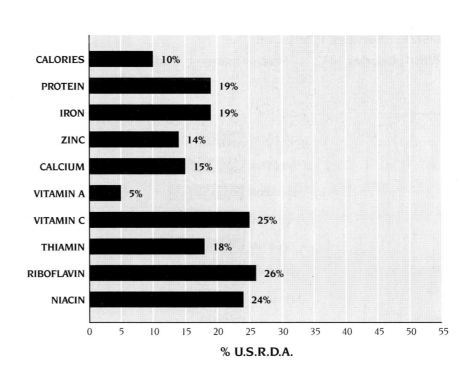

JAMAICAN CHICK-PEA FRITTERS

INGREDIENTS

2 CLOVES GARLIC, MINCED
1 SMALL ONION, 1 CUP CHOPPED
1 CAN GARBANZO BEANS (16 OZS.) (CHICK-PEAS), DRAINED
2 EGGS
½ CUP WHOLE WHEAT PASTRY FLOUR
1 TEASPOON HOT RED PEPPER SAUCE

¼ TEASPOON FRESHLY GROUND BLACK PEPPER
½ TEASPOON LIGHT SALT (OPTIONAL)
½ CUP FRESH PARSLEY, CHOPPED
1 TABLESPOON OLIVE OIL OR PEANUT OIL
FILIPINO DIPPING SAUCE OR NORWEGIAN HOT MUSTARD

DIRECTIONS

Chop garlic and onion in food processor or blender. Add drained garbanzos, eggs, flour, pepper sauce, black pepper, and salt, if used. Blend until combined.

Pour into a small mixing bowl. Stir in parsley. Cover and refrigerate until cooking time or up to 48 hours.

Heat oil in large nonstick skillet. Drop heaping tablespoons of garbanzo mixture into hot oil, forming eight patties. Flatten slightly. Reduce heat to medium and sauté 10 to 12 minutes until golden brown. Turn over and brown other side.

SERVING SUGGESTION: Serve with Filipino Dipping Sauce or Norwegian Hot Mustard Sauce. Or try them falafel-style in a pita pocket.

SERVING SIZE: 4 Servings, 2 Patties Each

PER SERVING: Calories 236   **Fiber:** 4 grams   **Sodium:** 452 mg.

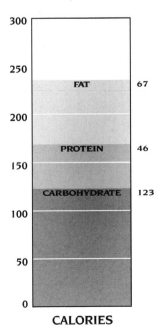

CALORIES

FAT 67
PROTEIN 46
CARBOHYDRATE 123

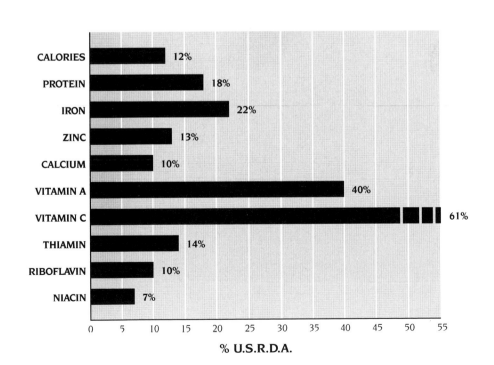

CALORIES 12%
PROTEIN 18%
IRON 22%
ZINC 13%
CALCIUM 10%
VITAMIN A 40%
VITAMIN C 61%
THIAMIN 14%
RIBOFLAVIN 10%
NIACIN 7%

% U.S.R.D.A.

PEKING SHRIMP

INGREDIENTS

1 TABLESPOON PEANUT OIL
3 SLICES FRESH GINGER (⅛-INCH EACH)
4 CLOVES GARLIC, MINCED
¼-½ TEASPOON CRUSHED RED PEPPER OR 1-2 DRIED CHINESE CHILES, SEEDED AND DICED
1 LB. LARGE SHRIMP (UNCOOKED)

Marinade

1 EGG WHITE
2 TABLESPOONS CORNSTARCH
1 TABLESPOON SOY SAUCE

Seasoning Sauce

2 TABLESPOONS SOY SAUCE
¼ CUP CIDER OR MALT VINEGAR
1½ TABLESPOONS SUGAR
2 TABLESPOONS DRY SHERRY OR SAKE
2 TABLESPOONS WATER

½ TEASPOON SESAME OIL (OPTIONAL)

DIRECTIONS

Heat 1 tablespoon peanut oil in a large nonstick skillet or wok. Add sliced ginger, minced garlic, and crushed red pepper. Sauté 1 minute, then turn heat off and allow flavors to blend while preparing shrimp.

Peel, devein, and wash shrimp. Spread on paper towels and blot dry.

Combine marinade ingredients in a medium bowl. Beat with fork to blend. Add shrimp and stir gently to coat. Chill until ready to cook.

In a small bowl combine seasoning sauce ingredients. Set aside.

When ready to cook, heat skillet with oil and spices until oil begins to smoke. Immediately add shrimp with marinade, spreading them out in a single layer.

Fry shrimp over high heat for 3 to 4 minutes until bottom side turns pink and coating begins to brown. Turn over, fry 2 to 3 minutes more until shrimp are pink and firm. Do not overcook.

Add seasoning sauce to skillet. Cook, stirring, 1 minute only. You should have about ½ cup of sauce in the pan now, do not cook off!

Turn into serving dish, sprinkle with a few drops of sesame oil and serve immediately. If you are serving rice, spoon remaining sauce over rice.

SERVING SIZE: ¼ Recipe

PER SERVING: Calories 177 **Fiber:** 0 **Sodium:** 796 mg.

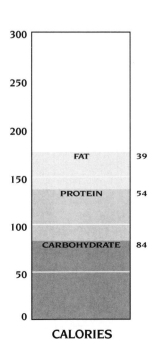

CALORIES

FAT	39
PROTEIN	54
CARBOHYDRATE	84

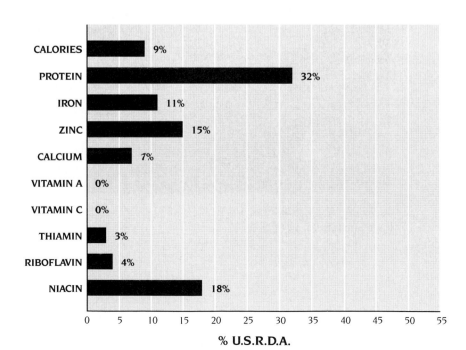

% U.S.R.D.A.

CALORIES 9%
PROTEIN 32%
IRON 11%
ZINC 15%
CALCIUM 7%
VITAMIN A 0%
VITAMIN C 0%
THIAMIN 3%
RIBOFLAVIN 4%
NIACIN 18%

SHRIMP EGG FU YUNG 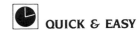 **QUICK & EASY**

China's answer to the quick supper omelet, egg fu yung is easy to make and inexpensive.
It's also a children's favorite, especially when served with fried rice.

INGREDIENTS

5 CUPS FRESH BEAN SPROUTS
½ BUNCH GREEN ONIONS, SLICED
¾ CUP SHRIMP, COOKED AND PEELED, OR 1 CAN
  (6 OZ.), DRAINED
4 EGGS
¼ TEASPOON BLACK PEPPER
½ TEASPOON LIGHT SALT
¼ TEASPOON GARLIC POWDER
2 TEASPOONS PEANUT OIL, DIVIDED

Sauce

1 TEASPOON CORNSTARCH
1 TEASPOON SUGAR
2 TEASPOONS SOY SAUCE
1 TEASPOON VINEGAR
1 CHICKEN BOUILLON CUBE DISSOLVED IN
  ½ CUP BOILING WATER

DIRECTIONS

Rinse bean sprouts and drain in colander.

Toss bean sprouts, green onions, and shrimp in large bowl.

In separate bowl or blender, beat eggs with pepper, light salt, and garlic powder. Pour over
  vegetables and toss together.

Heat 1 teaspoon of oil in large, heavy skillet. Spoon half of egg and vegetable mixture into hot
  skillet, forming three large patties.

Fry over low heat for 3 to 4 minutes until brown. Turn and fry 3 to 4 minutes on other side.

Repeat with remaining oil and sprout mixture.

While patties are cooking, make sauce: Combine cornstarch, sugar, soy sauce, and vinegar in a
  small saucepan. Add dissolved bouillon. Cook over medium-low heat, stirring constantly,
  until thick and bubbly, about 3 to 5 minutes. Spoon over patties when serving.

VARIATION: Pork Egg Fu Yung. Instead of shrimp, use ½ cup finely diced, cooked lean ham,
  or roast pork. Other shellfish or chicken work well too.

SERVING SIZE: 6 Servings, 1 Patty Each

PER SERVING: Calories 131   **Fiber:** 2 grams   **Sodium:** 310 mg.

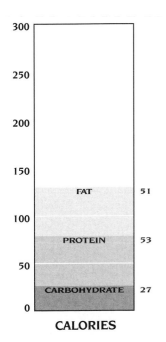

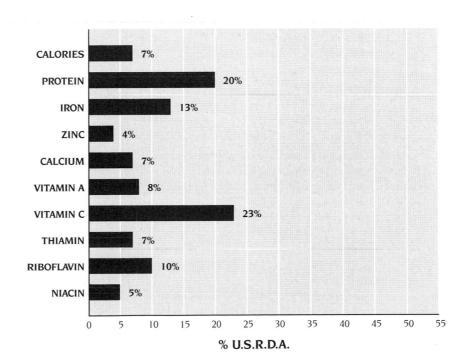

SHRIMP CREOLE

True to the form of any well-loved dish, there are as many versions of shrimp creole as there are chefs in Louisiana. This winning combination of shrimp and a peppery tomato sauce is served over mounds of steamed rice. While most recipes include ham, bacon, or bacon drippings, ours achieves the traditional smokiness from lean turkey ham. An interesting entree for relaxed entertaining.

INGREDIENTS

1 LB. COOKED SHRIMP
1 TABLESPOON BUTTER
3 CLOVES GARLIC, MINCED
2 LARGE ONIONS, CHOPPED
2 LARGE STALKS CELERY, THINLY SLICED
1 BELL PEPPER, CHOPPED
2 BAY LEAVES
½ LB. TURKEY HAM, OR CANADIAN BACON, CUT IN ¼-INCH CUBES

¼ TEASPOON THYME
½ TEASPOON HOT PEPPER SAUCE
1½ TEASPOONS CHICKEN BOUILLON GRANULES DISSOLVED IN ½ CUP BOILING WATER
4 LARGE TOMATOES, PEELED AND CUT IN BITE-SIZED CHUNKS
4 TABLESPOONS FRESH PARSLEY, CHOPPED
SCALLIONS, FOR GARNISH
STEAMED BROWN RICE

DIRECTIONS

If using raw shrimp, peel, devein, and boil or steam until bright pink.

Heat butter in a large nonstick skillet. Sauté garlic, onion, celery, and bell pepper with bay leaves and thyme over medium heat for about 15 minutes, until vegetables are tender.

Add cubed meat and sauté another 5 minutes until vegetables begin to brown.

Add hot pepper sauce, dissolved bouillon, and tomatoes. Simmer 5 minutes more.

Stir in parsley and cooked shrimp. Heat through. Serve over steamed brown rice. Garnish with sliced scallions.

VARIATION: Add 1 to 2 teaspoons curry powder along with the bay leaves and thyme.

SERVING SIZE: ⅙ Recipe

PER SERVING: Calories 207 **Fiber:** 3 grams **Sodium:** 794 mg.

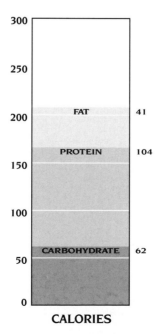

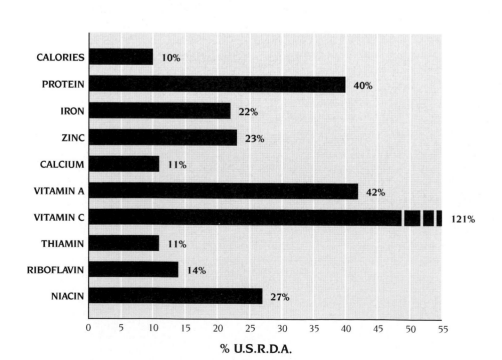

SHRIMP CURRY

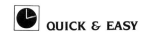 **QUICK & EASY**

This quick curry is best made with freshly steamed shrimp, but the pungently delicious sauce works wonders with precooked shrimp meat when time is of the essence.

INGREDIENTS

1 LB. COOKED SHRIMP	1 TEASPOON LIGHT SALT
1 TABLESPOON BUTTER OR OIL	¼ TEASPOON CHILI POWDER
½ ONION, CHOPPED	3 TABLESPOONS WHITE FLOUR
1 SMALL CAN GREEN CHILES, DICED	1½ CUPS NONFAT MILK
1-2 TEASPOONS CURRY POWDER	1 TABLESPOON LEMON JUICE
⅛ TEASPOON GINGER	STEAMED RICE
⅛ TEASPOON WHITE PEPPER	

DIRECTIONS

If using raw shrimp, peel, devein, and boil or steam until bright pink.

Heat butter or oil in a large nonstick skillet and sauté onion over medium heat until golden, about 15 minutes. Add chiles, curry powder, ginger, white pepper, light salt, and chili powder. Sauté, stirring constantly, until mixture sizzles, 3 to 5 minutes.

Sprinkle on flour and stir constantly until dispersed and beginning to brown.

Add milk all at once. Stir until thickened and bubbly.

Add cooked shrimp. Heat just until heated through.

Add lemon juice and serve immediately over steamed rice.

SERVING SIZE: ¼ Recipe

PER SERVING: Calories 234 **Fiber:** 1 gram **Sodium:** 539 mg.

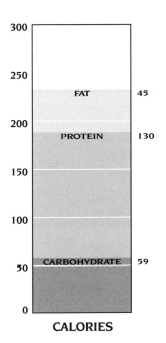

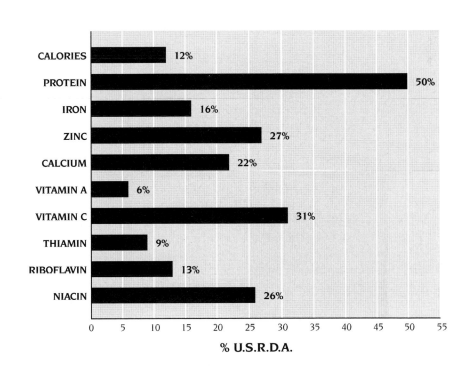

SHRIMP GUMBO

This Creole gumbo is traditionally served over rice with mixed greens and sweet potatoes on the side.

INGREDIENTS

- 1 LB. COOKED SHRMP
- 3 SLICES LEAN, SMOKED BACON, DICED
- 1 LARGE ONION, CHOPPED
- 3 CLOVES GARLIC, MINCED
- 2-3 CUPS FRESH OKRA, SLICED ½-INCH THICK, OR FROZEN OKRA, THAWED AND DRAINED
- 1 LARGE BELL PEPPER, CHOPPED
- 2 LARGE TOMATOES, CHOPPED

- ½ TEASPOON COARSELY GROUND BLACK PEPPER
- ½ TEASPOON HOT PEPPER SAUCE
- 2 BAY LEAVES
- 1 CUP BOILING WATER
- 1 CUP CATSUP
- LIGHT SALT TO TASTE

DIRECTIONS

If using raw shrimp, peel, devein and boil or steam until bright pink.

Sauté diced bacon over medium heat in a large nonstick skillet until crisp. Remove bacon and sauté onion and garlic in bacon fat for 5 to 10 minutes until tender.

Add sliced okra and sauté 5 to 10 minutes more.

Add bell pepper, tomatoes, black pepper, hot sauce, bay leaves, and boiling water.

Cover and simmer for 15 minutes until okra is tender. Remove lid and cook off excess liquid, if needed, until mixture has consistency of a thick sauce.

Add catsup and simmer 5 minutes more.

Stir in shrimp and cooked bacon. Add light salt if desired. Heat through and serve.

SERVING SIZE: 6 Servings, 1 Cup Each

PER SERVING: Calories 176   **Fiber:** 5 grams   **Sodium:** 549 mg.

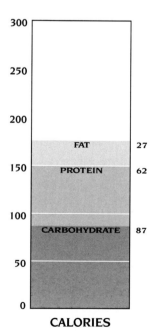

FAT 27
PROTEIN 62
CARBOHYDRATE 87

CALORIES

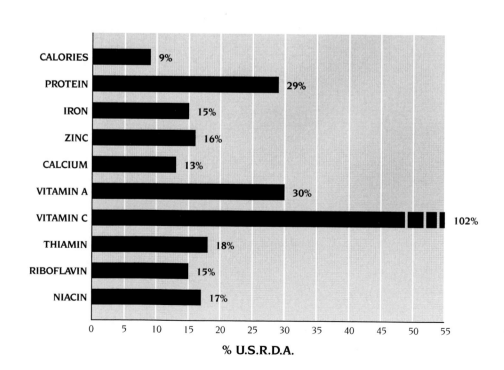

	% U.S.R.D.A.
CALORIES	9%
PROTEIN	29%
IRON	15%
ZINC	16%
CALCIUM	13%
VITAMIN A	30%
VITAMIN C	102%
THIAMIN	18%
RIBOFLAVIN	15%
NIACIN	17%

CLASSIC SCALLOP SAUTÉ

 QUICK & EASY

A wonderful supper dish straight from San Francisco's North Beach. Serve with plain pasta, a crisp green salad, and a crusty loaf of bread. Perfect when the hour is late—but the night is young.

INGREDIENTS

    2 LB. FRESH SCALLOPS
    2 TABLESPOONS OLIVE OIL
6-12 CLOVES GARLIC, MINCED
  ¼ CUP WHITE FLOUR
  ½ TEASPOON FRESHLY GROUND BLACK PEPPER
  ½ TEASPOON LIGHT SALT
   2 TABLESPOONS SHERRY

DIRECTIONS

Rinse scallops in cold water. Drain and blot dry on paper towels. Cut large ones in half but leave small scallops (½- ¾-inch) whole. Chill.

Heat olive oil in a large nonstick skillet. Add minced garlic and turn off heat.

Combine flour, pepper, and light salt in a large bowl.

Five minutes before serving time, reheat oil and garlic. Toss the scallops in the flour mixture.

When garlic oil is quite hot, add scallops. Keeping heat fairly high, sauté scallops for 4 to 5 minutes, just until firm and opaque.* Add sherry, heat through, and serve immediately.

SERVING SIZE: ⅙ Recipe

PER SERVING: Calories 181 **Fiber:** 0 **Sodium:** 218 mg.

*Fresh scallops, cooked quickly and served immediately, are an epicurean delight. Overcooked scallops, on the other hand, are reminiscent of fishy rubber. Do not overcook.

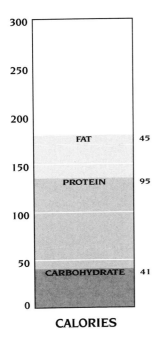

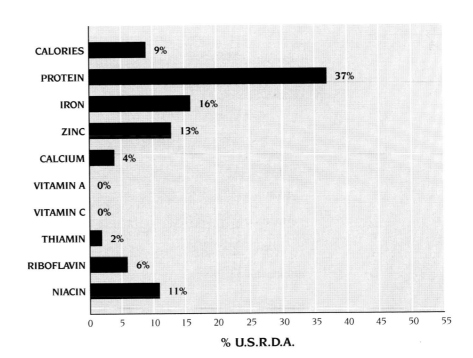

SOUTHERN FRIED CHICKEN

"Crispy on the outside, juicy on the inside"—good old-fashioned fried chicken! Our food photographer refused to believe that this rich golden-brown, pan-fried chicken could actually be low fat until he photographed the procedure. After he saw that the entire bird requires only a single tablespoon of fat for frying, he could not wait to finish the shoot—so we could eat! The trick lies in using chicken fat for that real fried chicken flavor. (Pictured on p. 40.)

INGREDIENTS

1 CHICKEN (3 LB.) CUT UP
1 TABLESPOON FAT FOR FRYING (CHICKEN FAT IS BEST)
⅓ CUP WHITE FLOUR
1 TEASPOON LIGHT SEASONED SALT

½ TEASPOON PAPRIKA
¼ TEASPOON POULTRY SEASONING
¼ TEASPOON ONION POWDER OR GARLIC POWDER
⅛ TEASPOON BLACK PEPPER
½ CUP WATER

DIRECTIONS

Select a large nonstick skillet with a closely fitting lid.

Remove all skin and visible fat from chicken.

If chicken fat is to be used for frying, fry the skins long enough to render 1 tablespoon fat, then discard skins. (If oil is used, omit this step.)

Combine flour and spices in plastic bag or bowl. Shake or roll chicken, one or two pieces at a time, in seasoned flour. Set aside on waxed paper. Coat all chicken with flour before heating fat.

Heat 1 tablespoon fat in the skillet, then add chicken, starting with breasts, then legs, thighs, wings, and back.

Brown over medium heat, about 10 to 12 minutes per side, until golden brown on all sides.

Add ½ cup water to chicken. Cover tightly, cook over low heat for 30 minutes.

Remove cover, turn up heat, and cook off any remaining liquid. Continue frying chicken until reddish-brown, 1 to 2 minutes.

SERVING SIZE: ¼ Recipe

PER SERVING: Calories 245 **Fiber:** 0 **Sodium:** 380 mg.

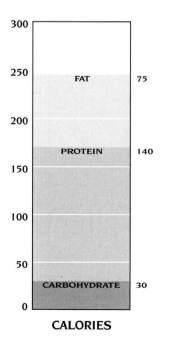

CALORIES

FAT	75
PROTEIN	140
CARBOHYDRATE	30

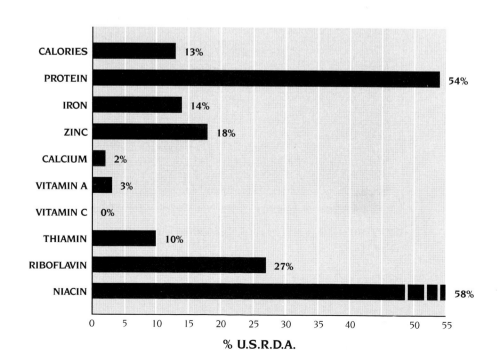

% U.S.R.D.A.

CALORIES	13%
PROTEIN	54%
IRON	14%
ZINC	18%
CALCIUM	2%
VITAMIN A	3%
VITAMIN C	0%
THIAMIN	10%
RIBOFLAVIN	27%
NIACIN	58%

CHICKEN AND CRUMBS

Oven baked chicken breasts with a crispy crumb coating—our answer to shaking and baking!

INGREDIENTS

6 LARGE CHICKEN BREASTS (2 LB.), SKINNED AND TRIMMED OF FAT
½ CUP WHOLE GRAIN CRACKER CRUMBS OR CORN FLAKE CRUMBS
1 TEASPOON LIGHT SEASONED SALT*
¼ TEASPOON BLACK PEPPER
½ TEASPOON ONION POWDER
¼ TEASPOON GARLIC POWDER
¼ TEASPOON THYME
½ TEASPOON PAPRIKA
½ TEASPOON SAGE

DIRECTIONS

Preheat oven to 400°.
Remove skin from chicken breasts and trim all visible fat. Rinse in cold water.
Combine remaining ingredients in a plastic bag or small bowl. Shake or roll chicken in crumb mixture to coat.
Place chicken in a 9-inch by 13-inch baking dish sprayed with nonstick cooking spray.
Bake uncovered for 35 to 45 minutes. Check after 30 minutes. If chicken is well browned, cover pan with foil for last 15 minutes baking time.

SERVING SIZE: 1 Chicken Breast, 6 Servings

PER SERVING: Calories 139 **Fiber:** 1 gram **Sodium:** 237 mg.

*Most of the sodium in this recipe comes from the 1 teaspoon seasoned light salt. Many seasoned salt substitutes are now available.

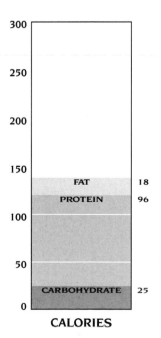

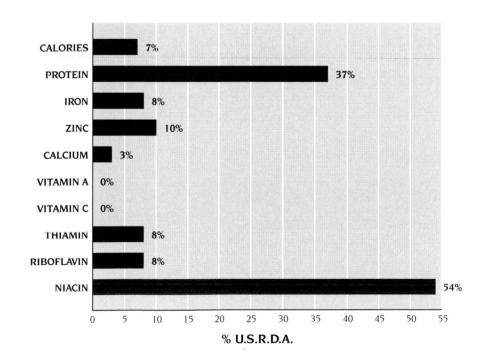

Eight Ways With Barbequed or Broiled Chicken

Making barbequed chicken low in fat is easy. Just remove all skin and fat before cooking and you literally pull off most of the fat and over half the total calories. The tricky part is making low-fat barbequed chicken that tastes wonderful and isn't dry. The secret lies in technique. Marinating is an important first step, so we've presented our top eight favorite marinades just to get you started. Barbequing and broiling procedures are presented separately and in great detail to include all the flavor and moisture-preserving tips.

INGREDIENTS

3 LB. CHICKEN LEGS, THIGHS, OR BREASTS
MARINADE (CHOOSE FROM THE FOLLOWING)

Mexican Lime Marinade

JUICE OF 3 LIMES
JUICE OF 1 LEMON
½ CUP DRY WHITE WINE
1 TEASPOON SUGAR
1 TEASPOON LIGHT SALT
¼ TEASPOON BLACK PEPPER
½ TEASPOON DRIED TARRAGON
1 CLOVE GARLIC, MINCED

Combine all ingredients.

Mustard Glaze

⅓ CUP GRAINY HOT MUSTARD
½ CUP UNSWEETENED APPLESAUCE
2 TABLESPOONS HONEY
2 TABLESPOONS CIDER VINEGAR

Stir all ingredients together in a small bowl.

Iranian Sauce

1 LARGE ONION, QUARTERED
6 TABLESPOONS LEMON JUICE OR JUICE OF 2
LEMONS
2 TEASPOONS LIGHT SALT
⅛ TEASPOON SAFFRON (OPTIONAL)

Puree all ingredients in blender or food processor to make a thin paste.

Hawaiian Sauce

1 CUP CANNED CHUNK OR CRUSHED PINEAPPLE
PACKED IN ITS OWN JUICE, WELL-DRAINED OR
FRESH PINEAPPLE, CUT IN CHUNKS
2 TABLESPOONS HONEY OR MOLASSES
2 TABLESPOONS DIJON MUSTARD
2 TABLESPOONS LEMON JUICE
¼ TEASPOON BLACK PEPPER
1 TEASPOON LIGHT SALT

Puree all ingredients in a blender or food processor.

Indonesian Sauce

1 ONION, QUARTERED
4 CLOVES GARLIC
3 TABLESPOONS HONEY
¼ CUP SALTED, ROASTED PEANUTS
1 TABLESPOON SOY SAUCE
1½ TEASPOONS COARSELY GROUND BLACK PEPPER
2 TABLESPOONS LEMON JUICE
¼ TEASPOON ALLSPICE
¼ TEASPOON CINNAMON
¼ TEASPOON CLOVES
¼ TEASPOON GROUND GINGER

Puree all ingredients in a blender or food processor.

Chinese Red Sauce

1 CAN (1 LB.) WHOLE TOMATOES
4 STALKS CELERY, 1⅓ CUPS CHOPPED
2 TABLESPOONS VINEGAR
2 TABLESPOONS SOY SAUCE
2 TABLESPOONS SHERRY
2 TEASPOONS SESAME OIL
BLACK OR RED PEPPER (OPTIONAL)

Puree all ingredients in blender or food processor.

Teriyaki Sauce

5 SMALL SCALLIONS, SLICED
½ CUP SOY SAUCE
⅓ CUP SHERRY
3 TABLESPOONS HONEY OR SUGAR SUBSTITUTE
3 CLOVES GARLIC, MINCED
2 TEASPOONS FRESH GINGER, MINCED OR
½ TEASPOON DRY
¾ CUP UNSWEETENED PINEAPPLE JUICE
¼ CUP FRESH LIME OR LEMON JUICE

Stir all ingredients together.

Oklahoma Barbeque Sauce, Salsa Cruda (Red Salsa), or Green Tomatillo Salsa (see Sauces, Chapter 2).

Using the sauces from Chapter 2 is a bit trickier, but the results are fantastic! Use just enough sauce to coat chicken when marinating. Don't use these sauces for basting because they will scorch. Set aside unused sauce to serve with chicken at the table. Sauce that has been in contact with raw chicken should not be served.

DIRECTIONS

Remove all skin and fat from chicken parts.

Place chicken in a bowl with marinade, turning to coat all pieces.

Marinate 4 to 48 hours in a covered dish in the refrigerator.

To Barbeque:

We recommend using chicken legs or thighs because dark meat, with its slightly higher fat content, holds its moisture better, but breasts also work well in a covered, kettle-type barbeque grill. Using uniformly sized pieces of chicken will simplify the barbeque chef's task, since all will cook at about the same speed. Skinned chicken requires more frequent basting than "unskinned," but the great advantage is that the flavors of the marinade or glaze go right into the meat.

For best results, use a covered barbeque pit or make a tent of heavy-duty aluminum foil. (This helps overcome one of the most common pitfalls of barbequed chicken: raw on the inside, burnt on the outside.) Set the grill 6 to 8 inches above coals for slow, even cooking. Keep fire fairly low and allow 50 to 60 minutes cooking time.

Just before barbequing, brush hot grill with oil to prevent sticking.

Drain marinated chicken and reserve marinade for basting.

Place chicken on oiled grill, cover, and barbeque for 25 to 30 minutes until one side is well browned. Turn and baste with marinade.

Cover and barbeque for 15 to 20 minutes to brown other side.

Turn chicken again and baste generously. Barbeque 5 minutes to set glaze. Turn meat again and repeat glazing procedure. Serve.

Heat any remaining marinade to boiling and serve alongside.

To Broil:

Legs, thighs, or breasts all broil beautifully. We suggest you choose one cut for even cooking.

Drain marinated chicken and reserve sauce.

Preheat oven to 450°.

Place drained chicken in a single layer in a greased 9-inch by 13-inch baking pan. Bake for 10 minutes.

Turn chicken, bake 10 minutes more.

Reduce oven to 350°. Baste meat with marinade and continue baking for 30 minutes. Brush with sauce two or three times during baking. At the end of 30 minutes drain off any pan juices and reserve them.

Once again, brush meat generously with marinade. Turn on oven broiling unit and place pan 6 inches below heat. Broil for 3 to 4 minutes until well browned. Repeat process on other side. Serve.

Remaining marinade and/or pan juices can be heated to boiling and served with chicken.

SERVING SIZE: Broiled Chicken Leg plus Thigh, 6 Servings

PER SERVING: Calories 178   **Fiber:** 0   **Sodium:** 88 mg.

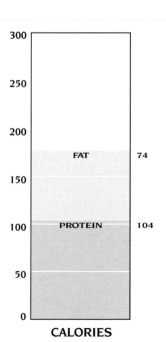

CALORIES

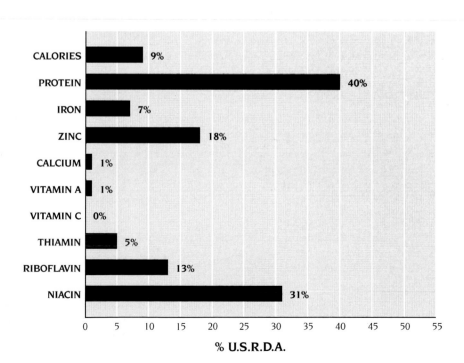

% U.S.R.D.A.

CHICKEN POT PIE

An old-fashioned country dinner pie has it all—meat, vegetables, starch, and even milk. The long list of ingredients may be intimidating at first glance, but don't dismay. By using canned chicken chunks and frozen peas and carrots, you can present an impressive entree with less than 30 minutes preparation time. Serve with a salad of fresh greens.

INGREDIENTS

1 TABLESPOON CHICKEN FAT OR OIL
1 ONION, CHOPPED
2 STALKS CELERY, CHOPPED
1 CAN (14 OZ.) CHICKEN BROTH
½ CUP NONFAT MILK
3 TABLESPOONS WHITE FLOUR
1½ CUPS COOKED CHICKEN OR TURKEY, CUT IN ½-INCH CUBES OR 1 CAN (15 OZ.) CHICKEN CHUNKS
1 CUP FRESH COOKED OR FROZEN GREEN PEAS
1 MEDIUM COOKED POTATO(1 CUP), CUT IN ½-INCH CUBES
½ CUP COOKED OR FROZEN CARROTS, CUT IN ½-INCH CUBES
4 TABLESPOONS FRESH PARSLEY, CHOPPED

¼ TEASPOON BLACK PEPPER
½ TEASPOON CURRY POWDER
1 TEASPOON POULTRY SEASONING
LIGHT SALT TO TASTE

Batter

3 EGG WHITES, STIFFLY BEATEN
1 CUP WHOLE WHEAT PASTRY FLOUR
1 TEASPOON BAKING POWDER
¼ TEASPOON LIGHT SALT
½ TEASPOON SUGAR
1 CUP NONFAT MILK
3 EGG YOLKS
2 TEASPOONS OIL

DIRECTIONS

Sauté onion and celery in fat in a large, heavy saucepan over medium heat until golden brown, about 10 to 15 minutes.

Add broth. Heat until simmering.

Mix milk with flour. Add to broth. Stir until thickened.

Add chicken cubes, peas, potatoes, and carrots. Heat through.

Add parsley, pepper, curry powder, poultry seasoning, and light salt to taste.

Turn into 9-inch by 13-inch baking dish or eight individual casserole dishes.

Preheat oven to 450°.
Make batter crust:
    Beat egg whites until stiff.
    Mix flour, baking powder, light salt, and sugar in a medium bowl.
    Mix milk, egg yolks, and oil in a larger bowl.
    Add dry to wet ingredients and stir only until blended.
    Fold in beaten egg whites. Spread crust evenly over filling before baking.
Bake for 5 minutes, turn heat down to 300° and bake for 20 minutes, or until crust is golden brown and set.

VARIATION: Use a rolled out biscuit dough instead of batter crust.

SERVING SIZE: ⅛ Recipe

PER SERVING: Calories 248   **Fiber:** 4 grams   **Sodium:** 398 mg.

Chicken Pot Pie (facing page)

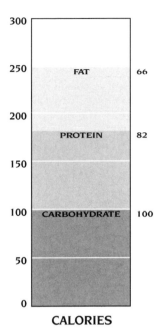

FAT 66
PROTEIN 82
CARBOHYDRATE 100

CALORIES

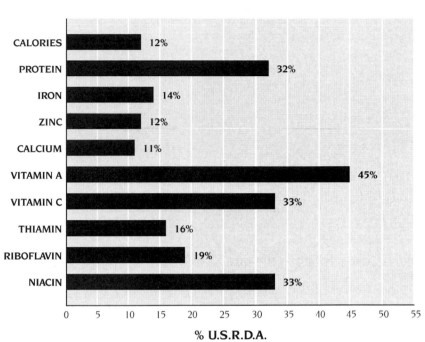

	% U.S.R.D.A.
CALORIES	12%
PROTEIN	32%
IRON	14%
ZINC	12%
CALCIUM	11%
VITAMIN A	45%
VITAMIN C	33%
THIAMIN	16%
RIBOFLAVIN	19%
NIACIN	33%

% U.S.R.D.A.

Chicken Enchiladas (p. 150)

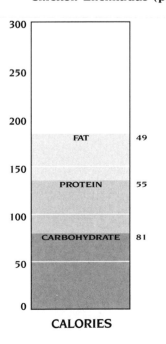

FAT 49
PROTEIN 55
CARBOHYDRATE 81

CALORIES

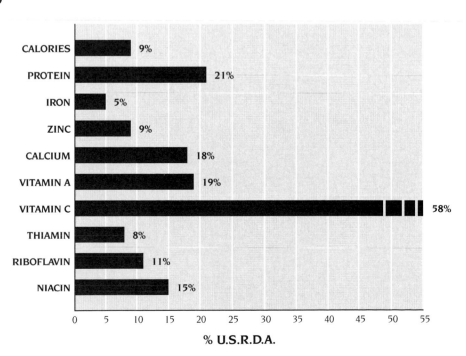

	% U.S.R.D.A.
CALORIES	9%
PROTEIN	21%
IRON	5%
ZINC	9%
CALCIUM	18%
VITAMIN A	19%
VITAMIN C	58%
THIAMIN	8%
RIBOFLAVIN	11%
NIACIN	15%

% U.S.R.D.A.

CHICKEN ENCHILADAS

These delicious enchiladas needn't occupy your entire day. The sauce, as well as the roast chicken, can be made (or even purchased) well ahead, so that actual assembly takes only 20 minutes. Refried beans, tortillas, and a marinated vegetable salad are excellent accompaniments.

INGREDIENTS

12 TORTILLAS, CORN OR WHOLE WHEAT

Sauce*

 1 TEASPOON OIL
1-2 CLOVES GARLIC, MINCED
 1 LARGE ONION, CHOPPED
 1 LB. FRESH TOMATOES OR 1 CAN (15 OZ.)
 1 CAN (8 OZ.) WHOLE GREEN CHILES, SEEDED
 ½ TEASPOON OREGANO
 1 CAN (8 OZ.) TOMATO SAUCE

Filling

 2 CUPS LEAN ROASTED CHICKEN OR TURKEY, SHREDDED, OR 3 CANS (6 OZ. EACH) CHUNKED CHICKEN
 ⅔ CUP NONFAT YOGURT
 ⅔ CUP LOW-FAT COTTAGE CHEESE
 ½ TEASPOON LIGHT SALT (OMIT IF USING CANNED MEAT)
 4 OZ. SHARP CHEDDAR CHEESE, SHREDDED, OR MEXICAN CHEESE, CRUMBLED
 1 TABLESPOON FRESH CILANTRO OR PARSLEY, CHOPPED

DIRECTIONS

Preheat oven to 350°.

Heat oil in a large nonstick skillet. Sauté garlic 1 minute, then add onion and sauté 2 minutes longer.

Finely chop tomatoes and seeded chiles in blender or food processor. Add to onion mixture along with oregano and tomato sauce.

Simmer for 20 to 30 minutes over low heat, until thick.

Thoroughly combine all filling ingredients and set aside.

In a 9-inch by 13-inch baking dish, evenly distribute half the prepared sauce.

To assemble enchiladas: Heat tortillas, one at a time in nonstick skillet, until softened. Place a spoonful of filling across each tortilla, roll the filled tortillas loosely and set side by side in the baking dish.

Cover enchiladas with remaining sauce. Bake for 20 to 25 minutes until heated through. Serve immediately.

SERVING SIZE: 12 Servings, 1 Enchilada Each

PER SERVING: Calories 185   **Fiber:** 3 grams   **Sodium:** 378 mg.

*A 20 oz. can or 2½ cups of prepared enchilada sauce can be substituted.

Graph on p. 149

CHICKEN IN ORANGE SAUCE

For a gracious dinner serve with Wild Rice Pilaf, brussels sprouts, and a fresh fruit salad.

INGREDIENTS

6 CHICKEN BREASTS (2 LB.), SKINNED
2 TEASPOONS PEANUT OIL

Sauce

2-3 TEASPOONS ORANGE RIND, SLIVERED
½ CUP FRESH ORANGE JUICE
2 TABLESPOONS FRESH LEMON JUICE
3 TABLESPOONS HONEY
¼ TEASPOON NUTMEG

¼ TEASPOON GINGER
¼ TEASPOON ALLSPICE
¼ TEASPOON LIGHT SALT
¼ TEASPOON WHITE PEPPER
¾ CUP WHITE WINE

DIRECTIONS

Preheat broiler. Set rack 6 inches below heat.
Remove skin and fat from chicken breasts.
Spread peanut oil in an 8-inch by 10-inch broiling pan. Place chicken breasts in the pan, meaty side down to coat with oil, then turn them over and arrange in a single layer, meaty side up.
Broil for 10 to 15 minutes, until lightly browned.
Meanwhile, prepare sauce: Remove peel, not rind from orange. Cut into thin slivers. Juice orange and lemon. Combine all sauce ingredients.

When chicken is browned, remove pan from oven. Reset oven temperature to 400°. Pour sauce evenly over chicken breasts, return to oven, and bake for 20 minutes.
Turn over and bake for 10 minutes longer.
Turn again, spoon sauce over meat. Change oven to broiler setting to brown chicken, about 2 to 3 minutes per side.

VARIATION: Cranberry-Orange Chicken. Substitute low-calorie cranberry juice cocktail for white wine.

SERVING SIZE: 1 Breast with Sauce, 6 Servings

PER SERVING: Calories 175 **Fiber:** 0 **Sodium:** 136 mg.

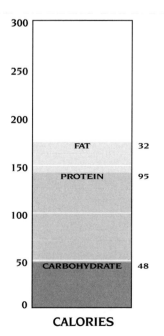

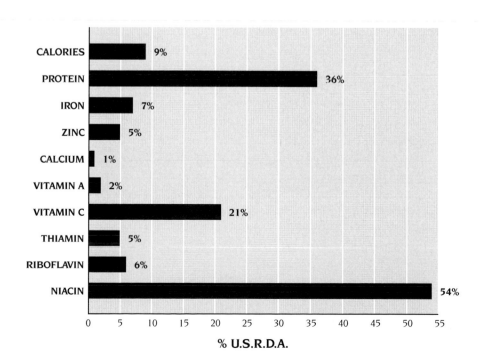

HERBED CHICKEN IN WINE SAUCE

Serve this elegant entree to your most highly esteemed guests and don't divulge its low-fat nature until you have collected the rave reviews. If you are really showing off, use tiny red-skinned potatoes, pearl onions, and whole baby carrots. To serve, arrange chicken and vegetables—artfully of course—on a heated platter and sprinkle with freshly chopped parsley. Strain the wine sauce into a warmed saucier to pass separately. A simple butter lettuce salad, fresh hot rolls, and steamed asparagus make lovely accompaniments.

INGREDIENTS

1 CHICKEN (3 LB.)
1 TABLESPOON OIL OR CHICKEN FAT
½ LB. FRESH MUSHROOMS
½ LB. SMALL BOILING (PEARL) ONIONS, OR 2 MEDIUM ONIONS
3 SMALL STALKS CELERY, WITH LEAVES
8 TINY NEW POTATOES OR 4 SMALL RED OR WHITE POTATOES
1 LARGE CARROT OR 6 WHOLE BABY CARROTS

12 OZ. DRY WHITE WINE 1½ CUPS (SAUTERNE WORKS WELL)
1 CLOVE GARLIC, MINCED
½ TEASPOON THYME
1 TEASPOON LIGHT SALT (OPTIONAL)
¼ TEASPOON BLACK PEPPER
2 BAY LEAVES
3 LARGE SPRIGS FRESH PARSLEY, WHOLE
2 TABLESPOONS FRESH PARSLEY, CHOPPED FOR GARNISH

DIRECTIONS

Preheat oven to 350°.

Cut up chicken. Remove all skin and visible fat.

Heat oil or chicken fat in a large nonstick skillet. Brown chicken parts well on all sides. Drain off fat, if any appears.

Wash mushrooms, slice thickly.

Peel onions. If using boiling onions, leave whole. If using medium onions, cut each into eighths.

Clean celery, cut each stalk in half.

Scrub potatoes. If new potatoes are used, leave whole. If larger potatoes are used, peel and cut each in half.

Peel carrot and cut into tiny (⅛-inch) cubes or julienne. (Leave baby carrots whole.)

Remove browned chicken pieces to a very large baking dish. Use the crispings in the skillet to make sauce by adding wine, garlic, thyme, light salt, if desired, and pepper to skillet. Simmer for 2 to 3 minutes, stirring with spatula.

Arrange prepared vegetables around chicken pieces in baking dish, then pour sauce over all. Tuck in bay leaves and whole parsley sprigs.

Bake, covered, for 1½ hours. Remove cover during last 20 minutes of baking to brown.

Just before serving, remove parsley sprigs and bay leaves.

Sprinkle with fresh chopped parsley.

VARIATION: Low-sodium version. Omit salt or use a salt substitute (112 mg sodium per serving).

SERVING SIZE: ⅙ Recipe

PER SERVING: Calories 250 **Fiber:** 4 grams **Sodium:** 294 mg.

Herbed Chicken in Wine Sauce (facing page)

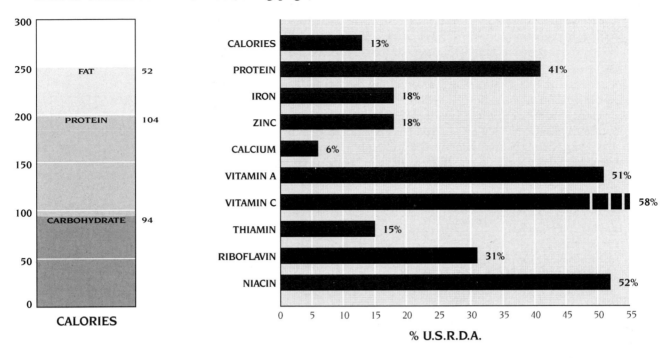

Mum's Chicken Curry (p. 154)

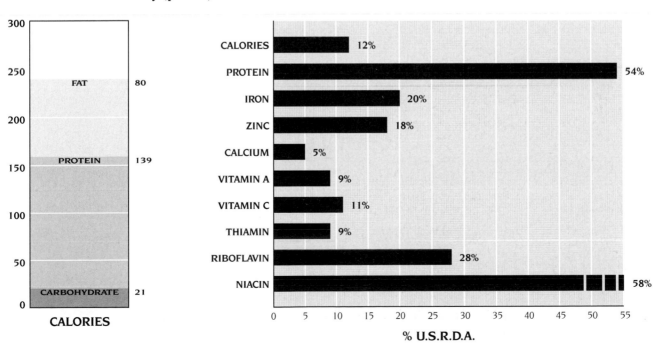

MUM'S CHICKEN CURRY

"Mum" is Analeen Stork. Raised in Ceylon (now Sri Lanka) and presently living in San Francisco, she is perhaps the best curry cook outside India. Her kitchen is jammed with hundreds of jars and bottles—filled with peculiar-looking spices, herbs, and condiments. Nothing is labeled, and there is not a measuring spoon on the premises. Mum cooks with her eyes, her nose, and the 76 years of experience behind her palate. Thanks to four generations of little Storks raised on Mum's spicy concoctions, some of her original recipes have now been committed to ink. This is our all-time favorite.

In India, biting down on a slice of ginger, a stick of cinnamon, or a whole cardamom seed while eating a curry is considered a bonus. If your palate is not accustomed to such intense bursts of flavor, watch for the whole spices and set them aside as you eat. Serve this curry dish with steamed rice, Dall, Singhalese Tomato Salad, and chutney.

INGREDIENTS

1	WHOLE CHICKEN (3 LB.)
1	ONION, MINCED
2-4	CLOVES GARLIC, MINCED
4	SLICES FRESH GINGER ROOT, ⅛-INCH THICK
1	SMALL HOT GREEN CHILI, CUT IN ¼-INCH ROUNDS
1	TABLESPOON OIL
1-2	TABLESPOONS VINEGAR
½	CUP WATER
1	TEASPOON LIGHT SALT
½	CUP COCONUT MILK (OPTIONAL BECAUSE IT IS HIGH IN FAT)
½	CUP NONFAT MILK (OPTIONAL)

Spices

1-2	SOFT-ROLLED CINNAMON STICKS,* 3-INCH, CRUMBLED
2	BAY LEAVES
4	WHOLE CARDAMOM PODS OR ¼ TEASPOON GROUND CARDAMOM
8	WHOLE CLOVES
½	TEASPOON POWDERED TURMERIC
2-3	TABLESPOONS (MADRAS-STYLE IS BEST) CURRY POWDER
½-1	TEASPOON CRUSHED RED CHILES

DIRECTIONS

Skin chicken, removing all visible fat, and cut into serving pieces.

Mince onion and garlic. Slice ginger root and chiles.

Measure all spices into a small bowl.

In a large stew kettle, heat oil until just below smoking. With fan running and a lid handy, add all spices to hot oil, stirring with a long-handled spoon. The spices will fume, sputter, and pop! Sauté for at least 2 minutes to develop full flavor, stirring constantly to prevent scorching.

Now add onion, garlic, ginger root, and chiles. Over low heat, stir-fry 5 minutes longer.

Add vinegar, water, light salt, and chicken. Stir well. Cover tightly, set at lowest possible heat and simmer for 60 to 90 minutes until meat is tender. There should be plenty of sauce in the pot.

Add additional light salt and chiles to taste.

Add coconut milk, if used, or, add nonfat milk if more liquid is desired. Heat through.

VARIATION: Mum's Meat Curry. Substitute 1½ lb. trimmed lean beef, cut in chunks, for the chicken. Simmer until very tender. Add a head of lettuce, shredded, during last 10 minutes of cooking.

SERVING SIZE: ¼ Recipe

PER SERVING: Calories 240   **Fiber:** 1 gram   **Sodium:** 388 mg.

*These cinnamon sticks are made of very thin sheets of cinnamon bark and look like rolled-up paper. They can be found in Mexican or Oriental grocery stores, in the gourmet foods section of larger supermarkets, or in spice shops or sections of many grocery stores.

Graph on p. 153

MEDITERRANEAN CHICKEN

Two confirmed eggplant haters, on two separate occasions, were taken in by the enticing aroma and savory richness of this dish. Both proclaimed it delicious and never guessed that the secret ingredient was eggplant. Serve over pasta with freshly grated parmesan cheese to taste. A green salad is the ideal accompaniment.

INGREDIENTS

1 CHICKEN (ABOUT 3 LB.), CUT UP
1 TEASPOON LIGHT SALT
¼ TEASPOON FRESHLY GROUND BLACK PEPPER
4 TEASPOONS OLIVE OIL, DIVIDED
1 LARGE ONION, CHOPPED
½ CUP CHICKEN BROTH

1 MEDIUM EGGPLANT, CUT IN ¼-INCH CUBES
2 LARGE TOMATOES, PEELED AND CHOPPED, OR 1 CAN (1 LB.)
¼ TEASPOON EACH BASIL, THYME, AND OREGANO
1 CAN (8 OZ.) TOMATO SAUCE

DIRECTIONS

Remove all skin and fat from chicken.

Sprinkle with light salt and pepper.

Heat 2 teaspoons olive oil in a large nonstick skillet. Add chicken, brown well over medium-high heat on all sides and remove from pan.

Heat remaining 2 teaspoons olive oil in the same skillet. Add chopped onion and sauté over medium heat until tender, about 10 to 12 minutes.

Add broth, stirring to scrape up pan crispings. Stir in eggplant, tomatoes, herbs, and tomato sauce.

Return browned chicken to sauce in skillet, spooning some sauce over each piece. Cover pan tightly, reduce heat to lowest possible setting. Cook for 45 minutes to 1 hour, stirring occasionally to prevent scorching.

SERVING SIZE: ⅙ Recipe

PER SERVING: Calories 217 **Fiber:** 4 grams **Sodium:** 556 mg.

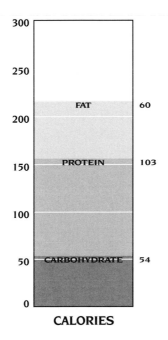

FAT 60
PROTEIN 103
CARBOHYDRATE 54

CALORIES

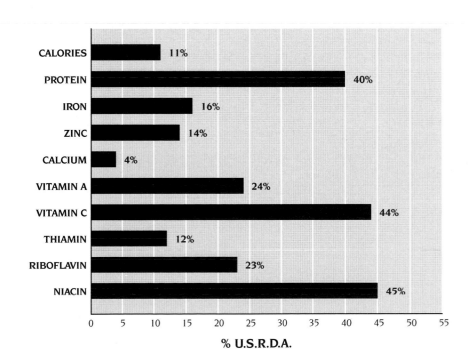

	%
CALORIES	11%
PROTEIN	40%
IRON	16%
ZINC	14%
CALCIUM	4%
VITAMIN A	24%
VITAMIN C	44%
THIAMIN	12%
RIBOFLAVIN	23%
NIACIN	45%

% U.S.R.D.A.

TURKEY, PEAS, AND MUSHROOMS

A main dish that combines the nutty flavor of sherry with sweet green peas and savory mushrooms. Despite the simplicity of this quick-fix skillet combination, there's nothing ho-hum about the finished entree. Serve it with a baked potato and lettuce salad, or over split cornbread squares with sweet potatoes and fruit compote for a heartier rendition.

INGREDIENTS

- 1 LB. GROUND TURKEY
- 12 OZ. FRESH MUSHROOMS, 3 CUPS THICKLY SLICED, OR 1 CAN (16 OZ.) SLICED MUSHROOMS, DRAINED
- 1 BUNCH GREEN ONIONS, 2 CUPS SLICED
- 1 CAN (14½ OZ.) CHICKEN BROTH
- 2 CUPS GREEN PEAS OR 1 BOX (10 OZ.) FROZEN
- ½ TEASPOON WHITE PEPPER

- 1 TEASPOON LIGHT SALT (OPTIONAL)
- 2 TABLESPOONS FLOUR
- ½ CUP COLD WATER
- ½ CUP DRY SHERRY
- 2 TABLESPOONS PLAIN NONFAT YOGURT FOR GARNISH
- ½ CUP FRESH PARSLEY, CHOPPED, FOR GARNISH

DIRECTIONS

Brown turkey oven medium heat in a nonstick skillet for 8 to 10 minutes. Drain fat, if any.

Add sliced mushrooms to meat. Sauté for 5 to 10 minutes until golden.

Add sliced green onions to meat mixture along with broth, peas, pepper, and light salt, if used.

Shake flour in jar with cold water to dissolve. Add flour-water and sherry to mixture. Simmer, stirring until thickened.

Top with yogurt and parsley.

SERVING SIZE: 6 Servings, ¾ Cup Each

PER SERVING: Calories 226 **Fiber:** 5 grams **Sodium:** 392 mg.

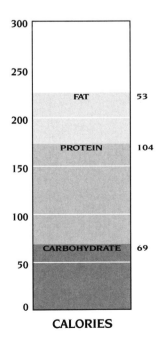

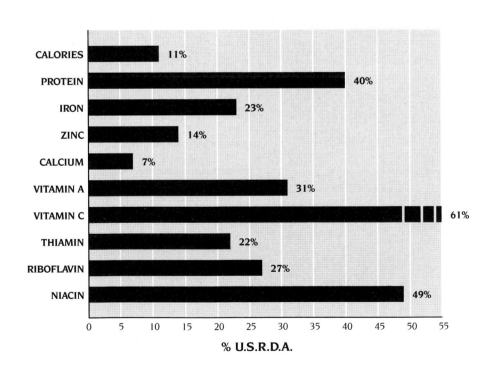

TURKEY LOAF

Low in calories and high in nutrients, this is a great stand-in for the traditional beef version.

INGREDIENTS

2 LB. GROUND TURKEY
2 TABLESPOONS CATSUP
2 TABLESPOONS SALSA OR DASH CAYENNE PEPPER
1 TABLESPOON WORCESTERSHIRE SAUCE
1 MEDIUM ONION, FINELY CHOPPED
1 STALK CELERY, FINELY CHOPPED

1 TEASPOON EACH ROSEMARY, THYME, AND SWEET BASIL
2 TABLESPOONS FRESH PARSLEY, CHOPPED
⅓ CUP OATMEAL, BRAN, OR BREAD CRUMBS
1 TEASPOON LIGHT SALT
¼ TEASPOON BLACK PEPPER

DIRECTIONS

Preheat oven to 325°.
Mix all ingredients thoroughly in a large bowl.
Turn into a loaf pan sprayed with nonstick cooking spray.
Bake uncovered at 325° for 1½ hours.
Drain accumulated liquid, if necessary, just before serving.

SERVING SIZE: 6 Servings, 1 Large Slice Each

PER SERVING: Calories 233   **Fiber:** 2 grams   **Sodium:** 333 mg.

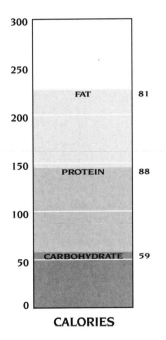

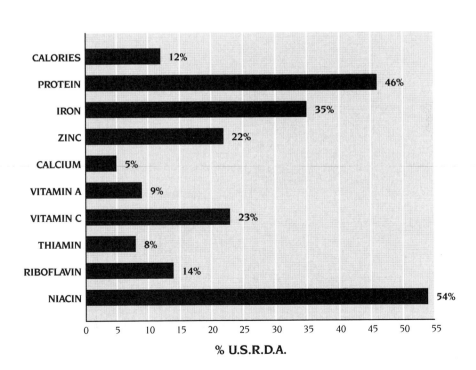

EVE'S TURKEY LOAF

Instead of trying to make ground turkey taste like ground beef, we accentuated its unique flavor with the traditional accoutrements of a holiday dinner. This might best be described as "turkey and dressing loaf." For a fast but festive supper, serve with English Peas, baked sweet potatoes, and Cranberry Orange Relish.

INGREDIENTS

2 LB. GROUND TURKEY
1 LARGE ONION, FINELY CHOPPED
3 LARGE STALKS CELERY, FINELY CHOPPED
1 LARGE GREEN APPLE, FINELY CHOPPED
8 SLICES WHOLE WHEAT BREAD, COARSELY CRUMBLED OR CUBED
2 TEASPOONS POULTRY SEASONING
¼ TEASPOON FRESHLY GROUND BLACK PEPPER

1 TEASPOON LIGHT SALT
½ TEASPOON MARJORAM
1 TEASPOON SAGE
1 TEASPOON THYME
4 TABLESPOONS FRESH PARSLEY, CHOPPED
4 EGGS
½ CUP LOW-CALORIE CRANBERRY JUICE OR OTHER FRUIT JUICE

DIRECTIONS

Preheat oven to 350°.

In a very large bowl mix turkey with all other ingredients until well blended.

Turn into large (3-quart) flat casserole dish, or two loaf pans sprayed with nonstick cooking spray.

Bake for 1½ to 2 hours, depending on size and thickness of loaf. Test for doneness by pricking center of loaf; when juices run clear, rather than pink, turkey is thoroughly cooked.

SERVING SIZE: 1 Slice, 10 Servings

PER SERVING: Calories 228   **Fiber:** 2 grams   **Sodium:** 290 mg.

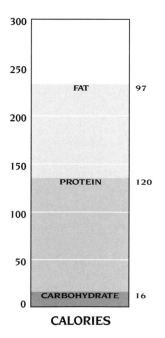

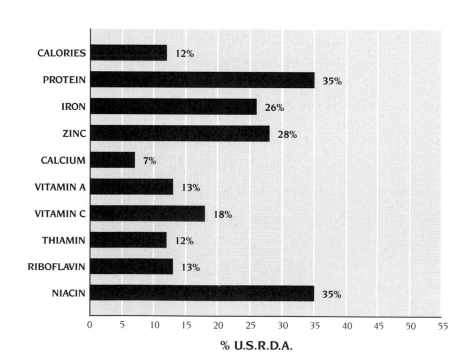

INSTANT TURKEY TOSTADAS

INGREDIENTS

6 WHOLE WHEAT FLOUR TORTILLAS

Filling

1 LB. GROUND TURKEY
2 ONIONS, CHOPPED
1 CAN (10 OZ.) ENCHILADA SAUCE
1 CAN (7 OZ.) DICED GREEN CHILES
2 TEASPOONS CUMIN
1 TABLESPOON FRESH CILANTRO, CHOPPED
  CRUSHED HOT RED CHILI TO TASTE

Toppings

1 SMALL HEAD ICEBERG LETTUCE, SHREDDED
2 TOMATOES, CHOPPED
1 SMALL ONION, CHOPPED
3 OZ. MOZZARELLA OR CHEDDAR CHEESE, GRATED
  DIET ITALIAN DRESSING
  HOT SAUCE OR SALSA
  FRESH LIME JUICE

DIRECTIONS

In a large nonstick skillet, brown ground turkey over medium heat for about 15 minutes.
Add chopped onions and sauté until onions are translucent.
Add enchilada sauce, diced green chiles, cumin, cilantro, and crushed red chili. Stir and
  simmer for a few minutes to blend flavors. (For a very smooth or fine topping, this mixture
  can be whirled briefly in a food processor.)
Warm tortillas in a nonstick skillet or over gas flame.
To assemble tostadas: Top each with one sixth of meat mixture, lettuce, tomatoes, onion, and
  grated cheese. Serve with diet Italian dressing, hot sauce or salsa, and fresh lime juice as
  accompaniments.

SERVING SIZE: 6 Servings, 1 Tostada Each

PER SERVING: Calories 300   **Fiber:** 5 grams   **Sodium:** 457 mg.

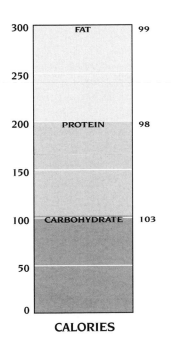

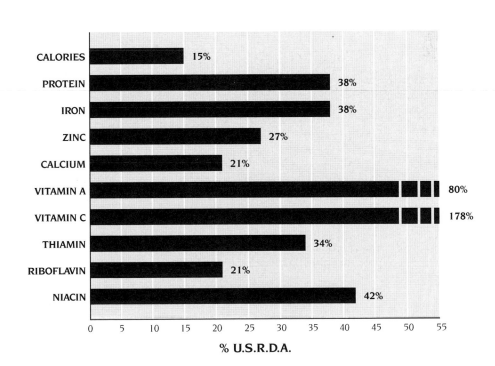

% U.S.R.D.A.

Beef, Pork, Veal & Lamb

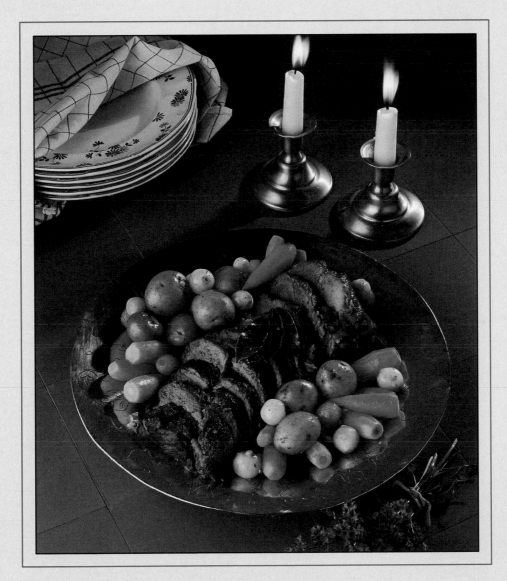

Old-Fashioned Pot Roast (p. 164)

PEPPER STEAK

A cosmopolitan blend of the best in low-fat cooking, combining juicy strips of beef with crisp-tender vegetables, similar to a stir-fry in its simplicity, but as rich and flavorful as a Hungarian pot roast!

INGREDIENTS

2 LB. ROUND STEAK, TRIMMED OF FAT
1 TEASPOON MEAT TENDERIZER
2 TABLESPOONS WATER
1½ LB. FRESH TOMATOES OR 1 CAN (28 OZ.) TOMATOES
1 TABLESPOON OIL
3 CLOVES GARLIC, MINCED

2 TEASPOONS BEEF BOUILLON GRANULES OR 2 CUBES BOUILLON DISSOLVED IN ½ CUP HOT WATER
2 TABLESPOONS WORCESTERSHIRE SAUCE
1 MEDIUM ONION, SLICED
4 LARGE GREEN OR RED BELL PEPPERS, CUT IN ½-INCH STRIPS

DIRECTIONS

Trim all fat from steak, and cut steak across the grain into ⅛-inch strips. Place in a bowl, sprinkle with meat tenderizer and about 2 tablespoons water. Set aside while preparing vegetables.

Peel and wedge fresh tomatoes or drain tomatoes, reserving liquid, and cut into wedges.

In a large nonstick skillet, brown meat strips in 1 tablespoon oil over high heat for about 5 to 6 minutes. Drain off excess fat.

Add garlic; sauté 1 minute. Add dissolved bouillon, Worcestershire sauce, sliced onions, and reserved tomato liquid. Cover and simmer until meat is tender, 30 to 40 minutes.

Six minutes before serving time, add tomato wedges and pepper strips to meat mixture. Cook over medium-high heat until crisp-tender and serve immediately. Best served with steamed rice.

SERVING SIZE: ⅛ Recipe

PER SERVING: Calories 175   **Fiber:** 6 grams   **Sodium:** 369 mg.

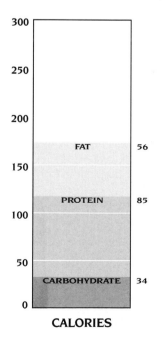

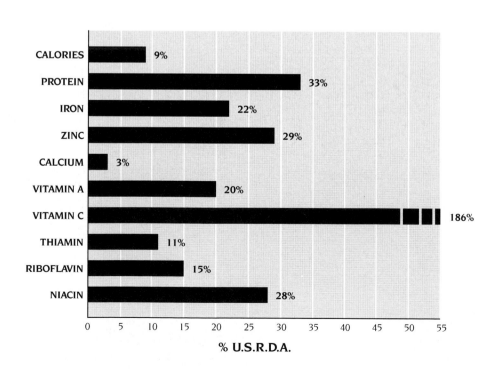

ANNE'S VINEGAR STEAK

Tender braised beef is smothered in sweet onion, with just enough vinegar for flavor balance. This hearty main dish requires minimal preparation but remember to allow 2 to 3 hours for slow simmering. Serve with steamed potatoes and a tossed green salad.

INGREDIENTS

1 LB. BONELESS ROUND STEAK, ½-INCH THICK, TRIMMED OF FAT
¼ CUP WHITE FLOUR
½ TEASPOON LIGHT SALT
¼ TEASPOON BLACK PEPPER
1 TABLESPOON OIL
2 LARGE RED ONIONS, SLICED INTO ½-INCH RINGS
3 TABLESPOONS VINEGAR
1 CUP WATER

DIRECTIONS

Trim all fat from meat and cut meat into four-serving-size pieces.

Combine flour, light salt, and pepper. Dredge meat in flour mixture and lay out on waxed paper.

Heat oil in a large, heavy skillet. (Using a cast iron skillet can increase the iron content of this dish by as much as eight-fold.) Add prepared meat. Brown on both sides over medium-high heat for about 8 to 10 minutes.

Distribute onion slices over top of well-browned meat. Sprinkle with vinegar and water. Cover tightly and simmer over very low heat for an hour.

Turn meat and onions so onions are under meat. Simmer another hour and turn again, redistributing onions on top of meat.

Simmer about 30 minutes longer, until meat is very tender. Remove lid to cook off any remaining liquid. Continue cooking until meat is just beginning to brown again.

Adjust seasonings, adding light salt and vinegar to taste.

SERVING SIZE: ¼ Recipe

PER SERVING: Calories 238 **Fiber:** 2 grams **Sodium:** 218 mg.

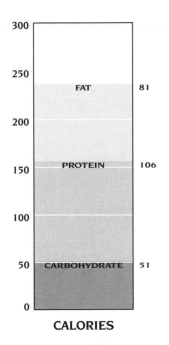

CALORIES

FAT	81
PROTEIN	106
CARBOHYDRATE	51

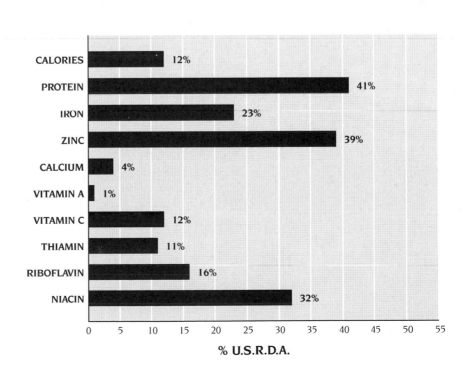

	% U.S.R.D.A.
CALORIES	12%
PROTEIN	41%
IRON	23%
ZINC	39%
CALCIUM	4%
VITAMIN A	1%
VITAMIN C	12%
THIAMIN	11%
RIBOFLAVIN	16%
NIACIN	32%

OLD-FASHIONED POT ROAST

Fork-tender braised beef, just like Mom used to make, with potatoes and vegetables simmered in the meat juices. Our special blend of seasonings gives this pot roast the flavor you remember, while careful trimming of the meat before browning cuts out half the old-fashioned calories.

INGREDIENTS

4 LB. BONELESS RUMP OR CROSS-RIB ROAST	3 BAY LEAVES
1 TABLESPOON RENDERED FAT OR OLIVE OIL	3 STALKS CELERY, SLICED
2 TEASPOONS LIGHT SALT	2 ONIONS, CHOPPED
1 TEASPOON CELERY SEED	2 CUPS WATER
1 TABLESPOON GROUND CORIANDER SEED*	6 LARGE CARROTS, CUT IN 2-INCH LENGTHS
3 CLOVES GARLIC, MINCED	6 MEDIUM POTATOES, QUARTERED
½-1 TEASPOON COARSELY GROUND BLACK PEPPER	

DIRECTIONS

Carefully trim all fat from roast. In a large, heavy cast iron skillet, fry the trimmings for a few minutes to render some fat. Reserve 1 tablespoon fat and discard the rest. (To reduce cholesterol, skip this step and use 1 tablespoon olive oil.)

Sear trimmed roast in the reserved fat, browning it well over medium heat, 5 to 8 minutes per side. Drain off fat.

Sprinkle light salt, celery seed, ground coriander, garlic, and pepper evenly over the meat in the pan. Turn meat so that seasonings are underneath. Brown 1 minute longer.

Remove meat to a very large kettle, dutch oven, or pressure cooker.† Add bay leaves, celery, and onions to original browning skillet. Sauté vegetables for 8 to 10 minutes to develop flavor and rich, brown color.

Add 2 cups water to skillet. Simmer for 2 to 3 minutes, stirring to scrape up browned meat juices from bottom of pan.

Pour contents of skillet over meat in kettle. Cover and simmer for 1½ hours until meat is barely tender.

Add carrots and potatoes. Cover and simmer 40 to 45 minutes longer until vegetables are tender and meat is very tender.

SERVING SIZE: ¹⁄₁₂ Recipe

PER SERVING: Calories 300   **Fiber:** 3 grams   **Sodium:** 326 mg.

*If ground coriander is unavailable, whole coriander seeds can be ground in a food processor, blender, or coffee grinder.
†To save time use a pressure cooker, following manufacturer guidelines for cooking times of meat and vegetables.

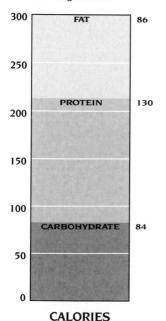

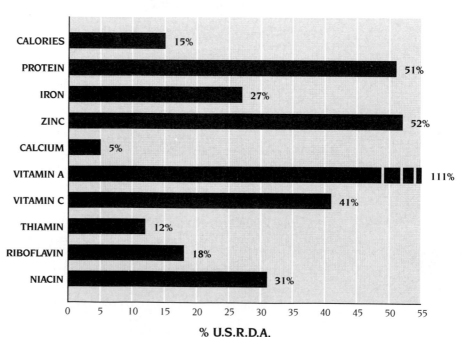

MARY'S RAGOUT

This superb recipe was contributed by Mary Fenton, who lost 13 pounds in 10 weeks, while attending our weight control classes. Mary, who is 77 years old, attached a note to the recipe stating simply that it came "from an old gas cookbook, circa 1940." Later we learned that she had been preparing this recipe for the past 45 years because it's quick and easy and her husband loves it. We tested the recipe and—not surprisingly our husbands (and children) loved it, too. Total preparation time is about 20 minutes, after which this one-dish meal cooks itself without further attention. By the way, if you wonder why a recipe combining two kinds of red meat is included in a low-fat cookbook, take a look at the spectacular nutrient profile.

INGREDIENTS

1 LB. ROUND STEAK, TRIMMED OF FAT
½ LB. CANADIAN BACON, THINLY SLICED
　　FRESHLY GROUND BLACK PEPPER
2 MEDIUM CARROTS, SLICED

3 MEDIUM ONIONS, SLICED
6 MEDIUM POTATOES, SLICED
　　LIGHT SALT (OPTIONAL)
1 CUP WATER

DIRECTIONS

Choose a large saucepan or Dutch oven with a tightly fitting lid or use a very large electric skillet.

Cut the trimmed beef across the grain into little strips 2 inches long and ½-inch wide.

Put sliced Canadian bacon in a layer on the bottom of the pan over medium-low heat. Layer steak strips on top of the bacon. Sprinkle with pepper.

Next, put in carrots and onions. Sprinkle with light salt, if desired, and pepper.

Distribute sliced potatoes evenly on top. Sprinkle with light salt, if desired, and pepper. Add 1 cup water.

Cook, tightly covered, over low heat for about 1 hour or until steak and vegetables are tender and liquid has been absorbed. If too much liquid remains, cook it off by removing lid during last 15 minutes.

SERVING SIZE: ⅙ Recipe

PER SERVING: Calories 296　　**Fiber:** 4 grams　　**Sodium:** 786 mg.

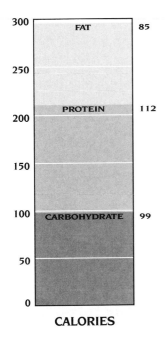

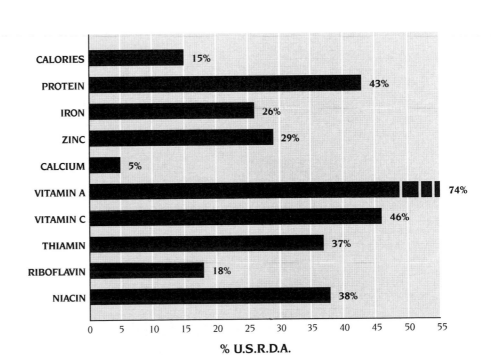

% U.S.R.D.A.

SWISS STEAK

There are many versions of this well-known dish. Some call for carrots and celery, others for bell peppers and pimento. This very basic rendition asks for only onions and tomatoes, yet our families unanimously voted it the best! Rice or noodles and steamed green beans are good complements.

INGREDIENTS

1 LB. ROUND STEAK
3 TABLESPOONS FLOUR
½ TEASPOON LIGHT SEASONED SALT
⅛ TEASPOON BLACK PEPPER
1 TABLESPOON OIL
6 LARGE TOMATOES, PEELED AND COARSELY CHOPPED OR 2 CANS (1 LB. EACH) TOMATOES
2 LARGE ONIONS, THINLY SLICED
WATER, AS NEEDED

DIRECTIONS

Trim meat carefully, removing all possible fat.
Combine flour, light seasoned salt, and pepper. Pound into meat with a meat mallet or rolling pin.
Heat oil in a large nonstick skillet and brown meat quickly on both sides over medium-high heat for about 3 to 4 minutes per side.
Add tomatoes and onions.
Cover and cook over very low heat for 1 to 1½ hours until quite tender. Check two or three times during cooking. Turn meat midway through cooking time, scraping crispings from skillet and adding water, if needed, to prevent scorching.

SERVING SIZE: ¼ Recipe

PER SERVING: Calories 280   **Fiber:** 4 grams   **Sodium:** 124 mg.

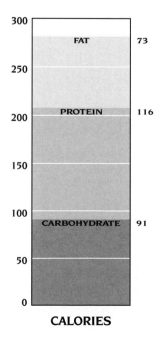

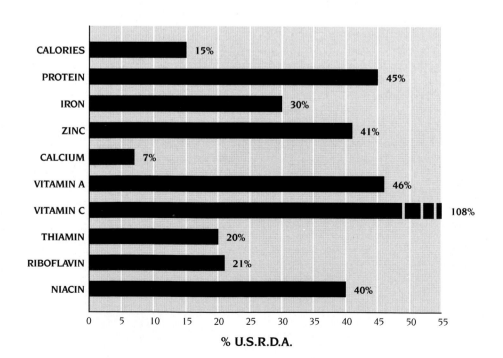

MICROWAVE MEATLOAF

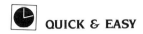 QUICK & EASY

With a food processor and a microwave, this meatloaf can be on the table in 25 minutes (29 if you start with frozen meat). Cook some potatoes in the microwave while you assemble the meatloaf ingredients, make a salad while it bakes, and—presto-whizzo—it's dinner!

INGREDIENTS

1 ONION, MINCED	1 TEASPOON LIGHT SEASONED SALT
1 LARGE CARROT, DICED OR SHREDDED	¼ TEASPOON BLACK PEPPER
1 BELL PEPPER OR 1 STALK CELERY, CHOPPED	1 TEASPOON WORCESTERSHIRE SAUCE
2 TABLESPOONS FRESH PARSLEY, CHOPPED	¼ CUP CATSUP OR BBQ SAUCE
2 EGGS	1 LB. EXTRA LEAN GROUND BEEF
⅔ CUP ROLLED OATS	2 TABLESPOONS CATSUP FOR GLAZE

DIRECTIONS

Prepare vegetables by hand or in a food processor. Do not overprocess.

Add eggs, rolled oats, light salt, pepper, Worcestershire sauce, and catsup. Mix or process just until blended.

Crumble in the raw ground beef and mix with a spoon or process just until mixed. Overprocessing will give you pâté.

Turn into a 9-inch by 5-inch by 3-inch loaf pan. Shape into flat loaf of even thickness (not domed in the center) so it will microcook evenly. Spread 2 tablespoons catsup over top.

Cover with waxed paper and microwave on 70% power (medium-high) for 15 minutes, rotating the dish every 5 minutes. Let stand 7 minutes.

SERVING SIZE: ⅙ Recipe

PER SERVING: Calories 193   **Fiber:** 2 grams   **Sodium:** 241 mg.

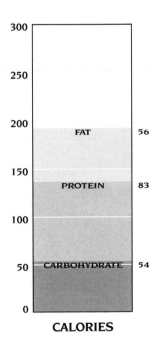

Calories

FAT 56
PROTEIN 83
CARBOHYDRATE 54

CALORIES

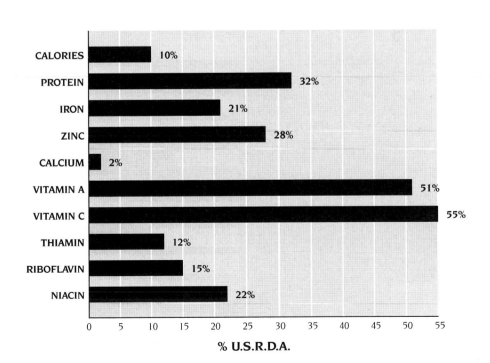

	% U.S.R.D.A.
CALORIES	10%
PROTEIN	32%
IRON	21%
ZINC	28%
CALCIUM	2%
VITAMIN A	51%
VITAMIN C	55%
THIAMIN	12%
RIBOFLAVIN	15%
NIACIN	22%

MARIN JOE'S SPECIAL

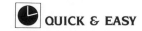 **QUICK & EASY**

Created by the famous Marin Joe during a midnight, "What can I cook?" emergency, this recipe has become an all-time favorite. Use it the next time you need something wonderful for dinner in 20 minutes. Check the nutrient profile of this fast and fabulous dish.

INGREDIENTS

1	LB. GROUND ROUND
3	MEDIUM ONIONS, CHOPPED
¾	LB. MUSHROOMS, 3 CUPS SLICED
1	TEASPOON LIGHT SALT
¼-½	TEASPOON GARLIC POWDER
⅛-¼	TEASPOON BLACK PEPPER
1	BUNCH FRESH SPINACH, CHOPPED OR 16 OZ. FROZEN CUT SPINACH, THAWED AND DRAINED
4	EGGS, LIGHTLY BEATEN

DIRECTIONS

Brown ground round in a large nonstick skillet over medium-high heat for 6 to 8 minutes. Drain off any fat.

Add chopped onions. Sauté over medium heat until onions are translucent and tender, about 10 to 12 minutes.

Add sliced mushrooms and seasonings. Sauté about 5 more minutes until mushrooms are tender and golden brown.

Meanwhile, cook fresh or frozen spinach. Drain off any water.

Add cooked chopped spinach to meat mixture. Mix thoroughly.

Add beaten eggs. Cook, stirring and turning constantly until eggs are set. Serve immediately.

SERVING SIZE: 6 Servings, 1⅓ Cups Each

PER SERVING: Calories 232　　**Fiber:** 3 grams　　**Sodium:** 329 mg.

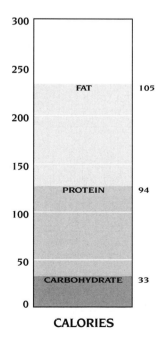

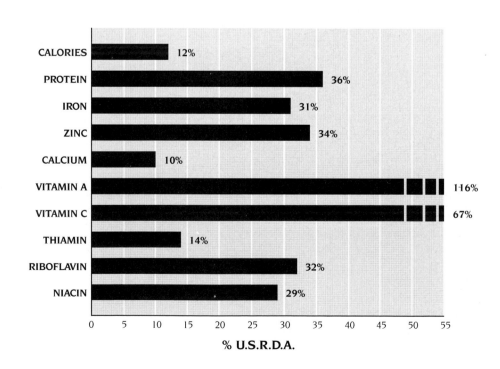

TEXAS HASH

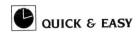 **QUICK & EASY**

This Tex-Mex dish tastes like stuffed peppers—except the peppers are chopped up and mixed with the rice, which makes things a good deal simpler.

INGREDIENTS

1 CUP UNCOOKED BROWN RICE
2½ CUPS WATER
½ TEASPOON LIGHT SALT
1 LB. GROUND ROUND
2 LARGE ONIONS, CHOPPED
2 LARGE BELL PEPPERS, CHOPPED
½-1 SMALL HOT GREEN CHILI, MINCED

1 CAN (8 OZ.) TOMATO SAUCE
2 LARGE TOMATOES, CHOPPED, OR 1 CAN (1 LB.), COARSELY CHOPPED
1 CUP FRESH CILANTRO LEAVES, CHOPPED
1-2 TABLESPOONS CHILI POWDER (OPTIONAL)
LIGHT SALT AND BLACK PEPPER TO TASTE

DIRECTIONS

Cook rice in 2½ cups water with ½ teaspoon light salt until tender, 45 to 60 minutes.

Brown meat in a large nonstick skillet over medium-high heat for 6 to 8 minutes, carefully draining fat.

Add onions, bell peppers, and green chili. Sauté 20 to 25 minutes until vegetables are tender.

Add tomato sauce and chopped tomatoes. Simmer, uncovered, for 10 minutes.

Add cooked rice and fresh cilantro. Taste and season with chili powder, light salt and black pepper as desired. Simmer, uncovered for 5 to 10 minutes to blend flavors and cook off any excess liquid.

SERVING SIZE: 8 Servings, 1 Cup Each

PER SERVING: Calories 210   **Fiber:** 5 grams   **Sodium:** 282 mg.

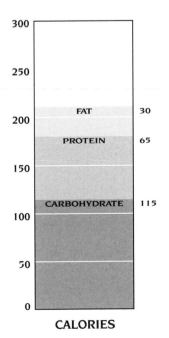

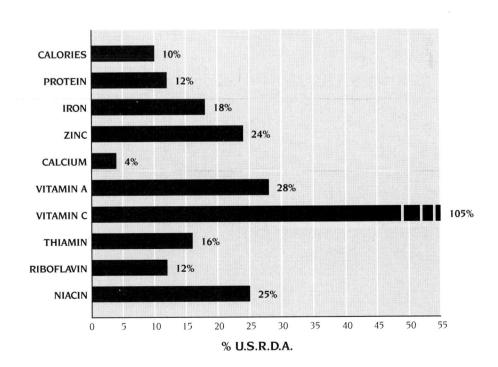

TACOS

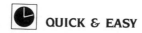 **QUICK & EASY**

People who believe tacos are born in deep vats of grease and come out into the world through drive-up windows naturally think of them as junk food. In fact, when properly prepared, tacos are the epitome of good nutrition! In addition to containing items from all four food groups, these tasty bundles of balanced nutrition are considered edible by children and teenagers.

INGREDIENTS

1 LB. GROUND ROUND
2 MEDIUM ONIONS, CHOPPED
1 CAN (7 OZ.) GREEN CHILES, DICED
1 TEASPOON CUMIN
½ TEASPOON LIGHT SALT
1 LB. CANNED TOMATOES
¼ TEASPOON GARLIC POWDER
2 TEASPOONS CHILI POWDER OR TO TASTE
1 TABLESPOON LEMON OR LIME JUICE

12 CORN TORTILLAS

Toppings

4 OZ. SHARP CHEDDAR CHEESE, 1⅓ CUPS GRATED
2 LARGE TOMATOES, DICED
1 ONION, MINCED
½ LARGE HEAD ICEBERG LETTUCE, SHREDDED
SALSA

DIRECTIONS

Brown ground round in a large nonstick skillet, over medium-high heat for 6 to 8 minutes. Drain fat.

Add onions, chiles, cumin, light salt, canned tomatoes, garlic powder, and chili powder to meat. Simmer for 10 to 15 minutes to blend flavors and cook off fluid. Break up the tomatoes as they simmer.

Add lemon or lime juice and adjust seasoning.

Prepare cheese, tomatoes, onion, and lettuce for final assembly.

Heat tortillas in an ungreased skillet for about 10 seconds on each side until warm and soft.

To assemble: Use ½ cup meat filling for each tortilla. Top with cheese, fresh tomatoes, onion, lettuce, and salsa. Fold tortillas around stuffing.

VARIATIONS: Crispy Tacos. Heat tortillas (flat) on two cookie sheets in 400° oven for 4 to 5 minutes until crisp. Cook meat mixture until quite dry, spread evenly over crisp tortillas. Sprinkle with cheese. Place under broiler until cheese melts. Serve with toppings, as above. For a finely textured taco meat, brown beef, drain, then chop briefly in food processor.

SERVING SIZE: 1 Taco

PER SERVING: Calories 181 **Fiber:** 4 grams **Sodium:** 219 mg.

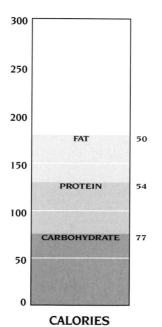

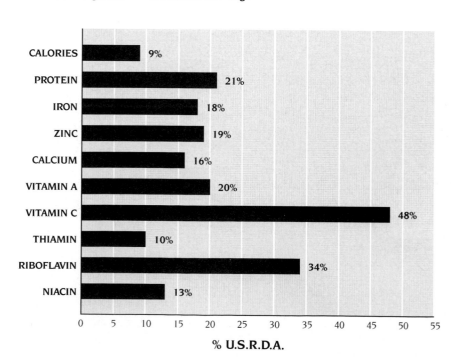

PICADILLO

Picadillo—in one form or another—is popular throughout Latin America. Each region has its own version of this sweet, spicy mixture of meats and fruits. Serve it with rice and beans or simply roll it up in warm tortillas.

INGREDIENTS

1 TABLESPOON OLIVE OIL
2 LB. LEAN STEW MEAT (SIRLOIN TIP OR THICK-CUT ROUND)
2 LARGE ONIONS, CHOPPED
2 CLOVES GARLIC, MINCED
2 CUPS HOT WATER
1 CINNAMON STICK
2 TEASPOONS LIGHT SALT
6 MEDIUM TOMATOES, PEELED AND CHOPPED, OR 2 CANS (1 LB. EACH), COARSELY CHOPPED

1 CAN (8 OZ.) GREEN CHILES, DICED
¼ CUP VINEGAR
2 TEASPOONS SUGAR
½ TEASPOON GROUND CINNAMON
2 DASHES GROUND CLOVES
2 TEASPOONS CUMIN
¾ CUP RAISINS
2 APPLES, DICED

DIRECTIONS

Trim all fat from meat and cut meat into large chunks.

Heat oil in a large cast iron skillet. Brown the beef chunks over medium heat for 10 to 12 minutes. Add onions and garlic. Sauté until golden, stirring often.

Add water, cinnamon stick, and light salt. Bring to a boil, reduce heat, cover, and simmer for 1½ to 2 hours until meat is tender enough to shred.

Remove cover and boil off liquid. Then, using two forks, shred meat into bite-sized pieces.

Add tomatoes, chiles, vinegar, sugar, ground cinnamon, cloves, and cumin. Cook, uncovered, over medium heat for 20 to 25 minutes to develop flavor and reduce liquid.

Add raisins and apples. Simmer for 15 minutes. Fruit should blend into the picadillo but not disintegrate.

VARIATION: Add up to 6 cups of banana, pear, or pineapple chunks.

SERVING SIZE: 8 Servings, 1 Cup Each

PER SERVING: Calories 282　　**Fiber:** 4 grams　　**Sodium:** 364 mg.

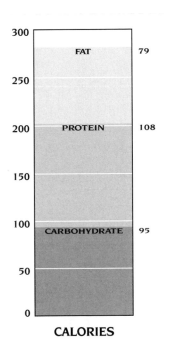

FAT	79
PROTEIN	108
CARBOHYDRATE	95

CALORIES

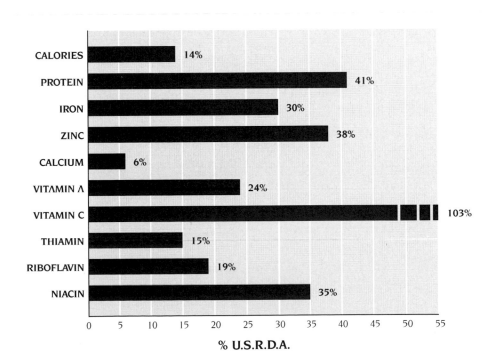

CALORIES 14%
PROTEIN 41%
IRON 30%
ZINC 38%
CALCIUM 6%
VITAMIN A 24%
VITAMIN C 103%
THIAMIN 15%
RIBOFLAVIN 19%
NIACIN 35%

% U.S.R.D.A.

SUKIYAKI

A careful blending of subtle flavors—the epitome of Japanese culinary art.

INGREDIENTS

2 LB. LEAN FLANK OR ROUND STEAK
½ CUP SOY SAUCE
1 BEEF BOUILLON CUBE DISSOLVED IN ½ CUP WATER
¼ CUP DRY SHERRY OR SAKE (RICE WINE)
2 TABLESPOONS SUGAR
¼ TEASPOON BLACK PEPPER

1 TABLESPOON OIL
2 LARGE STALKS CELERY, SLICED DIAGONALLY ⅛-INCH THICK
1 BUNCH GREEN ONIONS, CUT IN 1-INCH LENGTHS
½ LB. FRESH MUSHROOMS, 2 CUPS SLICED ⅛-INCH THICK
1 CAN (8 OZ.) BAMBOO SHOOTS, DRAINED

DIRECTIONS

Trim all fat from meat and cut across the grain in slices ⅛-inch thick.

Mix soy sauce, dissolved bouillon, sherry, sugar, and pepper in a medium bowl. Stir in sliced meat and marinate while preparing vegetables.

Heat oil in a wok or large nonstick skillet until it smokes. Drain marinade off meat and reserve it. Add well-drained meat to wok and stir-fry over high heat until meat is browned and moisture

has cooked off, about 10 minutes. Remove meat to a platter.

Put ½ cup of the reserved marinade in wok. Add celery, onions, mushrooms, and bamboo shoots. Stir-fry until celery is crisp-tender, 3 to 5 minutes.

Add meat and any remaining marinade to wok. Heat through and serve with pan juices over rice or noodles.

SERVING SIZE: 10 Servings, 1 Cup Each

PER SERVING: Calories 171   **Fiber:** 2 grams   **Sodium:** 859 mg.

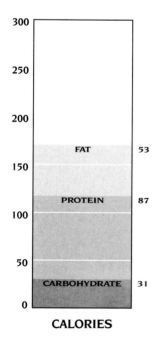

CALORIES

FAT 53
PROTEIN 87
CARBOHYDRATE 31

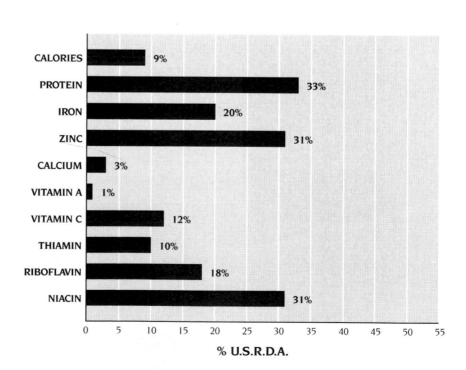

% U.S.R.D.A.

CALORIES 9%
PROTEIN 33%
IRON 20%
ZINC 31%
CALCIUM 3%
VITAMIN A 1%
VITAMIN C 12%
THIAMIN 10%
RIBOFLAVIN 18%
NIACIN 31%

BEEF WITH BROCCOLI

A favorite stir-fry combination from the subtly seasoned Cantonese cuisine. Meat and vegetables in one, this dish is simple to prepare and requires nothing more than steamed rice as an accompaniment.

INGREDIENTS

1 LB. LEAN FLANK STEAK OR TOP ROUND, TRIMMED
1 LARGE BUNCH (ABOUT 2 LB.) BROCCOLI
2 CLOVES GARLIC, MINCED
2 TEASPOONS PEANUT OIL
2 TABLESPOONS WATER

Marinade

2 TEASPOONS SAKE (RICE WINE) OR SHERRY
½ TEASPOON BAKING SODA
2 TABLESPOONS SOY SAUCE
1½ TEASPOONS CORNSTARCH
2 TEASPOONS SESAME OIL
½ TEASPOON SUGAR

Sauce

2 TEASPOONS CORNSTARCH
1 CUP CHICKEN BROTH
1 TEASPOON SOY SAUCE
¼-½ TEASPOON WHITE OR BLACK PEPPER

DIRECTIONS

Trim beef of all fat, then slice across the grain into ⅛-inch strips.

Combine marinade ingredients in medium bowl. Add beef strips and mix well. Let stand 20 to 30 minutes to tenderize.

Trim tough stems and leaves from broccoli. Break tops into bite-sized florets and cut stems into ½-inch slices.

Combine sauce ingredients in small bowl and set aside.

Heat a large nonstick skillet or wok until very hot. Add beef strips with marinade. Stir-fry over high-est possible heat until lightly browned. Remove beef from skillet and set aside.

Heat the 2 teaspoons peanut oil in the same skillet. Add minced garlic and prepared broccoli. Stir-fry over high heat for 3 to 5 minutes until broccoli is crisp-tender. Add 2 tablespoons water, cover tightly, and steam over medium heat for 3 minutes.

Remove lid. Add sauce ingredients. Stir until sauce bubbles. Add beef, heat through and serve immediately.

VARIATION: Low-Sodium Beef with Broccoli. Use low-sodium soy sauce and chicken broth.

SERVING SIZE: ¼ Recipe

PER SERVING: Calories 273 **Fiber:** 3 grams **Sodium:** 887 mg.

Graph on p. 174

Beef with Broccoli (p. 173)

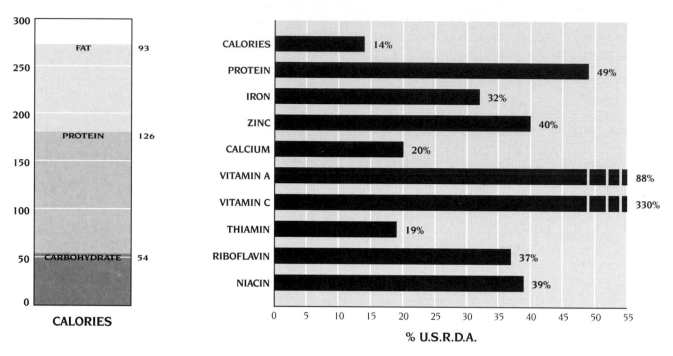

FAT	93
PROTEIN	126
CARBOHYDRATE	54

CALORIES

	% U.S.R.D.A.
CALORIES	14%
PROTEIN	49%
IRON	32%
ZINC	40%
CALCIUM	20%
VITAMIN A	88%
VITAMIN C	330%
THIAMIN	19%
RIBOFLAVIN	37%
NIACIN	39%

Veal Scaloppine (facing page)

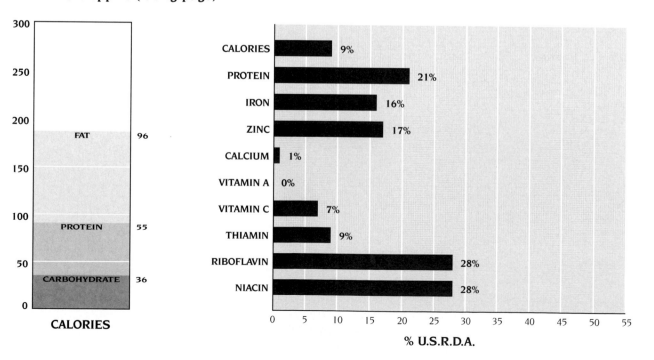

FAT	96
PROTEIN	55
CARBOHYDRATE	36

CALORIES

	% U.S.R.D.A.
CALORIES	9%
PROTEIN	21%
IRON	16%
ZINC	17%
CALCIUM	1%
VITAMIN A	0%
VITAMIN C	7%
THIAMIN	9%
RIBOFLAVIN	28%
NIACIN	28%

VEAL SCALOPPINE

Veal, the tender meat of young calf, is very soft, fine-grained meat with practically no fat in the tissue. Scaloppine, escalope, collop, and cutlet are various names for boneless pieces of veal cut from either the rib-eye muscle or the loin. Veal round steaks, cut ¼-inch thick, work equally well in a cutlet recipe. Many veal recipes are European in origin, and most call for a lot of added fat to compensate for the fact that veal is not "marbelized." Instead of finding ways to undo veal's natural leanness, why not capitalize on it?

Our scaloppine is pounded, dredged with flour and sautéed in olive oil to achieve the flavor and texture unique to this classic Italian dish. But our technique eliminates 90% of the fat called for in the original recipe. Since this recipe yields an abundant portion of rich mushroom sauce, the perfect accompaniments are plain, boiled pasta or steamed potatoes and a simple vegetable or salad.

INGREDIENTS

- 8 OZ. FRESH MUSHROOMS, 2 CUPS SLICED
- ⅛ TEASPOON BLACK PEPPER
- ½ CUP DRY WHITE WINE
- 4 VEAL CUTLETS (½ LB.) ¼-INCH THICK
- ½ TEASPOON LIGHT SALT (OPTIONAL)

- 2 TABLESPOONS FLOUR
- 1 TABLESPOON OLIVE OIL
- ¾ CUP WHITE ONION, VERY FINELY CHOPPED
- 1 CUP CHICKEN BROTH

DIRECTIONS

Place mushrooms, pepper, and wine in a small saucepan. Simmer uncovered for about 10 minutes until mushrooms are tender.

Pound the veal with flat side of meat mallet or with a rolling pin to half the original thickness. Sprinkle with light salt, if desired, then dredge with flour.

Heat olive oil in a large nonstick skillet over high heat. Add onion and shake pan to distribute onion evenly.

Arrange breaded cutlets on bed of onion in skillet and cook for 1 or 2 minutes over high heat until meat begins to brown. Turn and cook 1 or 2 minutes to brown other side.

Reduce heat to low, add broth, and simmer for 2 minutes.

Turn veal and add the mushroom mixture. Increase the heat and cook for 3 to 5 minutes until fluid is reduced, and sauce is slightly thickened.

VARIATION: Turkey Scaloppine. Substitute turkey cutlets (sliced raw breast meat) for veal.

SERVING SIZE: 1 Cutlet

PER SERVING: Calories 187   **Fiber:** 2 grams   **Sodium:** 273 mg.

BARBEQUED PINEAPPLE PORK AND ONIONS

Enjoy a simple, but spectacular summer barbeque. Keep in mind that meat should be marinated a day ahead for best flavor.

INGREDIENTS

6 LEAN CENTER-CUT PORK LOIN CHOPS (2 LB.)
1 FRESH PINEAPPLE, SLICED, OR 1 CAN (1 LB.) SLICED PINEAPPLE, DRAINED
2 LARGE, SWEET ONIONS (WALLA WALLA, MAUI, OR OTHER MILD VARIETY), SLICED INTO ½-INCH RINGS

Marinade

1 CUP ORANGE JUICE
¼ CUP WHITE VINEGAR
1 TABLESPOON HONEY
3 TABLESPOONS SOY SAUCE
¼ TEASPOON BLACK PEPPER

DIRECTIONS

Trim chops of all fat. Do not remove bone.

Mix marinade ingredients in a dish large enough to hold the meat.

Add trimmed pork chops and refrigerate, covered, overnight.

To barbeque allow about 30 minutes cooking time.* If possible, use a covered barbeque unit. Heat coals or adjust flame to result in a low, steady fire. Set grill 4 to 6 inches from flame, since pork chops should cook through and brown evenly rather than sear.

Grill marinated pork chops, basting occasionally to brown one side thoroughly—about 10 minutes. Turn them over, and place one slice pineapple on each chop, slightly off-center. Move the chops to one side of the grill, to make space for grilling onions, and continue cooking chops for 10 to 20 minutes to brown other side and cook through.

Meanwhile, brush the open grill with oil. Lay onion slices on oiled grill and brush with marinade. Barbeque onion rings 3 to 5 minutes per side, until they have nice brown stripes and are limp but not mushy. Place one cooked onion ring on top of each pork chop, overlapping pineapple slice.

Serve meat topped with pineapple and grilled onion slices.

SERVING SIZE: 6 Servings, 1 Chop Each

PER SERVING: Calories 268   **Fiber:** 2 grams   **Sodium:** 476 mg.

*Quick tip: Since pork should be cooked through to well-done stage, you can save time and worry by precooking marinated meat in microwave or standard oven, then finishing on the barbeque pit.

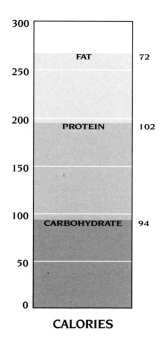

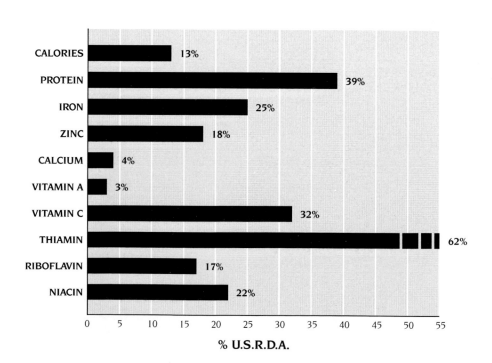

CHILE VERDE

The complete name for this dish is "adobo verde de lomo cerdo" which means, "pork loin smothered with a very thick sauce made of green chiles." Whatever you call it, if you try it once, you will cook it again and share it with friends. The green chili salsa transforms plain pork loin into a dish worthy of any gourmet's table. Garnish with white onion slices, radishes, and small inner leaves of romaine lettuce. Serve with refried beans and warmed flour tortillas.

INGREDIENTS

2 LB. TRIMMED LOIN OF PORK*
1 ONION, CHOPPED
2 TEASPOONS LIGHT SALT
2 CUPS WATER
   BLACK PEPPER TO TASTE
2 TABLESPOONS FRESH ORANGE JUICE

Sauce

6-7 FRESH TOMATILLOS (MEXICAN GREEN TOMATOES) (½ LB.) OR 1 CAN (6½ OZ.) "TOMATILLOS ENTEROS"
1 ONION, CUT IN CHUNKS
2 CLOVES GARLIC
3 LARGE OR 6 SMALL GREEN ONIONS, CUT IN 3-INCH SLICES
2 CANS (7 OZ.) DICED GREEN CHILES
¼ CUP FRESH CILANTRO (6 SPRIGS WITH STEMS REMOVED), OR 1 TABLESPOON DRIED CORIANDER LEAF
¼-½ TEASPOON CRUSHED RED CHILI TO TASTE
6 LARGE OUTSIDE LEAVES OF ROMAINE LETTUCE

DIRECTIONS

Cut trimmed pork loin into 1-inch cubes.

Put the pork, chopped onion, and 1 teaspoon light salt in large, heavy kettle or cast iron skillet. Add water to barely cover the meat, about 2 cups. Bring to a boil, reduce heat, cover, and simmer for 45 to 60 minutes until barely tender.

While meat is cooking, remove brown husks from fresh tomatillos and then wash them. (They should be firm, with color ranging from bright green to a softer yellow-green.) If using canned tomatillos, measure half a can, or ¾ cup, tomatillos with their liquid.

In blender or food processor puree onions, garlic, green onions, tomatillos with their liquid, green chiles, and cilantro leaves. Add desired amount red chili.

Wash romaine leaves; shake dry. With blender or food processor running, add romaine leaves one at a time until all are pureed. You will have about 6 cups of bright green sauce.

After 45 minutes, check pork. If fork tender, remove lid, turn up flame, and cook off any remaining liquid. If not, continue cooking until tender.

Pour sauce over meat cubes and cook, uncovered, over lowest possible flame for 15 minutes to develop flavor and reduce liquid.

Season to taste with additional hot chili, light salt, and black pepper.

Continue cooking over very low flame, stirring often to prevent scorching, 10 to 15 minutes longer until sauce is very thick.

Just before serving add orange juice and stir to combine.

SERVING SIZE: ⅛ Recipe

PER SERVING: Calories 253   **Fiber:** 2 grams   **Sodium:** 374 mg.

*Buy a 4-lb. pork loin roast to yield 2 pounds lean meat after trimming off bones and fat.

Graph on p. 178

Chile Verde (p. 177)

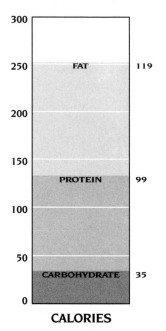

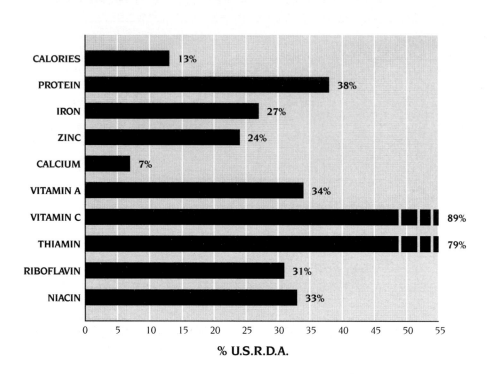

Imperial Pork with Green Beans (facing page)

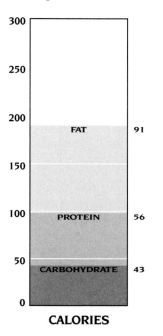

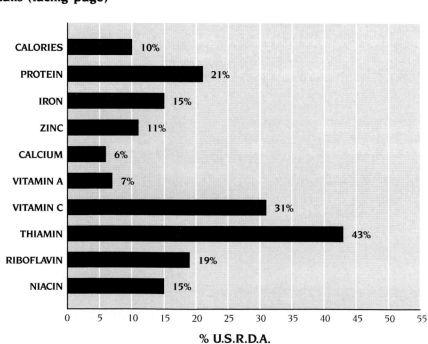

IMPERIAL PORK WITH GREEN BEANS QUICK & EASY

INGREDIENTS

- 2 LARGE PORK LOIN CHOPS OR
  8 OZ. TRIMMED PORK LOIN
- 2 LARGE OR 4 SMALL DRIED CHINESE MUSHROOMS
- ½ CUP HOT WATER
- 2 CUPS FRESH GREEN BEANS
- 1 STALK CELERY
- 4 GREEN ONIONS
- 1 CAN (8 OZ.) BAMBOO SHOOTS, DRAINED
- 1 TABLESPOON OIL

- 2 CLOVES GARLIC, MINCED
- 1 TEASPOON FRESH GINGER ROOT, MINCED, OR
  ¼ TEASPOON POWDERED GINGER
- 2 TEASPOONS SOY SAUCE
- 1 TEASPOON RICE WINE (SAKE)
- ¼ TEASPOON SUGAR
- 1¼ CUPS DOUBLE-STRENGTH CHICKEN BROTH
- 2 TEASPOONS CORNSTARCH
- 1 TABLESPOON COLD WATER
- 1 TABLESPOON SHERRY

DIRECTIONS

Trim pork of all fat. Cut lean meat across the grain into ⅛-inch strips.

Pour ½ cup boiling water over dried mushrooms in small bowl. Soak for 10 to 15 minutes to soften. Remove tough stems, then slice tender caps into thin strips.

Slice green beans lengthwise as thinly as possible.

Slice celery and green onions thinly, on the diagonal.

Cut bamboo shoots lengthwise into thin matchsticks.

Heat oil in wok or large, heavy skillet.

Add garlic and ginger. Stir-fry for 30 seconds until lightly browned.

Add pork strips and stir-fry over high heat until meat whitens and cooks through, 3 to 5 minutes.

Add mushrooms, green beans, soy sauce, rice wine, and sugar. Stir-fry for 5 minutes.

Add celery, green onions, bamboo shoots, and chicken broth. Bring to a boil, then reduce heat, cover, and cook for 5 minutes.

Stir together cornstarch, water, and sherry. Add to pan and stir until thickened.

SERVING SUGGESTION: Serve with steamed rice and additional soy sauce for those who desire it. For a larger meal, precede with Egg Flower Soup or Hot and Sour Soup, and finish with melon or tropical fruit.

VARIATION: Low-sodium version. Without soy sauce and chicken broth, the sodium content of this dish is 46 mg per serving. Using low-sodium substitutes for these two ingredients will significantly reduce total sodium content.

SERVING SIZE: ¼ Recipe

PER SERVING: Calories 190   **Fiber:** 4 grams   **Sodium:** 765 mg.

Graph on facing page

SWEET AND SOUR PORK

Despite the lengthy ingredient list, this delicious stir-fry assembles quickly and easily. Flavor is best if meat is marinated overnight.

INGREDIENTS

1½ LB. LEAN PORK, TRIMMED OF FAT
2 MEDIUM ONIONS, CHOPPED IN 1-INCH CHUNKS
2 THIN CARROTS, CUT DIAGONALLY IN ¼-INCH SLICES
2 STALKS CELERY, CUT DIAGONALLY IN ⅛-INCH SLICES
1 BEEF BOUILLON CUBE
½ CUP BOILING WATER
3 TEASPOONS OIL
1 CAN (20 OZ.) JUICE-PACKED PINEAPPLE CHUNKS, DRAINED, RESERVE JUICE
1 BELL PEPPER, SEEDED AND CUT IN 1-INCH PIECES
1 CAN (4 OZ.) MUSHROOMS, DRAINED (OPTIONAL)
1 CAN (8 OZ.) BAMBOO SHOOTS, DRAINED (OPTIONAL)

Marinade

3 TABLESPOONS SOY SAUCE
3 TABLESPOONS DRY WHITE WINE
2 CLOVES GARLIC, MINCED
1 INCH PIECE FRESH GINGER, PEELED AND MINCED

Sauce

⅓ CUP BROWN SUGAR
4 TEASPOONS CORNSTARCH
⅓ CUP CIDER VINEGAR
1 CUP RESERVED PINEAPPLE JUICE
1 TABLESPOON SOY SAUCE

DIRECTIONS

Mix marinade ingredients in a medium bowl.

Trim fat from pork and cut meat into small shreds.

Stir meat into marinade. Cover and refrigerate at least 30 minutes or overnight, if possible.

Before beginning to cook:

Combine all sauce ingredients in a small bowl. Set aside.

Cut up onions, carrots, celery, and bell pepper.

Dissolve bouillon in boiling water for broth. Set aside.

Heat 2 teaspoons of the oil in a wok or a large, heavy skillet. When oil is smoking hot, add meat and marinade and stir-fry for 5 to 7 minutes or until all moisture is gone and meat begins to brown. Remove meat from pan.

Put remaining 1 teaspoon oil in pan. When it is smoking hot, add onions, carrots, and celery. Stir quickly to coat vegetables with oil. Then add the broth. Stir-fry for 5 minutes until vegetables are crisp-tender.

Return meat to pan. Add pineapple and bell pepper, plus mushrooms and bamboo shoots, if used. Stir-fry 2 more minutes.

Add sauce, heat through, and serve.

SERVING SIZE: 8 Servings, 1 Heaping cup each

PER SERVING: Calories 298   **Fiber:** 2 grams   **Sodium:** 632 mg.

Graph on facing page

Sweet and Sour Pork (facing page)

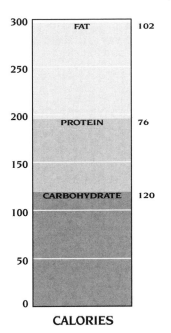

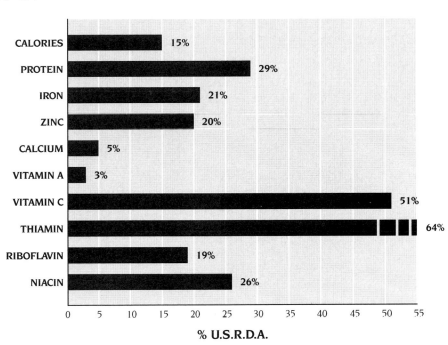

Stuffed Cabbage Rolls (Golobki) (p. 182)

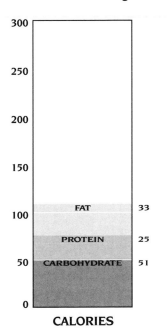

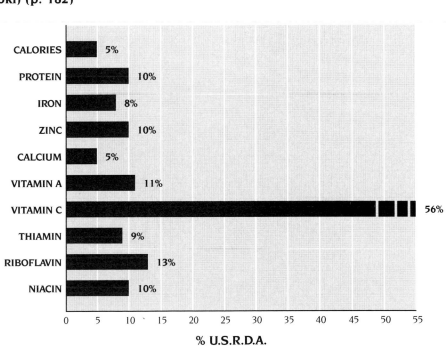

STUFFED CABBAGE ROLLS (GOLOBKI)

Polish people take leaves from the most pedestrian of vegetables—simple green cabbage—roll them up with a savory beef and rice stuffing, then call the dish golobki, which means "little doves." Why? Because the neat little packages, glazed with a sweet and tangy sauce, vaguely resemble another highly regarded delicacy—stuffed breast of dove.

If you think making golobki is a bit of a procedure, you're right. Allow 3 hours total cooking time, an hour of which will be spent in actual food preparation. If you wonder whether cabbage rolls can be worth the trouble, rest assured that they are. Besides, unless you are feeding eight hungry people, you should have enough left over to freeze for another dinner. Serve with boiled potatoes and pickled beets.

INGREDIENTS

- 1 LARGE HEAD CABBAGE*
- 2 STRIPS RAW BACON, DICED (2 OZ.)
- 2 SMALL OR 1 LARGE ONION, MINCED
- 2 SMALL OR 1 LARGE STALK CELERY, DICED
- 2 SLICES WHOLE WHEAT BREAD
- ½ CUP CHICKEN BROTH OR BOUILLON
- 2 TABLESPOONS DRIED ITALIAN OR JAPANESE DRIED MUSHROOMS, OR 1 CAN (8 OZ.) REGULAR MUSHROOMS, OR 4 OZ. FRESH MUSHROOMS
- ½ CUP HOT WATER (IF USING DRIED MUSHROOMS)
- ½ LB. LEAN GROUND ROUND
- 1 EGG

- 1 CUP COOKED BROWN RICE
- 1 TEASPOON LIGHT SALT
- ½ TEASPOON BLACK PEPPER
- ¼ TEASPOON ALLSPICE
- ½ TEASPOON SAGE

Sauce

- 2 CANS (8 OZ. EACH) TOMATO SAUCE
- 2 TABLESPOONS WHITE FLOUR
- 2 TABLESPOONS BROWN SUGAR
- 3 TABLESPOONS VINEGAR

DIRECTIONS

Cook rice if necessary.

In your largest pot, bring to a boil enough salted water to completely submerge the large head of cabbage. (The looser the head, the easier the job of separating each leaf.) Put cabbage in boiling water, cover, turn off heat, and leave for 30 minutes.

Sauté bacon, onions, and celery in a large, heavy skillet.

In a small bowl soak bread in bouillon until soft and mushy. If using dried mushrooms, soak in ½ cup hot water. When softened, chop finely.

In a large bowl mix ground round, egg, cooked brown rice, soaked bread with bouillon, diced mushrooms, and all seasonings. Add sautéed bacon and vegetable mixture. Mix well.

Remove cabbage from water and drain. Remove one leaf at a time from the head, trying not to tear it. With a sharp knife, cut off back of main stem, so leaf will roll.

Put about ⅓ cup of filling on each leaf, spread a bit so it covers bottom half of leaf.

Start rolling at base (stem end) of leaf. Roll halfway, fold in sides of leaf, finish rolling.

Place cabbage rolls in tightly packed layers in a large, heavy kettle or Dutch oven.

Combine sauce ingredients and pour over cabbage rolls.

Cover kettle and simmer on low 2 hours, adding water if necessary to prevent scorching, or cover Dutch oven and bake 2 hours at 350°.

To freeze: Arrange golobki in a single layer on a sheet of heavy foil. Drizzle with sauce, wrap tightly and freeze. To reheat, place foil package in 350° oven or unwrap and heat in a saucepan over low heat, adding water as needed. For microwave reheating, freeze in plastic bags.

SERVING SIZE: 15 Servings, 1 Roll Each

PER SERVING: Calories 109 **Fiber:** 2 grams **Sodium:** 279 mg.

*Choose a head of cabbage with loose, rather than tightly wrapped, leaves, or leaves will be difficult to separate.

Graph on p. 181

LAMB SHISH KEBAB

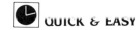 QUICK & EASY

A deliciously different entree for the barbeque or broiler, the ingredient list is short, and the preparation is eminently simple. Keep in mind that marinating overnight requires a bit of preplanning. Serve with Rice Pilaf and Middle Eastern Cucumber Relish.

INGREDIENTS

    2 LB. LEAN LEG OF LAMB OR BEEF SIRLOIN TIP
    2 LARGE ONIONS, CUT IN EIGHTS

Marinade

    2 LARGE ONIONS
    4 TABLESPOONS LEMON JUICE
    3 TEASPOONS CUMIN
    ½ CUP NONFAT PLAIN YOGURT
    1 TEASPOON FRESHLY GROUND BLACK PEPPER
    1 TEASPOON LIGHT SALT (OR TO TASTE)

DIRECTIONS

Trim meat of fat and cut into 1-inch cubes.

Puree onions, lemon juice, cumin, yogurt, light salt, and pepper in blender or food processor.

Place cubed meat in a glass bowl or casserole dish and pour the onion mixture over it.

Using two forks, pierce meat at ¼-inch intervals to tenderize and introduce marinade. Cover and allow to marinate in the refrigerator overnight.

Before cooking, cut the other 2 onions into eighths.

On six skewers, alternate meat and onion. Broil or barbeque over charcoal until meat is brown, basting once or twice with marinade.

Heat—but do not boil—remaining marinade in saucepan or microwave to use as a dipping sauce.

SERVING SIZE: 6 Servings, 1 Shish Kebab Each

PER SERVING: Calories 229   **Fiber:** 2 grams   **Sodium:** 300 mg.

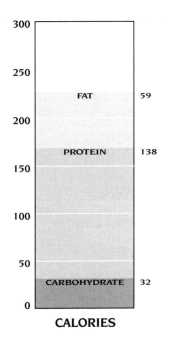

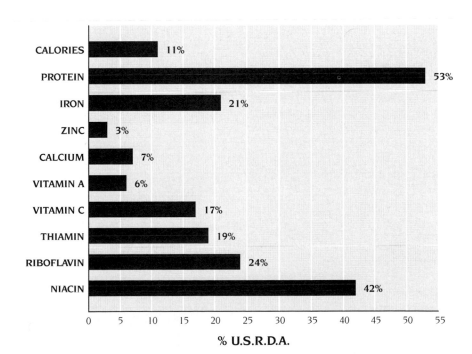

LIVER AND ONIONS

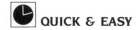 QUICK & EASY

Don't try this recipe using polar bear liver. Unless you are planning an Arctic expedition, polar bears and their parts may be low on your list of dietary concerns, but you might enjoy this bit of nutrition trivia. In America, where many people glibly risk nutrient toxicity every day by taking unnaturally high doses of vitamins and minerals in capsule form, nutrition scientists have identified only one food which *naturally* contains enough vitamin A to be dangerous: polar bear liver! Of course, there is a reason. The liver serves as a storehouse for extra nutrients. What makes the bears' different is that they live at the very top of a carnivorous food chain. When they eat a seal, for instance, they get all the vitamins and minerals stored in the seal's liver; and that seal got all the vitamins and minerals stored in the fish livers—and the big fish ate the little fish, and so on. It seems the bears can handle this high concentration of vitamin A without problems, but the early Arctic explorers, at least those who were fond of polar bear liver, ended up with vitamin A toxicity! With supermarket varieties of liver there's no need to worry about a nutrient overdose, and a single serving provides 10 days' worth of vitamin A! In fact, a glance at the overall nutrient profile will explain why mothers tell their children that liver is delicious.

INGREDIENTS

3 TEASPOONS BUTTER OR MARGARINE
1 LARGE ONION, SLICED IN RINGS
1 LB. CHICKEN, PORK, OR CALF LIVER
½ TEASPOON LIGHT SALT

DASH BLACK PEPPER
2 TEASPOONS VINEGAR
1 TEASPOON WORCESTERSHIRE SAUCE
2 TABLESPOONS WATER

DIRECTIONS

Melt 2 teaspoons of the butter in a nonstick skillet. Add onion slices and sauté over medium heat until transparent and golden, about 10 to 15 minutes.

Remove onions from skillet. Melt remaining 1 teaspoon butter and add sliced pork or calf liver or whole chicken livers. Sprinkle with light salt and pepper. Brown over medium heat about 3 minutes per side.

Distribute onions evenly over browned liver in skillet.

In a small bowl combine vinegar, Worcestershire sauce, and water, then pour over the liver and onions.

Cook over medium heat for 2 to 3 minutes until most of the liquid is gone, then serve.

SERVING SIZE: ¼ Recipe

PER SERVING: Calories 184 **Fiber:** 1 gram **Sodium:** 306 mg.

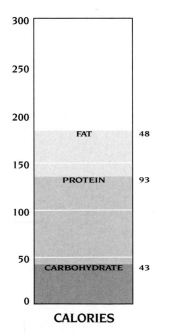

FAT	48
PROTEIN	93
CARBOHYDRATE	43

CALORIES

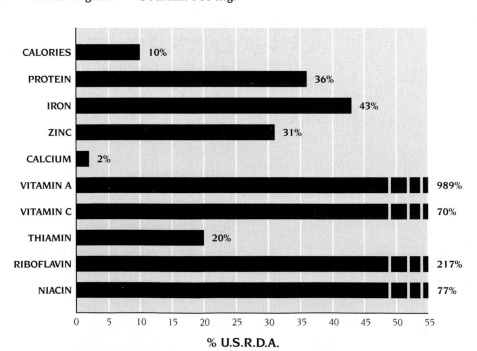

	% U.S.R.D.A.
CALORIES	10%
PROTEIN	36%
IRON	43%
ZINC	31%
CALCIUM	2%
VITAMIN A	989%
VITAMIN C	70%
THIAMIN	20%
RIBOFLAVIN	217%
NIACIN	77%

% U.S.R.D.A.

BIGOS—A HUNTER'S STEW

A pungently delicious robust dish, best on the coldest of winter nights. The original bigos, or hunter's stew, was made of sauerkraut and smoked meats, so that it could be carried along on a hunting trip without fear of spoilage. Each night, the pot of bigos was heated over the campfire, where hunters gathered to warm their weary bones and to pass the flask of cognac. To this day, in the hunting lodges of Eastern Europe, steaming bowls of bigos are typically accompanied by straight shots of good cognac and large chunks of coarse black bread.

INGREDIENTS

½ LB. POLISH SAUSAGE (KIELBASA)
2 OZ. BACON, 2 SLICES CUT INTO SHREDS
3 MEDIUM ONIONS, CHOPPED
¾ LB. TURKEY HAM OR LEAN HAM, CUT IN ½-INCH CUBES
¼ LB. CANADIAN BACON, CUT IN ½-INCH CUBES
½ LB. LEAN COOKED ROAST BEEF, CUT IN ½-INCH CUBES

2 JARS (32 OZ. EACH) OR 2 CANS (28 OZ. EACH) SAUERKRAUT
8 CUPS WATER
1 LARGE APPLE, DICED
1 CUP CATSUP
1 CUP RED WINE
3 BAY LEAVES
1 TEASPOON CRACKED BLACK PEPPER OR WHOLE PEPPERCORNS

DIRECTIONS

Cut Polish sausage into quarters, lengthwise, then into ½-inch slices. Brown sausage well in a large, heavy skillet over low heat for about 15-20 minutes. Drain off fat and discard. Remove sausage to paper towel to drain.

Place bacon shreds and onions in the same heavy skillet. Sauté over low heat for 15 to 20 minutes until bacon is cooked and onion is limp.

In a large (5-quart) nonaluminum pot, combine cooked sausage, sautéed bacon and onion, turkey ham, Canadian bacon, and roast beef.

Drain sauerkraut, rinse with fresh water, and drain again. Add to meat with 8 cups water, apple, catsup, wine, bay leaves, and black pepper.

Simmer, covered, over low heat for 1 to 2 hours to blend flavors. Bigos can be served at this point, but it actually improves each time it is reheated and stores well in the refrigerator for up to 2 weeks.

SERVING SIZE: 12 Servings, 1 Cup Each

PER SERVING: Calories 195 **Fiber:** 4 grams **Sodium:** 1243 mg.

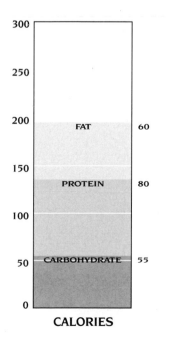

CALORIES

FAT 60
PROTEIN 80
CARBOHYDRATE 55

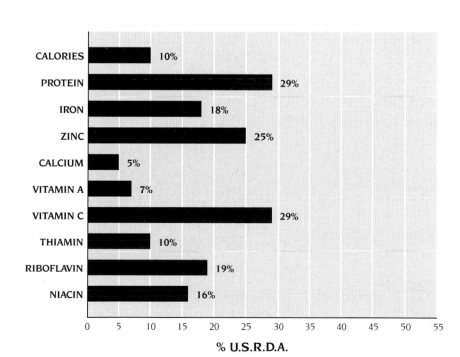

% U.S.R.D.A.

	%
CALORIES	10%
PROTEIN	29%
IRON	18%
ZINC	25%
CALCIUM	5%
VITAMIN A	7%
VITAMIN C	29%
THIAMIN	10%
RIBOFLAVIN	19%
NIACIN	16%

SAUSAGES

If you love sausage but consider it a sin, that could be because it is loaded with saturated fat, calories, and salt—plus various additives with fluctuating status on the G.R.A.S.* list. Here's some good news. You can have that Sunday morning flavor, sans guilt, by making your own sausage from very lean ground meat. Don't worry—it's easy. All you need is a little help from your friendly meat man.

We suggest you try pork—it gives the most traditional flavor—but turkey or veal or a combination can be very good, since sausages are, by nature, highly seasoned. (See graphs below for nutrient profiles of these meats.) To get truly lean ground pork, select a large roast, such as a leg, butt, or loin. Ask the butcher to trim it of all visible fat before grinding. You will have to pay for the entire roast, including the fat, but you'll save yourself the trouble of trying to cook and drain and blot it out later. A leg of pork will yield 6 to 8 pounds of lean ground meat. The seasonings listed are for 2-pound batches, but the recipes can easily be increased. Sausage keeps well, uncooked, in the freezer for 6 to 8 months.

INGREDIENTS

Country (Breakfast Sausage)

- 2 LB. LEAN GROUND PORK, TURKEY, OR VEAL
- 2½ TEASPOONS DRIED SAGE
- ½ TEASPOON DRIED THYME
- ¼-½ TEASPOON CAYENNE PEPPER
- ¾ TEASPOON BLACK PEPPER
- ¼ TEASPOON GARLIC POWDER
- ⅛ TEASPOON CELERY SEED
- ¼ BAY LEAF
- 1½-3 TEASPOONS LIGHT SALT OR SALT SUBSTITUTE

Italian Sausage

- 2 LB. LEAN GROUND PORK, TURKEY, OR VEAL
- 1 TEASPOON BLACK PEPPER
- 1 TEASPOON DRIED BASIL
- 1 TEASPOON ONION POWDER
- 2 TEASPOONS GARLIC POWDER
- 3 TEASPOONS THYME
- 2 TEASPOONS ANISE SEED
- 2 TEASPOONS LIGHT SALT OR SALT SUBSTITUTE

*G.R.A.S. is the Food and Drug Administration's list of food additives "generally recognized as safe."

Pork Sausage

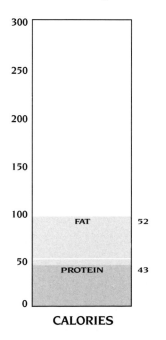

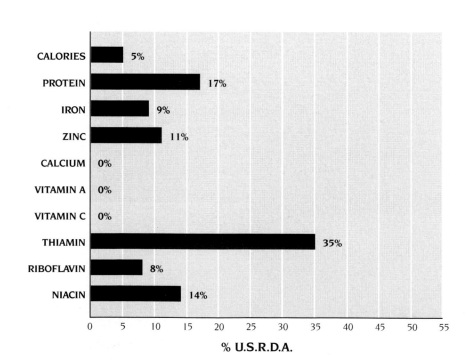

DIRECTIONS

Grind seasonings together well in blender, food processor, or grinder.

Thoroughly mix ground meat with seasonings.

Form into 16 patties.

Place in a large nonstick skillet. Add ½ cup water, cover, and cook for about 10 minutes over medium heat.

Remove lid. Allow remaining liquid to cook off, then finish sausages by browning, 2 to 3 minutes on each side.

SERVING SIZE: 1 Patty, 2 oz. Each

PER SERVING: (For Pork, Turkey, and Veal) **Calories** 95, 90, 90   **Fiber:** 0   **Sodium:** 40, 38, 51 mg.

Turkey Sausage

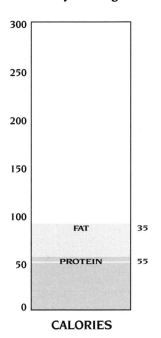
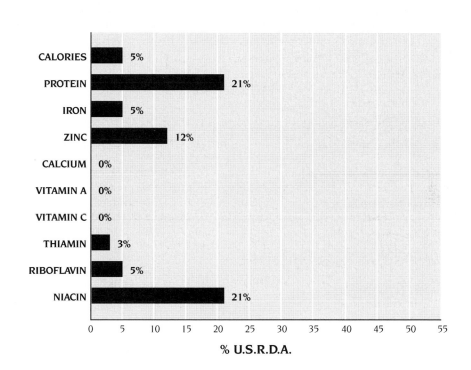

Veal Sausage

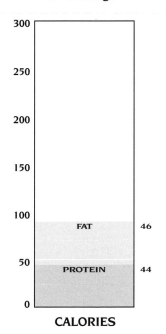
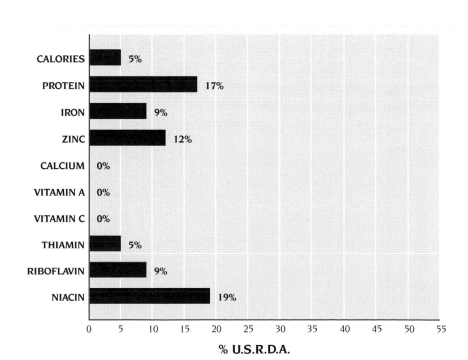

Cheese & Egg Dishes

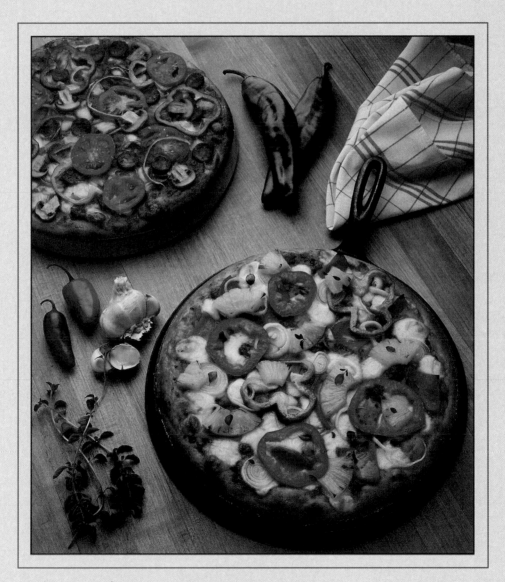

Quick Homemade Pizza, Hawaiian Pizza (pp. 190-191)

ABOUT PIZZA

Before you call this wonderful dish junk food—consider these facts: it contains all four of the food groups, provides vegetables in a format which children consider edible, and is liked by practically everyone. The trouble with homemade pizza is that it's a lot of trouble. The trouble with take-out pizza is that it can pack up to 450 calories per slice for one eighth of a "family size," 16-inch pizza—and you can't eat just one slice. To solve the pizza lover's dilemma, we have two easy pizzas, Presto Snack Pizza and Joe's Homemade Pizza. Both decadently delicious, but heroically high in nutrients and, unbelievably, low enough in fat for living lean.

JOE'S HOMEMADE PIZZA

When our friend Joe Legman, owned a wonderful pizza place in New York City, he used to say, "You can't make great pizza without a brick oven. See, what you do is, you get this oven up to about 800°, then you slide your pizza right onto those hot bricks, and that gets your crust all nice and crisp on the bottom!" When Joe sold his restaurant—and his brick oven—he couldn't say that anymore because he figured out a way to make his incredible pizza, crisp crust and all, in his perfectly normal kitchen. He dedicated a cookie sheet to this cause by cutting off one edge, so he could bake his pizza until firm, then slide it off the cookie sheet directly onto the oven rack. This rack is set in the lowest possible position in the oven, which has been preheated to the highest possible temperature (usually about 500°). Joe's wife, Linda, confides that his system is foolproof as long as the heat is coming from below the pizza, not from a broiling element above. (Pictured on p. 189.)

INGREDIENTS

Whole Wheat Crust

- 1 PACKAGE QUICK-RISING DRY YEAST
- 1 CUP HOT WATER (110°-115°)
- 1 TEASPOON SUGAR OR HONEY
- 1 TEASPOON LIGHT SALT
- 2-2½ CUPS WHOLE WHEAT FLOUR
- 2 TEASPOONS OLIVE OIL
- 1 TABLESPOON POLENTA (COARSE GROUND CORNMEAL)

Sauce

- 1 CAN (6 OZ.) TOMATO PASTE
- ½ TEASPOON DRIED ROSEMARY
- ¼ TEASPOON EACH OREGANO, BASIL, AND THYME
- 1 CLOVE GARLIC, MINCED
- ¼ TEASPOON COARSELY GROUND BLACK PEPPER

Toppings

- ½ LB. LOW-FAT ITALIAN SAUSAGE
- ½ LB. LOW-FAT MOZZARELLA CHEESE, SHREDDED
- 1 LARGE RED ONION, THINLY SLICED
- 1 LARGE BELL PEPPER, THINLY SLICED
- 4-5 LARGE MUSHROOMS, SLICED
  GRATED PARMESAN CHEESE FOR GARNISH (OPTIONAL)
  CRUSHED RED PEPPER FOR GARNISH (OPTIONAL)

DIRECTIONS

Dissolve yeast in hot water in a large mixing bowl. Add sugar, light salt, and 1 cup flour. Beat 100 strokes. Allow to stand at least 5 minutes or up to 1 hour.

Beat in additional 1 cup flour until dough is smooth and elastic.

Add ¼ cup more flour to make a stiff dough. Turn out on a floured board. Knead 1 to 2 minutes, just until smooth. Let rest 5 minutes.

Grease 1 large pizza pan or cookie sheet with 2 teaspoons olive oil, then sprinkle evenly with cornmeal.

With oiled hands, stretch, roll and pat dough on floured board to fit pan. The dough will be elastic and will tend to spring back. Just keep pushing the heel of your hand into the thick spots, until the dough is distributed evenly. Transfer dough to prepared pan. If it won't stay put, leave

Continued

it alone for 10 minutes or so, while you prepare the sauce and vegetables. When you return to the dough, you'll find it has softened and risen a bit from continued yeast activity and will be much easier to handle.

Preheat oven to 450°.

In a small bowl, mix all sauce ingredients well. Spread evenly over pizza dough.

Slice cooked low-fat Italian sausage (see meats, Chapter 8) or cook ½ lb. commercial Italian sausage over low heat until well done to remove as much fat as possible. Slice thinly.

Sprinkle grated cheese evenly over sauce. Distribute sausage, then onions, peppers, and mushrooms over top.

Place pizza in preheated oven on lowest rack. Bake for 12 to 15 minutes. For an extra-crisp crust, slide pizza from pan directly onto rack during the last 5 minutes of baking.

Serve with grated parmesan if desired and pass crushed red pepper on the side.

VARIATIONS: Quick Homemade Pizza. Use frozen bread dough (thawed) for crust and canned pizza sauce. Top as desired.

Extra-Quick Homemade Pizza. Buy a take-and-bake cheese pizza with a whole wheat crust. Add your own vegetable toppings and lean meat at home. This is a useful idea when each of your children has a different pizza preference. Let each family member dress his own corner of the pizza with favorite toppings.

Hawaiian Pizza. Replace Italian sausage and mushrooms with Canadian bacon and pineapple.

SERVING SIZE: ¹/₁₂ Pizza

PER SERVING: Calories 187 **Fiber:** 2 grams **Sodium:** 201 mg.

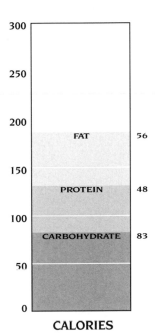

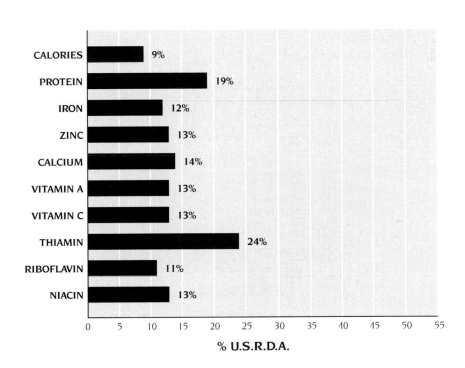

PRESTO SNACK PIZZA

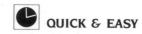 **QUICK & EASY**

INGREDIENTS

- 2 SANDWICH-SIZE (2 OZ.) WHOLE WHEAT FRENCH ROLLS
- ½ CUP ITALIAN TOMATO SAUCE
- 2 TABLESPOONS PARMESAN CHEESE, GRATED
- 2 OZ. LOW-FAT MOZZARELLA CHEESE, ⅔ CUP SHREDDED
- ½ SMALL ONION, VERY THINLY SLICED
- 1 SMALL TOMATO, THINLY SLICED

DIRECTIONS

Preheat oven to 400°.

Split the French rolls lengthwise and spread with a thin layer of Italian tomato sauce.

Sprinkle evenly with parmesan, then mozzarella.

Arrange sliced tomatoes, then onions, on top.

Bake for 4 to 6 minutes until cheese begins to melt. Finish under broiler to brown top.

VARIATIONS: Whole grain English muffins or pita bread work well in place of French bread.
Vary toppings, but keep these tips in mind as you do:

1. Take care not to load the pizza with too many vegetables at once. They release water when heated, and large quantities can make a pizza soggy. A quick trick to compensate for extra vegetables is to spread the sliced onions, bell peppers, mushrooms, zucchini, or whatever in a single layer on a microproof dish and microwave uncovered on high for 3 to 5 minutes or sauté in a nonstick skillet. This will reduce water content tremendously and precook the vegetables.

2. Keep in mind that fatty meats such as pepperoni, salami, and other sausages can really drive up the calorie count. Use sparingly and precook to reduce fat content or choose leaner meats such as Canadian bacon, turkey ham, or our homemade low-fat sausage.

SERVING SIZE: 2 Servings, 2 Halves Each

PER SERVING: Calories 287 **Fiber:** 3 grams **Sodium:** 341 mg.

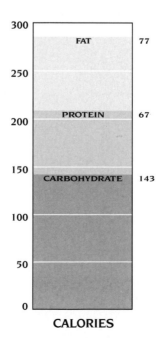

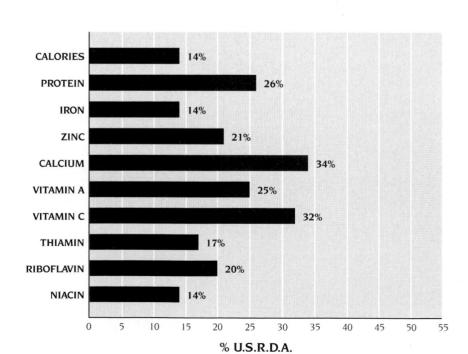

SPINACH GNOCCHI

Gnocchi are small Italian dumplings. These delectably light, savory morsels come in a variety of shapes, colors, and flavors. Potato gnocchi are probably the most familiar, but we think these spinach gnocchi are the best! The biggest mystery about gnocchi, aside from pronunciation (nyok-kee) is why the Italian people would give this name to such a delightful food. The direct translation of gnocchi is lumps.

INGREDIENTS

1 CUP SPINACH (1 LARGE BUNCH) COOKED AND DRAINED OR
1 PACKAGE (10 OZ.) FROZEN CHOPPED SPINACH, THAWED AND DRAINED
½ LB. DRY CURD COTTAGE CHEESE*
¼ TEASPOON FRESHLY GROUND BLACK PEPPER

⅛ TEASPOON NUTMEG
1 OZ. PARMESAN CHEESE, ⅓ CUP GRATED
2 EGGS
¼ CUP WHOLE WHEAT PASTRY FLOUR
1 OZ. PARMESAN CHEESE, ⅓ CUP GRATED FOR TOPPING

DIRECTIONS

Cook spinach until tender, drain well in colander, then squeeze dry. Chop very finely or puree in food processor.

Place spinach in small heavy saucepan. Add cottage cheese (or ricotta), pepper, and nutmeg. Cook, stirring constantly, over low heat for 4 to 5 minutes until well combined and rather dry.

Remove from heat. Beat in ⅓ cup parmesan, eggs, and flour. Allow mixture to cool until firm enough to handle.

With well-floured hands, roll heaping teaspoonfuls of dough into 1-inch balls (20 to 24). Set on waxed paper.

Twenty minutes before serving time, heat 4 to 6 quarts water to a boil.

Gently lower half the gnocchi into the boiling water. Simmer 6 to 8 minutes. When gnocchi puff up and float to the top, lift out with a slotted spoon, drain quickly, and keep warm while cooking the second batch.

Serve immediately, topped with remaining parmesan.

SERVING SIZE: 4 Servings, 5 to 6 Gnocchi Each

PER SERVING: Calories 200 **Fiber:** 2 grams **Sodium:** 290 mg.

*If dry curd cottage cheese is not available, use low-fat ricotta cheese (adds 45 calories per serving).

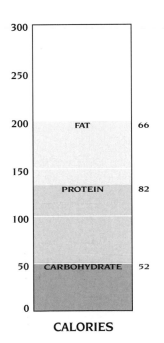

CALORIES

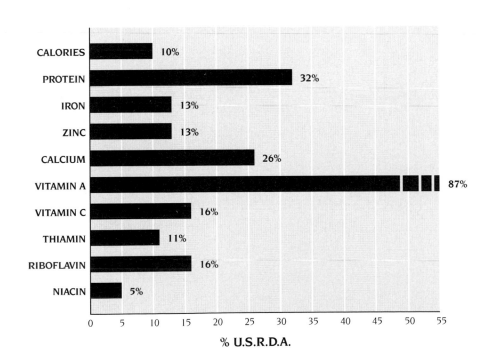

% U.S.R.D.A.

COTTAGE CHEESE PANCAKES 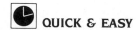 QUICK & EASY

INGREDIENTS

3 EGGS
1 CUP LOW-FAT COTTAGE CHEESE
1 TEASPOON VANILLA
⅓ CUP WHOLE WHEAT PASTRY FLOUR
¼ TEASPOON LIGHT SALT (OPTIONAL)
    DASH CINNAMON (OPTIONAL)
2 TEASPOONS BUTTER

DIRECTIONS

Using blender, food processor, or mixer, beat eggs, cottage cheese, and vanilla until smooth.

Add flour along with light salt and cinnamon, if used. Mix just until combined.

Melt 1 teaspoon butter in a large nonstick skillet, dispersing it evenly. Drop batter into skillet by rounded tablespoonfuls to form 8 to 10 small (2-inch) pancakes. Use about half the batter.

Cook over medium heat until bubbles appear on surface of pancakes. Turn and brown other side.

Repeat process with remaining batter and second teaspoon of butter.

Serve, topped with applesauce, fruit puree, or syrup.

SERVING SIZE: 3 Servings, 5 to 6 Small Pancakes Each

PER SERVING: Calories 214   **Fiber:** 1 gram   **Sodium:** 403 mg.

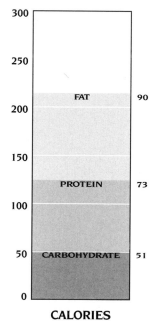

CALORIES

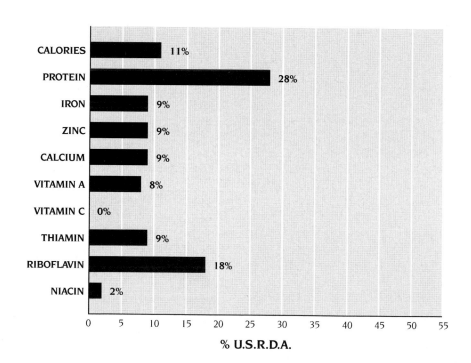

% U.S.R.D.A.

MIRACLE VEGETABLE PIE

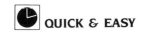 QUICK & EASY

The crust forms as you bake this amazing pie. Filled with the goodness of whole grain flour, fresh vegetables, and eggs, this dish is fun, quick, and appetizing.

INGREDIENTS

- 2 CUPS ZUCCHINI OR 3 CUPS MUSHROOMS
- 1 CUP TOMATO, CHOPPED
- ½ CUP ONION, DICED, OR ½ CUP GREEN ONION, SLICED
- ⅓ CUP PARMESAN CHEESE, GRATED
- 1½ CUPS NONFAT MILK

- ¾ CUP WHOLE WHEAT PASTRY FLOUR
- 3 EGGS
- 1 TEASPOON LIGHT SALT
- ¼ TEASPOON BLACK PEPPER
- 1 TABLESPOON OIL
- 1 TABLESPOON BAKING POWDER

DIRECTIONS

Preheat oven to 400°.

Cut zucchini in half lengthwise, then slice ¼-inch thick. If using mushrooms, slice ¼-inch thick.

Spray 10-inch quiche pan or 9-inch pie plate with nonstick cooking spray.

Sprinkle zucchini or mushrooms, then tomato, onion, and cheese into prepared pan.

Beat together milk, flour, eggs, light salt, pepper, oil, and baking powder until smooth.

Pour over other ingredients in pan.

Bake until a knife inserted in the center comes out clean, about 50 minutes.

Cool for 5 minutes and serve.

SERVING SIZE: ⅛ Pie

PER SERVING: Calories 129 **Fiber:** 3 grams **Sodium:** 332 mg.

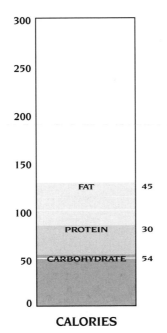

FAT 45
PROTEIN 30
CARBOHYDRATE 54

CALORIES

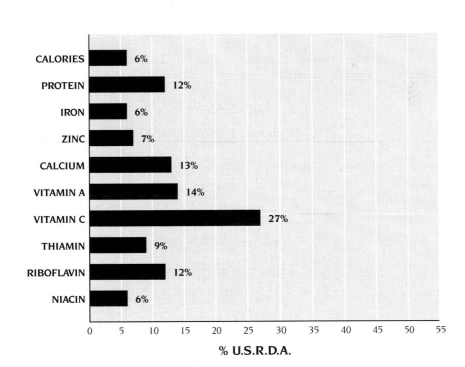

CALORIES 6%
PROTEIN 12%
IRON 6%
ZINC 7%
CALCIUM 13%
VITAMIN A 14%
VITAMIN C 27%
THIAMIN 9%
RIBOFLAVIN 12%
NIACIN 6%

% U.S.R.D.A.

FRITTATA

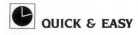 **QUICK & EASY**

Frittata is like crustless quiche. Italians like to serve it at room temperature, but it's also wonderful hot!

INGREDIENTS

2 EGGS
½ CUP LOW-FAT COTTAGE CHEESE
1⅓ CUPS NONFAT MILK
2 TABLESPOONS ONION, MINCED
2 TABLESPOONS FRESH PARSLEY, CHOPPED

1 OZ. PARMESAN CHEESE, ⅓ CUP GRATED
½ CUP WHOLE GRAIN CORNFLAKE CRUMBS
½ TEASPOON LIGHT SALT
⅛ TEASPOON EACH GARLIC POWDER, ROSEMARY, THYME, AND BLACK PEPPER
¾ LB. FRESH GREEN BEANS OR 1 PACKAGE (10 OZ.) FROZEN FRENCH-CUT GREEN BEANS

DIRECTIONS

Preheat oven to 350°.

Wash and string beans. French cut beans—slice diagonally as thinly as possible. Boil or steam sliced beans for 12 minutes, just until crisp-tender. If using frozen French-cut beans, thaw and drain, but do not cook.

Mix eggs, cottage cheese, and milk in blender or processor.

In a medium bowl toss together onion, parsley, grated cheese, cornflake crumbs, and seasonings.

Add blended egg mixture. Stir.

Spray a 9-inch or 10-inch pie plate or quiche pan with nonstick cooking spray.

Spread drained green beans evenly in bottom of plate. Pour egg mixture over beans.

Bake for 35 minutes until browned and set.

SERVING SIZE: 6 Servings, Side Dish; 3 Servings, Main Dish

PER SERVING (Side Dish): Calories 115 **Fiber:** 6 grams **Sodium:** 325 mg.

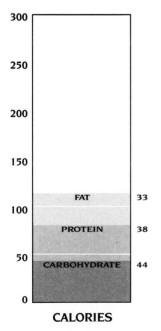

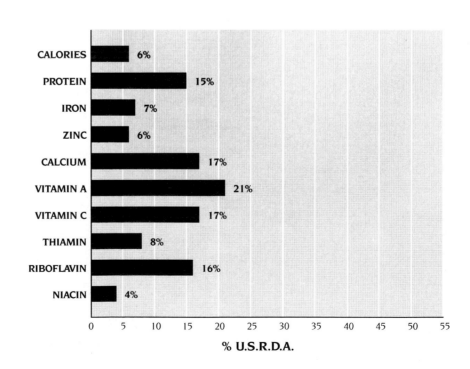

CHILE RELLENO CASSEROLE 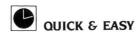 QUICK & EASY

The perfect party casserole—it assembles in minutes, freezes and reheats beautifully, and improves with standing time. A low-fat rendition of the classic chile relleno.

INGREDIENTS

1 LARGE CAN (1 LB. 11 OZ.) WHOLE GREEN CHILES OR 4 CANS (7 OZ. EACH)
12 OZ. SHARP CHEDDAR CHEESE, ABOUT 3 CUPS GRATED
3 EGGS
3 CUPS NONFAT MILK
1 CUP WHOLE WHEAT PASTRY FLOUR
1 TEASPOON BAKING POWDER
½ TEASPOON LIGHT SALT
½ TEASPOON BLACK PEPPER

DIRECTIONS

Preheat oven to 350°.
Spray large (3-quart) flat casserole dish with nonstick cooking spray.
Place half of the chiles in a single layer in the dish and sprinkle with half of the cheese.
  Repeat the layers.
In blender or processor, combine eggs, milk, flour, baking powder, light salt, and pepper.
  Blend until smooth.
Pour batter over cheese and chiles.
Bake, uncovered, for 1 hour until top is golden brown and batter is set.

SERVING SIZE: ¹/₁₂ Recipe

PER SERVING: Calories 209   **Fiber:** 2 grams   **Sodium:** 312 mg.

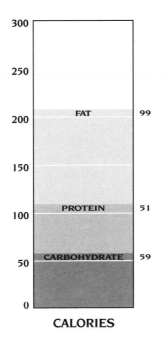

FAT 99
PROTEIN 51
CARBOHYDRATE 59

CALORIES

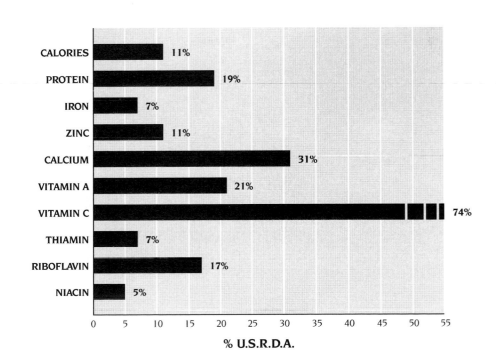

	%
CALORIES	11%
PROTEIN	19%
IRON	7%
ZINC	11%
CALCIUM	31%
VITAMIN A	21%
VITAMIN C	74%
THIAMIN	7%
RIBOFLAVIN	17%
NIACIN	5%

% U.S.R.D.A.

EGGPLANT PARMESAN

One of the reasons we now have "truth-in-menu" laws is eggplant. For years, budget-minded restauranteurs managed successfully, if somewhat unscrupulously, to substitute eggplant for abalone or veal in high-priced entrees. Its meaty texture and mild flavor also allow eggplant to impersonate various high-fat foods for a fraction of the calories. The bold flavors of Italian herbs, tomatoes, and cheeses combine with the subtle richness of eggplant in this favorite vegetarian entree. Serve with polenta or pasta and a green salad.

INGREDIENTS

1 TEASPOON OLIVE OIL
1 MEDIUM ONION, 1 CUP FINELY CHOPPED
4 CLOVES GARLIC, MINCED
2 TEASPOONS ITALIAN HERBS OR 1 TEASPOON
 BASIL, ½ TEASPOON OREGANO, AND
 ½ TEASPOON THYME
½ LB. FRESH MUSHROOMS, 2 CUPS SLICED
1 SMALL RED OR GREEN BELL PEPPER,
 FINELY CHOPPED

2 LB. TOMATOES, 4 CUPS PEELED AND CHOPPED
 OR 2 CANS (1 LB. EACH)
1 LARGE EGGPLANT (1½ LB.)
4 TEASPOONS OLIVE OIL
2 OZ. PARMESAN CHEESE, GRATED
 FRESHLY GROUND BLACK PEPPER
2 OZ. MOZZARELLA CHEESE, SHREDDED
 FRESHLY GRATED PARMESAN CHEESE, CAPERS,
 OR ANCHOVY FILLETS FOR GARNISH (OPTIONAL)

DIRECTIONS

Preheat oven to 350°.

In a large nonstick skillet, heat 1 teaspoon olive oil. Sauté onion and garlic over medium heat until tender, about 5 minutes.

Add herbs, mushrooms, and bell pepper. Sauté 5 minutes longer.

Add chopped tomatoes, reduce heat, and simmer, uncovered, for 10-15 minutes.

Meanwhile, slice eggplant into rounds, ½-inch thick.

Heat 1 teaspoon olive oil in another large nonstick skillet. Distribute oil evenly, then quickly place half the slices in the skillet. (Eggplant absorbs oil like a regular little sponge, so all the slices

need to hit the pan at about the same time.) Fry eggplant slices over low heat until golden brown, 6 to 8 minutes. Turn them over, then drizzle another teaspoon of olive oil around edges of pan and between slices to brown other side.

Remove fried eggplant to greased 8-inch by 10-inch baking dish and repeat process with second half of eggplant. When all eggplant slices are browned, arrange them in the baking dish, sprinkle evenly with grated parmesan, then pour sauce over top.

Bake for 40 minutes. Sprinkle with black pepper and mozzarella. Return to oven for 3 to 5 minutes, just until cheese has melted.

SERVING SIZE: ⅙ Recipe

PER SERVING: Calories 170   **Fiber:** 6 grams   **Sodium:** 210 mg.

Eggplant Parmesan (facing page)

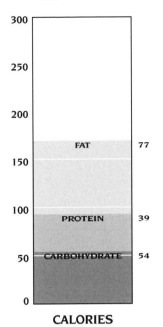

CALORIES

FAT 77

PROTEIN 39

CARBOHYDRATE 54

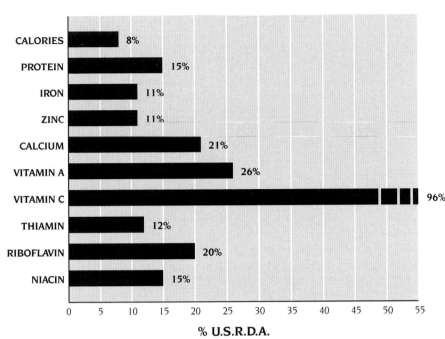

	% U.S.R.D.A.
CALORIES	8%
PROTEIN	15%
IRON	11%
ZINC	11%
CALCIUM	21%
VITAMIN A	26%
VITAMIN C	96%
THIAMIN	12%
RIBOFLAVIN	20%
NIACIN	15%

Chilequiles (p. 200)

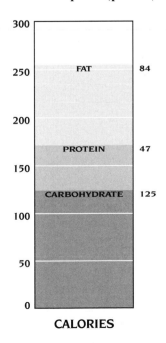

CALORIES

FAT 84

PROTEIN 47

CARBOHYDRATE 125

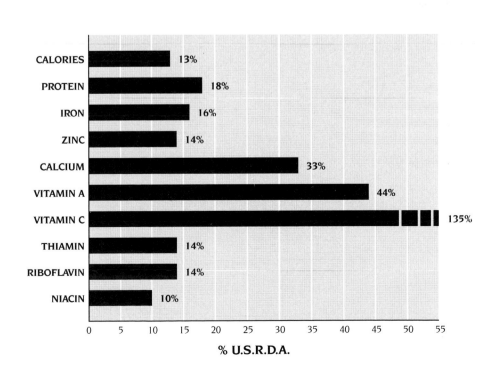

	% U.S.R.D.A.
CALORIES	13%
PROTEIN	18%
IRON	16%
ZINC	14%
CALCIUM	33%
VITAMIN A	44%
VITAMIN C	135%
THIAMIN	14%
RIBOFLAVIN	14%
NIACIN	10%

CHILEQUILES

Have you ever gone to a Mexican restaurant for breakfast? If not, chilequiles may be one of those great dining experiences still awaiting you. In Mexico this combination of tortillas, vegetables, and cheese is as typical to the breakfast menu as our eggs and toast. The popularity of this dish has been attributed to its simplicity and its delicious flavor. We suspect the real reason it appears on so many breakfast tables is that thrifty cooks and restauranteurs recognize an ingenious use for leftover tortillas when they see one! Traditional accompaniments in Mexico would include refried beans, fresh tortillas, and salsa. A glass of freshly squeezed orange juice or a "plata de frutas" (fruit plate of three or four fresh seasonal fruits cut in large chunks or slices) would typically be served as a starter.

INGREDIENTS

    1 TABLESPOON OLIVE OIL OR CORN OIL
    6 CORN TORTILLAS, CUT IN EIGHTHS
 1½ LB. RIPE TOMATOES (4 LARGE) OR 1 CAN (28 OZ.), PEELED AND CHOPPED
    1 LARGE ONION, 2 CUPS CHOPPED
    1 CAN (4 OZ.) DICED GREEN CHILES
    1 TABLESPOON FRESH CILANTRO, CHOPPED
  ¼ TEASPOON FRESHLY GROUND BLACK PEPPER
    LIGHT SALT (OPTIONAL)
    4 OZ. LOW-FAT MOZZARELLA CHEESE, 1 CUP GRATED

DIRECTIONS

Heat oil in a large nonstick skillet.

Add the cut up tortillas all at once and toss them around to distribute oil.

Fry over medium-heat for about 10 minutes, stirring frequently, until tortillas are golden brown and beginning to crisp.

Scald, peel, and chop fresh tomatoes or coarsely chop canned tomatoes.

When tortilla chips are done, remove to paper towels to drain. Add chopped onions to hot skillet. Increase heat to medium high and "deep fry" onions 5 to 10 minutes until golden brown. Stir frequently and be sure onions do brown; this is important to the flavor of this dish.

Add chopped tomatoes, chiles, cilantro, and pepper. Simmer 5 to 10 minutes to blend flavors and reduce liquid. Adjust seasonings and add light salt, if desired.

Add tortilla chips to sauce in skillet and stir until thoroughly combined. Sprinkle cheese evenly over top. Turn off heat and let stand 2 to 3 minutes until cheese melts.

VARIATIONS: Substitute sliced green onions for white.

Add some sliced mushrooms to fried onions and sauté about 2 minutes before adding tomatoes.

Use tomatillos in place of tomatoes.

Substitute cheddar cheese for mozzarella or use Mexican-style fresh cheese crumbled over top.

SERVING SIZE: ¼ Recipe

PER SERVING: Calories 256   **Fiber:** 6 grams   **Sodium:** 188 mg.

Graph on p. 199

TACOS CON PAPAS
(CHEESE AND POTATO TACOS)

In the United States, when a tortilla is filled with beef, we call it a taco; with beans, we call it a burrito. In Mexico a taco can be filled with almost anything, much like a sandwich. Potato-cheese tacos are not only authentic Mexican fare, they are also quite delicious.

INGREDIENTS

5 SMALL RED POTATOES, UNPEELED AND BOILED	1 HEAD LETTUCE OR CABBAGE, FINELY SHREDDED
⅔ CUP SWEET RED ONION, FINELY CHOPPED	SOUR CREAM MIXED WITH PLAIN YOGURT FOR
1 CUP FARMERS OR MEXICAN CHEESE*, CRUMBLED	TOPPING (OPTIONAL)
1 TABLESPOON CUMIN (OPTIONAL)	FRESH CILANTRO, CHOPPED, FOR GARNISH
12 CORN OR WHOLE WHEAT FLOUR TORTILLAS	(OPTIONAL)
SALSA CRUDA OR GREEN TOMATILLO SALSA (SEE CHAPTER 2)	

DIRECTIONS

Chop boiled potatoes into small cubes and put in a medium-sized bowl.

Add onion, cheese and cumin, if used. Mix well.

Warm tortillas in a hot nonstick skillet. Spoon one-twelfth of the mixture into each warmed tortilla.

Top with shredded lettuce or cabbage and salsa. Add sour cream with yogurt and cilantro, if desired, and serve.

VARIATION: Tacos Con Papas Enchilada-Style. Preheat oven to 350°. Place filled tortillas in a large, flat baking dish. Cover tightly and bake for 15 to 25 minutes or until heated through. Top with salsa and serve.

SERVING SIZE: 6 Servings, 2 Tacos Each

PER SERVING: Calories 300   **Fiber:** 8 grams   **Sodium:** 397 mg.

*Fresh Mexican cheese is like a dry cottage cheese, but with a stronger, sharper flavor. If unavailable, substitute ¾ cup drained cottage cheese plus 1 oz. blue cheese.

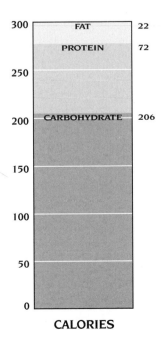

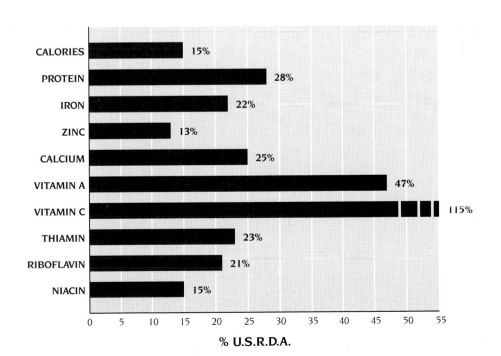

Pasta, Rice & Grains

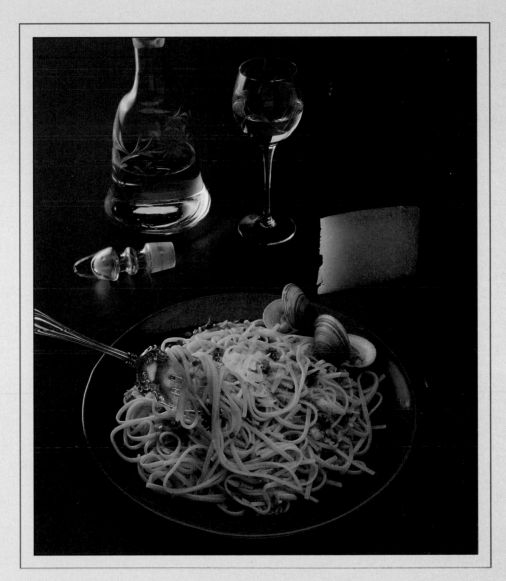

Linguine With Clam Sauce (p. 207)

SPAGHETTI CARBONARA

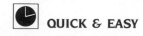 QUICK & EASY

Sonoma County in the heart of California's wine country is almost as famous for its Italian restaurants as it is for its wineries. It was in one of these that we were introduced to a northern Italian dish called spaghetti carbonara. This artful combination of freshly grated cheese, homemade pasta, virgin olive oil, and spicy Italian prosciutto was heavenly—but hardly our idea of low-fat fare. Determined to include it in our book, we proceeded to cook (and eat) numerous versions. This recipe finally emerged as the closest to the original gastronomic delight.

INGREDIENTS

2 TABLESPOONS OLIVE OIL OR BUTTER
1 CUP ONION, DICED
3 CLOVES GARLIC, MINCED
4 OZ. CANADIAN BACON (8 SMALL SLICES), DICED
½ CUP NONFAT MILK

2 EGGS
¼ TEASPOON FRESHLY GROUND BLACK PEPPER
½ LB. THIN WHOLE GRAIN SPAGHETTI
4 TEASPOONS PARMESAN CHEESE

DIRECTIONS

Prepare all ingredients before beginning to cook.

In a large saucepan heat 4 to 5 quarts of water to a rolling boil. Add spaghetti and cook "al dente," 7 to 9 minutes. Do not overcook.

Meanwhile, in a 2-quart nonstick saucepan, heat oil. Add onion and garlic and sauté over medium heat for 5 minutes until onion is translucent. Add bacon and cook, stirring constantly, for about 3 minutes. Reduce heat to low.

In small bowl beat milk and eggs together. *Very slowly* pour egg mixture into saucepan, stirring constantly. Cook and stir over low heat until mixture thickens, about 2 to 3 minutes. Add pepper.

Check the pasta, which should by now be "al dente," or just tender. Drain pasta quickly, toss with sauce, sprinkle with parmesan, and serve.

SERVING SIZE: 4 Servings, 1 Heaping Cup Each

PER SERVING: Calories 300 **Fiber:** 5 grams **Sodium:** 435 mg.

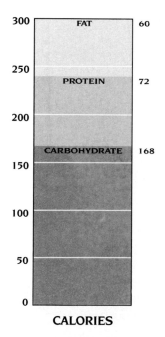

FAT	60
PROTEIN	72
CARBOHYDRATE	168

CALORIES

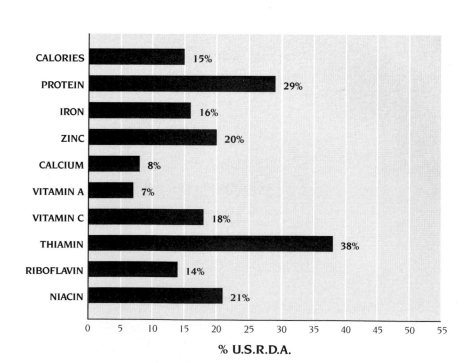

CALORIES 15%
PROTEIN 29%
IRON 16%
ZINC 20%
CALCIUM 8%
VITAMIN A 7%
VITAMIN C 18%
THIAMIN 38%
RIBOFLAVIN 14%
NIACIN 21%

% U.S.R.D.A.

VEGETARIAN SPAGHETTI

A full-flavored vegetarian pasta sauce for the gourmet palate. The lentils and pasta together make a complete protein. This sauce can also be served over polenta, gnocchi, rice, or any other grain to achieve the same high-protein quality.

INGREDIENTS

1 CUP LENTILS
1 BAY LEAF
2½ CUPS WATER
1 TABLESPOON OLIVE OIL
5-6 CLOVES GARLIC, MINCED
1 LARGE ONION, CHOPPED
2 STALKS CELERY, CHOPPED
1 LB. MUSHROOMS, 4 CUPS THICKLY SLICED

1 CUP WATER
3 CUPS TOMATO PUREE OR 1 CAN (1 LB., 12 OZ.) TOMATOES, PUREED
¼ CUP PARSLEY, CHOPPED
1 TEASPOON EACH OREGANO, MARJORAM, AND THYME
1 TEASPOON LIGHT SALT
1 LB. WHOLE GRAIN SPAGHETTI

DIRECTIONS

Sort and rinse lentils. Put them in a large pot with 2½ cups water and the bay leaf. Bring to boil, turn down heat, and simmer 30 minutes.

Heat the olive oil in a nonstick skillet. Add garlic and onion and sauté over medium heat for 5 to 10 minutes until onions are limp and translucent.

Add chopped celery and sliced mushrooms. Sauté 5 minutes more. Turn off heat, add 1 cup water to skillet to dissolve pan juices.

When lentils have simmered 30 minutes, add sau-

téed vegetables, tomato puree, parsley, herbs, and light salt.

Bring to a boil, then reduce heat and simmer, uncovered, for 1½ hours until sauce is reduced to desired consistency.

Ten minutes before serving, drop spaghetti into 4 quarts rapidly boiling water; cook 7 to 10 minutes, just until tender. Drain and serve immediately!

SERVING SIZE: ⅒ Recipe

PER SERVING: Calories 278   **Fiber:** 7 grams   **Sodium:** 215 mg.

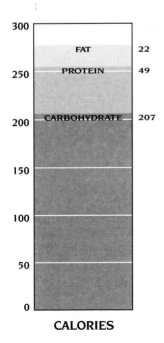

FAT	22
PROTEIN	49
CARBOHYDRATE	207

CALORIES

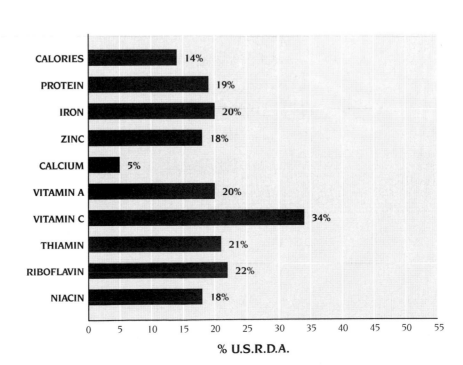

CALORIES 14%
PROTEIN 19%
IRON 20%
ZINC 18%
CALCIUM 5%
VITAMIN A 20%
VITAMIN C 34%
THIAMIN 21%
RIBOFLAVIN 22%
NIACIN 18%

% U.S.R.D.A.

PASTA AL PESTO

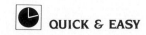 **QUICK & EASY**

Fresh basil is available only in the warm-weather months. When it's in season, we make pesto sauce and freeze it to enjoy during the winter.

INGREDIENTS

 2 TABLESPOONS OLIVE OIL
8-12 CLOVES GARLIC, MINCED
 1 OZ. PECANS, WALNUTS, OR PINE NUTS, ABOUT ¼ CUP FINELY CHOPPED
 1 LARGE BUNCH FRESH BASIL, 3-4 CUPS LEAVES, FIRMLY PACKED
 ½ LB. WHOLE WHEAT SPAGHETTI
 1 OZ. CHUNK PARMESAN CHEESE, ⅓ CUP GRATED

DIRECTIONS

In a large kettle bring 4 to 5 quarts water to a rolling boil.

Meanwhile, in a small, heavy skillet, gently heat oil with minced garlic and chopped nuts for 6 to 8 minutes, until garlic is barely golden. Remove from heat.

Wash basil. Pick leaves from stems. You should have 3 to 4 cups basil leaves. Chop the leaves into thin strips. Toss with oil and garlic in skillet, but do not heat until just before serving.

Grate the parmesan cheese.

Eight to 10 minutes before serving time, drop spaghetti into rapidly boiling water. Cook until just tender (al dente). Drain well. Toss with pesto sauce, sprinkle with parmesan, and serve.

SERVING SIZE: ⅙ Recipe

PER SERVING: Calories 264   **Fiber:** 4 grams   **Sodium:** 387 mg.

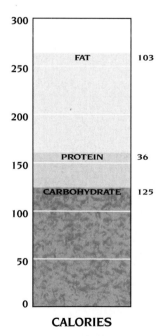

CALORIES

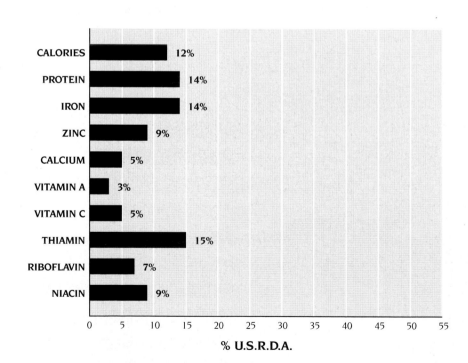

% U.S.R.D.A.

LINGUINE WITH CLAM SAUCE QUICK & EASY

Linguine is flat spaghetti, and linguine with clam sauce is a slice of heaven! The secret to success with this dish is timing. Our Italian friends have taught us that dinner is served when the pasta is done, so we've timed the directions rather precisely. If you wish your pasta "al dente" (Italian translation is "to the tooth," meaning the pasta retains some firmness and character), then use the minimum cooking times. This simple entree goes beautifully with Caesar Salad, a loaf of fresh bread, and a white Italian dinner wine. (Pictured on p. 203.)

INGREDIENTS

½ LB. WHOLE WHEAT OR WHITE LINGUINE
2 TEASPOONS LIGHT SALT
1 TABLESPOON OLIVE OIL
4 CLOVES GARLIC, MINCED
2 TABLESPOONS FRESH PARSLEY, CHOPPED

4 SMALL GREEN ONIONS, THINLY SLICED
1 CAN (10 OZ.) BABY CLAMS, LIQUID RESERVED
½ CUP DRY WHITE WINE
GRATED PARMESAN, ROMANO OR MITZETHRIA CHEESE FOR TOPPING

DIRECTIONS

In a large pot bring 4 quarts of water with 2 teaspoons light salt to a rolling boil.

If you are cooking whole grain linguine, allow 15 to 18 minutes cooking time; for white pasta allow 7 to 8 minutes cooking time. Pasta should be added to rapidly boiling water, cooked until just tender, drained, and served immediately with the sauce.

Sauté garlic in olive oil over low heat in a medium skillet, until golden, about 2 to 3 minutes. Set aside.

Prepare parsley and green onions. Drain the clams and reserve the juice.

Five minutes before serving time, add the clam juice and the wine to the garlic and oil. Heat for 4 minutes to blend flavors and reduce liquid to half of original volume.

Add clams, parsley, and green onions. Heat through.

Toss hot linguine with the sauce. Serve immediately, passing grated cheese on the side.

SERVING SIZE: ¼ Recipe

PER SERVING: Calories 300 **Fiber:** 5 grams **Sodium:** 585 mg.

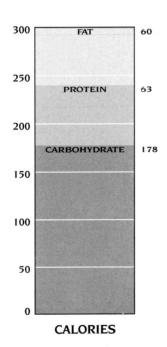

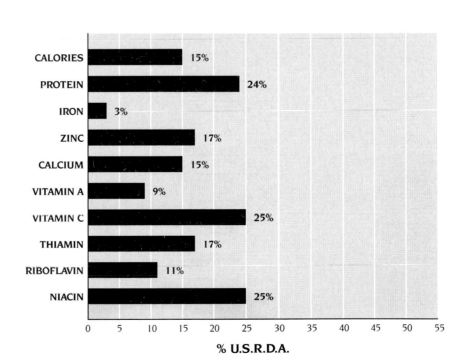

ZUCCHINI LINGUINE

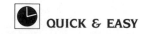 **QUICK & EASY**

Our hospitable friend, Lois Johansen, created this simple, perfectly delicious dish for unexpected guests, using the bounty of her husband's vegetable garden. It was such a hit that when winter came, she had to adapt the recipe to work with canned tomatoes! Take a tip from Lois—when vine-ripened tomatoes aren't available, you can use canned, simply cut back on added salt and cook off excess fluid. Lois insists, however, that freshly grated parmesan is mandatory year-round.

INGREDIENTS

- 1 TABLESPOON OLIVE OIL
- 1 ONION, CHOPPED
- 4-5 CLOVES GARLIC, FINELY CHOPPED
- 8 MEDIUM ZUCCHINI, 8 CUPS CUT IN HALF LENGTHWISE AND CHOPPED IN ¼-INCH SEGMENTS
- ¾ LB. LINGUINE

- 8 TOMATOES, PEELED AND CHOPPED, OR 1 CAN (1 LB. 12 OZ.)
- 1½ TEASPOON LIGHT SALT
  FRESHLY GROUND BLACK PEPPER
  FRESHLY GRATED PARMESAN CHEESE FOR TOPPING

DIRECTIONS

Heat oil in a large nonstick skillet. Add chopped garlic and onion and sauté over low heat until golden, 4 to 5 minutes.

Add sliced zucchini and sauté until tender, but not soggy, 20 to 30 minutes.

In a large saucepan, bring 4 to 5 quarts water to a rolling boil.

Ten minutes before serving time, add linguine, return to boil, and cook 8 to 12 minutes, just until al dente.

Add tomatoes to zucchini, season to taste with light salt and pepper. Heat through for 4 to 5 minutes.

Drain linguine and turn on to a large platter. Pour sauce over top and serve immediately.

Pass freshly grated parmesan.

SERVING SIZE: 8 Servings, 1 Cup Sauce and 1 Cup Pasta

PER SERVING: Calories: 245 **Fiber:** 11 grams **Sodium:** 215 mg.

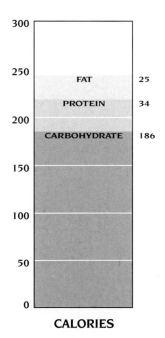

FAT	25
PROTEIN	34
CARBOHYDRATE	186

CALORIES

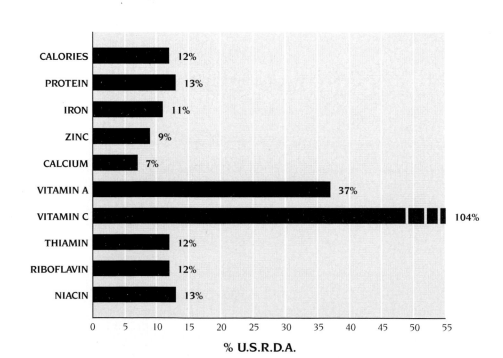

	% U.S.R.D.A.
CALORIES	12%
PROTEIN	13%
IRON	11%
ZINC	9%
CALCIUM	7%
VITAMIN A	37%
VITAMIN C	104%
THIAMIN	12%
RIBOFLAVIN	12%
NIACIN	13%

% U.S.R.D.A.

LASAGNA

Everybody loves lasagna, and no two cooks make it alike. The secret to a great lasagna is great sauce and lots of cheese.* If you are a purist, your sauce will start with vine-ripened tomatoes, imported Italian wood mushrooms, and fresh herbs from your window box. If you are "too busy to cook," you know that a wide selection of Italian sauces is available at the grocery store. Once the sauce is made or purchased, this lasagna can be prepared in 30 minutes and eaten an hour later. It freezes well, especially unbaked, so we suggest you double it and freeze one pan for a busy evening. (Disposable aluminum baking pans are nice for freezing, that way you don't take your favorite baking dish out of circulation.)

INGREDIENTS

½ LB. WHOLE WHEAT OR WHITE LASAGNA NOODLES
½ LB. GROUND ROUND OR EXTRA LEAN GROUND BEEF
1 MEDIUM ONION, DICED
2 CLOVES GARLIC, MINCED
1 BUNCH FRESH SPINACH, CHOPPED, COOKED, AND DRAINED, OR 1 PACKAGE (10 OZ.) FROZEN CHOPPED SPINACH, THAWED AND DRAINED
½ TEASPOON LIGHT SALT

⅛ TEASPOON BLACK PEPPER
2 EGGS, BEATEN
1 LB. DRY CURD COTTAGE CHEESE OR 1 LB. LOW-FAT RICOTTA
½ LB. FRESH MUSHROOMS, SLICED (2 CUPS), OR 1 CAN (8 OZ.), DRAINED
4 CUPS OF SPAGHETTI SAUCE, HOMEMADE OR CANNED
6 OZ. PART-SKIM MOZZARELLA CHEESE, 1½ CUPS GRATED
⅓ CUP PARMESAN CHEESE, GRATED PARMESAN FOR TOPPING

DIRECTIONS

Preheat oven to 350°

Bring 4 quarts water to full boil in a large pot. Slowly add lasagna noodles and stir *gently* to separate them. Boil for 10 to 15 minutes just until tender, but not mushy. Drain in a colander and rinse with cold water. Leave noodles in colander to drain.

Meanwhile, in a heavy skillet, brown meat over medium high heat for 6 to 8 minutes and drain off any fat.

Add onion, garlic, and mushrooms. Sauté for 5 minutes.

Add spinach, light salt, pepper, eggs, and cottage cheese (or ricotta). Stir to mix well and remove from heat.

Combine mozzarella and parmesan cheeses.

In a large flat 9-inch by 13-inch baking dish, assemble the lasagna from the bottom up in this order: a fourth of spaghetti sauce (about ¼-inch in bottom of dish), a single layer of noodles, half of meat-spinach-cheese mixture, half of mozzarella and parmesan, and half of mushrooms. Repeat. Cover with a fourth of the sauce and a third layer of noodles. End with a top layer of sauce.

Bake, uncovered, for 50 minutes. Let stand for 10 minutes before cutting. Cut into 12 pieces. Garnish with parmesan and serve.

SERVING SIZE: ¹⁄₁₂ Recipe

PER SERVING: Calories 232 **Fiber:** 3 grams **Sodium:** 678 mg.

*As for "lots of cheese," we solve the high-fat problem by using dry curd cottage cheese, which is made from skim milk. It looks just the way it sounds—like cottage cheese without the liquid. If it is not available in your area, use low-fat ricotta cheese instead and add 30 calories per serving.

Graph on p. 210

CARLA'S JAMBALAYA

INGREDIENTS

1½ CUPS UNCOOKED LONG GRAIN BROWN RICE
1 LB. HOT ITALIAN SAUSAGE
1 LARGE CLOVE GARLIC, MINCED
1 LARGE ONION, CHOPPED
1 RED OR GREEN BELL PEPPER, CHOPPED

2 CANS (1 LB. EACH) GREEN LIMA BEANS, RESERVE
½ CUP LIQUID
1 CAN (1 LB.) TOMATOES, RESERVE LIQUID
½ CUP HOT CATSUP
HOT PEPPER SAUCE FOR TOPPING (OPTIONAL)

DIRECTIONS

Cook, but do not overcook, the brown rice.

Remove sausage from casings and brown in a large kettle over medium heat for 15 to 20 minutes. Elevate one edge of pot to drain fat off meat. (You will remove about ⅓ cup fat.) Do not wash kettle.

When meat is browned and drained, crumble or chop it well or whirl it briefly in a processor. Set meat aside in a separate bowl.

Using the same kettle, sauté garlic, onion, and bell pepper over medium heat for 10 to 12 minutes until tender.

Add green lima beans along with ½ cup of their liquid. Discard remaining liquid.

Add canned tomatoes and their liquid and simmer, uncovered, for about 15 minutes.

Stir in catsup, cooked rice, and crumbled meat. Heat through and serve. For those who want a spicier dish, serve with hot pepper sauce on the side.

SERVING SIZE: 12 Servings, 1 Cup Each

PER SERVING: Calories 229 **Fiber:** 5 grams **Sodium:** 470 mg.

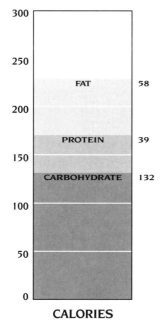

FAT	58
PROTEIN	39
CARBOHYDRATE	132

CALORIES

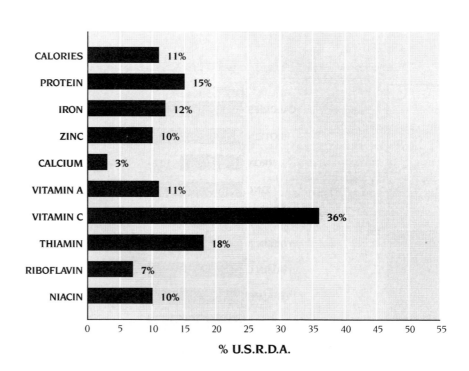

CALORIES 11%
PROTEIN 15%
IRON 12%
ZINC 10%
CALCIUM 3%
VITAMIN A 11%
VITAMIN C 36%
THIAMIN 18%
RIBOFLAVIN 7%
NIACIN 10%

% U.S.R.D.A.

SHRIMP JAMBALAYA

A wonderfully rich and spicy dish, shrimp jambalaya can be ordered by the bowlful in almost any cafe in New Orleans. Whether you visit Louisiana or not, you shouldn't miss this Cajun delight. For a spectacular "company" entree, use freshly steamed jumbo shrimp, arranging them on the rice mixture at the very last minute. A bowl of collard greens, some spicy red beans, and a basket of cornbread will round out your Cajun feast.

INGREDIENTS

1 LB. LOUISIANA HOT SMOKED SAUSAGE (BOUDIN) OR POLISH SAUSAGE (KIELBASA) AND RED PEPPER
2 LARGE ONIONS, CHOPPED
2 CLOVES GARLIC, MINCED
1 LARGE BELL PEPPER, CHOPPED
5 CUPS TOMATOES, PEELED AND DICED
2 TABLESPOONS WORCESTERSHIRE SAUCE

½ TEASPOON THYME
¼-½ TEASPOON CAYENNE PEPPER
LIGHT SALT (OPTIONAL)
4 CUPS COOKED BROWN RICE
3 CUPS COOKED FRESH SHRIMP (1½ LB.)
2 TABLESPOONS PARSLEY, CHOPPED, FOR GARNISH

DIRECTIONS

Cook brown rice.

Meanwhile, remove sausage from casing. Crumble it into a large saucepan, brown over medium heat for 10 to 12 minutes, and drain off fat. If you are using a cooked, smoked sausage like Polish, cut it into ½-inch cubes and brown. Drain fat.

Add onion, garlic, and bell pepper. Sauté for 10 to 12 minutes until tender, stirring occasionally.

Add tomatoes, Worcestershire, and thyme. Stir.

Add cayenne and light salt, if desired. Cover, turn heat to low, and simmer for 20 minutes to blend flavors.

Add cooked rice. Simmer uncovered for about 10 minutes until rice is hot and excess liquid has cooked off.

Add cooked shrimp and heat through. Garnish with chopped parsley and serve.

SERVING SIZE: ⅛ Recipe

PER SERVING: Calories 288   **Fiber:** 5 grams   **Sodium:** 746 mg.

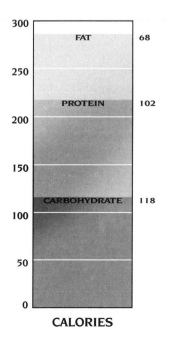

FAT 68
PROTEIN 102
CARBOHYDRATE 118

CALORIES

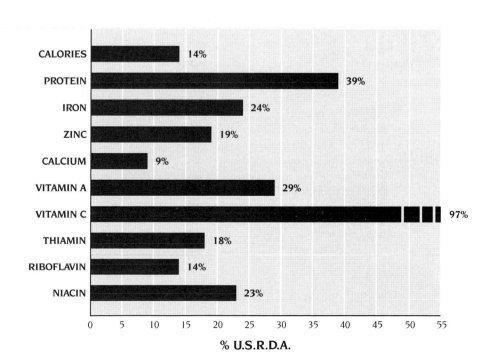

	% U.S.R.D.A.
CALORIES	14%
PROTEIN	39%
IRON	24%
ZINC	19%
CALCIUM	9%
VITAMIN A	29%
VITAMIN C	97%
THIAMIN	18%
RIBOFLAVIN	14%
NIACIN	23%

SPINACH RICE CASSEROLE 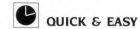 QUICK & EASY

INGREDIENTS

1 CUP BROWN RICE
3 CUPS WATER
1 EGG
1 TABLESPOON FLOUR
2 CUPS LOW-FAT COTTAGE CHEESE
1 PACKAGE (10 OZ.) FROZEN CHOPPED SPINACH,
  THAWED AND WELL DRAINED

¾ LB. MUSHROOMS, 3 CUPS QUARTERED OR SLICED
½ CUP ONION, CHOPPED
¼ CUP PARSLEY, CHOPPED
2 CLOVES GARLIC, MINCED
1½ TEASPOONS THYME
1 TEASPOON LIGHT SALT
2 TABLESPOONS GRATED PARMESAN CHEESE
2 TABLESPOONS SLICED ALMONDS

DIRECTIONS

Cook rice over low heat in 3 cups water until tender, about 45 minutes. Set aside.
Preheat oven to 375°.
In a large bowl, mix egg, flour, and cottage cheese. Stir in cooked rice, well-drained spinach,
  mushrooms, onion, parsley, garlic, thyme, and light salt. Mix well.
Pour mixture into a 13-inch by 9-inch baking dish which has been sprayed with nonstick
  cooking spray.
Sprinkle cheese and almonds over top. Bake, uncovered, for 30 minutes. Serve.

SERVING SIZE: 8 Servings, ¾ Cup Each

PER SERVING: Calories 190 **Fiber:** 5 grams **Sodium:** 420 mg.

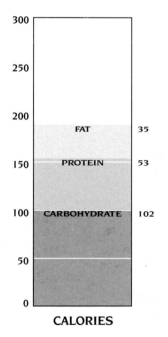

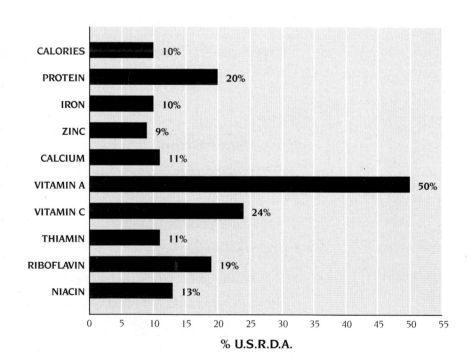

CRAB RICE SQUARES

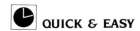 **QUICK & EASY**

INGREDIENTS

3 CUPS COOKED BROWN RICE
8 OZ. COOKED CRABMEAT
1 CUP NONFAT MILK
4 OZ. EXTRA SHARP CHEDDAR CHEESE, GRATED
3 EGGS, LIGHTLY BEATEN
¼ CUP PARSLEY, MINCED
½ CUP GREEN ONION TOPS, MINCED
1 RED BELL PEPPER, MINCED, OR 1 JAR (2 OZ.)
   CHOPPED PIMENTO
2 STALKS CELERY, MINCED

¼ TEASPOON WHITE OR BLACK PEPPER
2 TEASPOONS WORCESTERSHIRE SAUCE
½ TEASPOON OLIVE OIL

Orange Curry Sauce

1 CAN (10½ OZ.) CONDENSED CREAM OF CELERY
   SOUP
¼ CUP NONFAT MILK
¾ TEASPOON CURRY POWDER
¼ CUP FRESH ORANGE JUICE

DIRECTIONS

Cook the rice.

Preheat oven to 350°.

In a large bowl, mix together cooked brown rice, crabmeat, milk, cheese, eggs, parsley, onion
   tops, red bell pepper (or pimento), celery, pepper, and Worcestershire.

Grease a 9-inch by 13-inch baking dish with the ½ teaspoon olive oil and turn rice mixture
   into dish.

Bake for 45 minutes to 1 hour until casserole is set in the center.

Just before serving, prepare Orange Curry Sauce: In a medium saucepan, heat together the
   soup, milk, and curry powder, stirring constantly until mixture bubbles. Remove from heat.
   Stir in orange juice and serve immediately over crab rice squares.

VARIATION: Low-Sodium Crab Rice Squares. Cook rice without salt; use fresh crabmeat, low-
   sodium cheese, and low-sodium soup.

SERVING SIZE: ⅑ Recipe

PER SERVING: Calories 210   **Fiber:** 3 grams   **Sodium:** 672 mg.

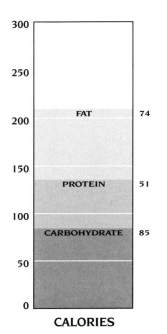

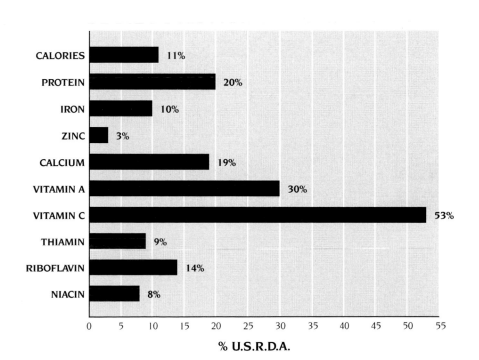

SHRIMP FRIED RICE

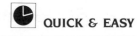 **QUICK & EASY**

Is this a side dish or entree? It's really just a matter of serving size. Paired with Oriental-style vegetables or Grand Egg Flower Soup, a steaming bowl of shrimp fried rice can be the main event. Add chopsticks, Chinese tea, and fortune cookies and turn this simple meal into a children's adventure.

INGREDIENTS

    1 TABLESPOON BACON FAT OR PEANUT OIL
    1 EGG
    2 TABLESPOONS SOY SAUCE
    3 CUPS COOKED BROWN RICE
    1 BUNCH GREEN ONIONS, 2 CUPS SLICED
    ¼ LB. MUSHROOMS, 1 CUP SLICED
    6 OZ. COOKED TINY SHRIMP, ABOUT ¾ CUP

DIRECTIONS

Cook the rice.
Heat oil in a large nonstick skillet.
Beat egg with soy sauce in a small bowl.
Pour egg into heated oil. Stir gently until egg is set.
Add cooked rice, green onions, and mushrooms. Stir-fry for 2 minutes over medium-high heat.
Add shrimp. Heat through and serve.

SERVING SIZE: 8 Servings, ½ Cup Each

PER SERVING: Calories 129   **Fiber:** 3 grams   **Sodium:** 430 mg.

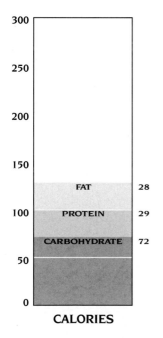

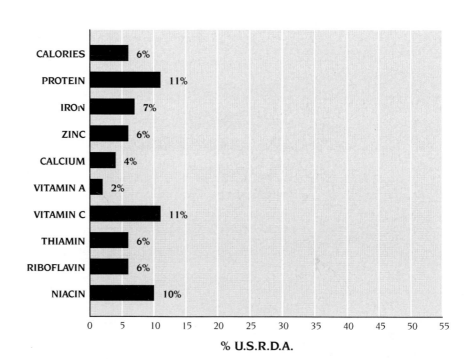

TOMATO RICE

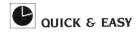 **QUICK & EASY**

INGREDIENTS

  1 CUP UNCOOKED LONG GRAIN BROWN RICE
1-2 ONIONS, CHOPPED
  1 TABLESPOON BUTTER
  3 LARGE TOMATOES, PEELED AND DICED
2½ CUPS CHICKEN BROTH*
⅛ TEASPOON BLACK PEPPER

DIRECTIONS

Brown rice and onions in butter in a large nonstick skillet for 5 to 10 minutes, stirring often.
Add remaining ingredients. Bring to a boil, cover, and simmer until liquid is absorbed and rice
   is tender, 1 to 1½ hours.† Serve.

SERVING SIZE: 4 Servings, 1 Cup Each

PER SERVING: Calories 248   **Fiber:** 7 grams   **Sodium:** 611 mg.

*To reduce sodium, substitute low-sodium broth (42 mg. sodium per serving).
†The acidity of the tomato juice tremendously increases the cooking time of rice.

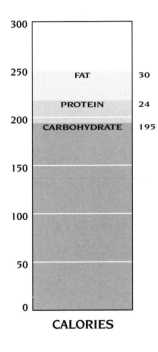

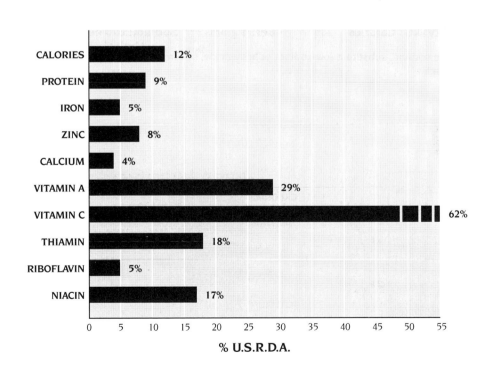

COUNTRY WHEAT PILAF

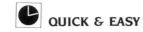 **QUICK & EASY**

Thirty minutes from start to finish, this dish entails about 5 minutes of actual work. Serve with carrots, coleslaw, and apple crisp; and for dinner in a serious hurry, baked apples and winter squash can be prepared in the microwave while the pilaf simmers.

INGREDIENTS

1 TABLESPOON BUTTER
½ CUP GREEN ONIONS, SLICED
2 CLOVES GARLIC, MINCED
1 BEEF BOUILLON CUBE DISSOLVED IN 3 CUPS WATER
1 TEASPOON OREGANO

⅛ TEASPOON BLACK PEPPER
1 CUP MEDIUM BULGAR WHEAT
8 OZ. COOKED TURKEY HAM, CUT IN BITE-SIZED PIECES
1 PACKAGE (10 OZ.) FROZEN GREEN BEANS

DIRECTIONS

Sauté green onions and garlic in butter over medium-high heat in a large nonstick skillet until tender, about 2 minutes.

Stir in 3 cups water with bouillon, oregano, and pepper.

Bring to a boil, stir in bulgar, and reduce heat. Cover and simmer 15 minutes.

Add turkey ham and green beans, cover, and simmer 10 minutes more until beans are heated through.

SERVING SIZE: 6 Servings, ¾ Cup Each

PER SERVING: Calories 247 **Fiber:** 6 grams **Sodium:** 529 mg.

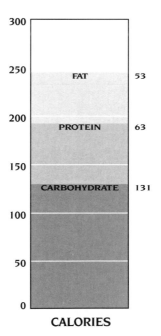

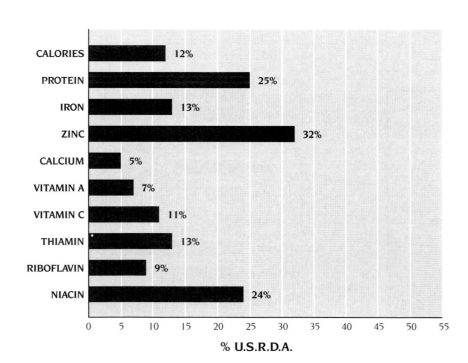

BLACK KASHA

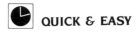 **QUICK & EASY**

Buckwheat—a dark, earthy, richly flavored grain. In Eastern Europe where both barley and buckwheat are common menu items, barley is called "white kasha," and buckwheat is called "black kasha." This buckwheat pilaf is the perfect accompaniment for wild game, roasted meat, or any similarly robust entree.

INGREDIENTS

    1 TABLESPOON OLIVE OIL
    2 LARGE ONIONS, DICED
    1 CUP BUCKWHEAT GROATS
    1 EGG
    2 CUPS BOILING WATER
    ½ TEASPOON LIGHT SALT

DIRECTIONS

Heat oil in large nonstick skillet. Add diced onions and sauté over medium heat until golden, about 15 minutes.

Mix buckwheat and egg together in a bowl.

Add buckwheat-egg mixture to onions and fry over high heat until dry and grains separate, about 2 to 3 minutes.

Add 2 cups boiling water and light salt. Cover and simmer about 30 minutes or until tender.

SERVING SIZE: 5 Servings, 1 Cup Each

PER SERVING: Calories 128   **Fiber:** 7 grams   **Sodium:** 126 mg.

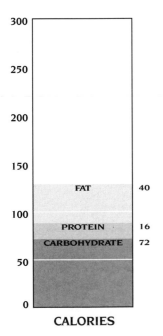

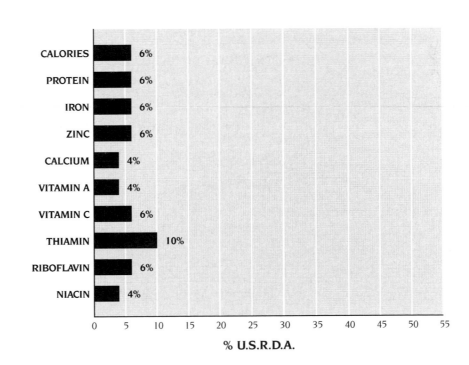

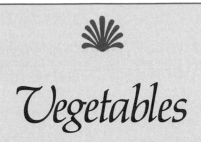

Vegetables

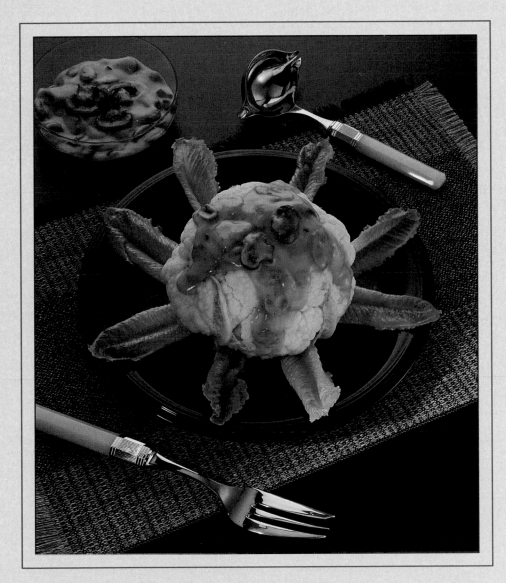

Cauliflower With Mushroom Cheese Sauce (p. 230)

When your mother's mother admonished, "Eat your greens, child!" she was handing down the knowledge that vegetables are critical to good nutrition. She may not have known that, along with fruits, they have the responsibility of providing ALL the vitamin C and most of the vitamin A in our diets. Scurvy, while one of the oldest diseases known, wasn't connected with nutrition until the 1700s, a time when men who signed onto sailing ships knew they had a 50% chance of dying from scurvy on a long voyage! It was not yet known that this dread disease resulted from the absence of fresh produce (thus, vitamin C) in the ships' provisions. In 1753, Dr. James Lind, a Scottish naval surgeon, discovered that citrus fruits cured scurvy, and in 1795 the British Navy began ordering its ships to add fresh limes to the sailors' provisions, thus earning them the nickname "limey's." Vitamin C itself wasn't identified until 1912.

A glance at the graphs included in this chapter will show the abundance of vitamin C in fresh vegetables, particularly those of the cabbage family—and the terrific vitamin A (carotene) content of dark green and yellow vegetables. Since nutrient profiles are so similar, portraying outstanding vitamin A and C content, graphs have been included for representative recipes only. While values for other nutrients appear low in contrast, notice that the calorie bar tends to be the lowest of all. Vegetables are so low in calories, the nutrient density (nutrients per calorie) is excellent, and the amounts of iron, zinc, calcium, and other "hard-to-get" nutrients provided by vegetables add significantly to the day's total. Soluble fiber content is another, more recently recognized, bonus for vegetable eaters. So "Eat your greens, child!"

STIR-FRY CABBAGE QUICK & EASY

INGREDIENTS

  2 TEASPOONS OIL (PEANUT OIL IS BEST)
  3 CUPS CABBAGE, SHREDDED
  1 CUP CELERY, CHOPPED
  1 ONION, THINLY SLICED
  ⅛ TEASPOON BLACK PEPPER
  1 TABLESPOON SOY SAUCE
    LIGHT SALT (OPTIONAL)

DIRECTIONS

Heat oil in a large skillet or a wok.
Add vegetables and cover tightly. Steam 5 minutes.
Season with pepper, soy sauce, and light salt, if desired.
Serve immediately!

SERVING SIZE: 4 Servings, 1 Cup Each

PER SERVING: Calories 64   **Fiber:** 4 grams   **Sodium:** 268 mg.

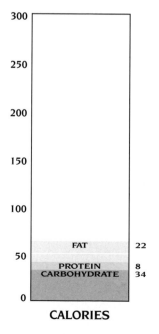

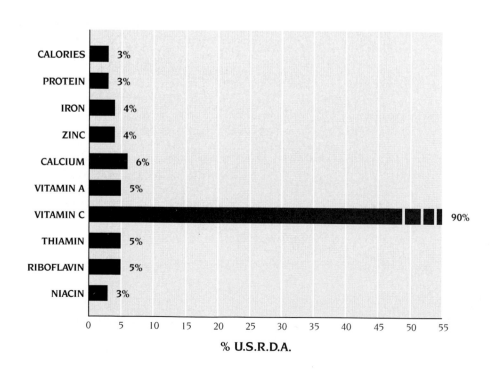

JAMAICAN CHOP SUEY

Our Jamaican friend, Faedeen Buchanan, followed her husband to California 4 years ago but still isn't sure it's okay to eat the food here. She cooks from her "back-home" recipes; and when you taste her chop suey, you'll know why. Don't be overwhelmed by the mountain of vegetables when you begin cooking. As Faedeen puts it, "they spring their own water and cook right down, you'll see."

INGREDIENTS

```
2 TABLESPOONS BUTTER
1½ TEASPOONS THYME
8 OZ. SMOKED TURKEY BREAST, CUT IN SMALL STRIPS
1 LARGE HEAD CABBAGE, SHREDDED
2 LARGE CARROTS, 3 CUPS SHREDDED
3 TOMATOES, DICED
1 MEDIUM ONION, CUT IN HALF AND THINLY SLICED
½ TEASPOON FRESHLY GROUND BLACK PEPPER
  LIGHT SALT TO TASTE
```

DIRECTIONS

Melt butter in a very large saucepan. Add thyme and turkey. Stir-fry over medium heat for 3 minutes.

Add cabbage, carrots, tomatoes, onion, and pepper. Toss to mix. Vegetables will cook down rapidly and reduce in volume.

Cover, turn heat to low, and simmer for 25 to 30 minutes, stirring occasionally. Vegetables will "spring their own water." Mixture becomes more tender with increased cooking time.

Season to taste with light salt, as desired.

SERVING SIZE: 10 Servings, 1 Cup Each

PER SERVING: Calories 112 **Fiber:** 7 grams **Sodium:** 403 mg.

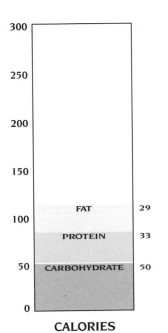

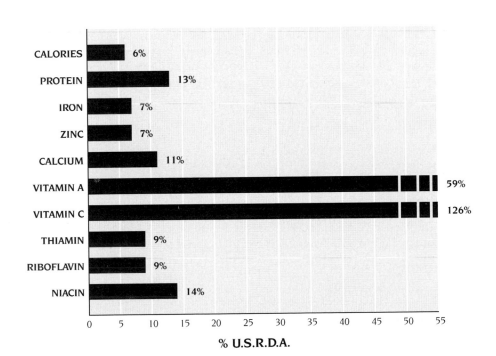

SWEET AND SOUR RED CABBAGE

QUICK & EASY

You'll welcome this addition to your list of great basics. It's quick and easy to make, teams up well with meat and potatoes, and is delicious!

INGREDIENTS

4 OZ. CANADIAN BACON, DICED
1 MEDIUM HEAD RED CABBAGE, QUARTERED, THEN SLICED OR CHOPPED
⅓ CUP VINEGAR

¼ CUP BROWN SUGAR
½ TEASPOON LIGHT SALT
¼ TEASPOON BLACK PEPPER

DIRECTIONS

Sauté diced Canadian bacon in a large saucepan over medium heat until crisp, 8 to 10 minutes. Remove bacon with slotted spoon, conserving any drippings or crispings left in the saucepan.

Add chopped cabbage to pan. Sauté over medium heat stirring frequently, for 5 to 10 minutes. Reduce heat, cover, and simmer in its own juices for 10 minutes more.

Add cooked bacon, vinegar, brown sugar, light salt, and pepper. Toss well. Cover and simmer about 15 minutes more or until cabbage is tender.

SERVING SIZE: ⅙ Recipe

PER SERVING: Calories 127 **Fiber:** 5 grams **Sodium:** 430 mg.

ORIENTAL CELERY AND ONIONS

QUICK & EASY

INGREDIENTS

3 SLICES LEAN BACON
1 LB. CELERY, CUT INTO 1-INCH PIECES
1 MEDIUM ONION, SLICED INTO RINGS

3 TABLESPOONS VINEGAR
1 TABLESPOON SUGAR
¼ TEASPOON BLACK PEPPER

DIRECTIONS

Fry bacon in a large nonstick skillet over medium heat until crisp, 6 to 8 minutes. Remove bacon and drain it on paper towels.

Remove all but 1 tablespoon bacon fat from skillet. Add celery and onion.

Sauté over medium heat for 5 minutes, stirring occasionally.

Reduce heat and cook, covered, for 12 to 15 minutes or until vegetables are crisp-tender.

Add vinegar, sugar, and pepper. Stir and heat through.

Put mixture in a serving dish, crumble bacon over the top, and serve.

SERVING SIZE: 6 Servings, 1 Cup Each

PER SERVING: Calories 86 **Fiber:** 3 grams **Sodium:** 147 mg.

STUFFED BAKED TOMATOES

An eye-catching side dish that you can serve with pride. For an especially fancy presentation, use a wedge-shaped garnish knife to create a zig-zag surface as you cut the tomatoes in half.

INGREDIENTS

3 LARGE FIRM TOMATOES
1½ TABLESPOONS FRESH PARSLEY, MINCED
½ TEASPOON DRIED BASIL, CRUSHED
¼ TEASPOON DRIED OREGANO
1 CLOVE GARLIC, MINCED

½ TEASPOON LIGHT SALT
FRESHLY GROUND BLACK PEPPER
3 TABLESPOONS PARMESAN CHEESE, GRATED
1½ SLICES WHOLE WHEAT BREAD, TOASTED AND CRUMBLED

DIRECTIONS

Preheat oven to 350°.

Slice tomatoes in half, crosswise. Scoop out pulp, leaving about ¼-inch of shell.

Place tomato pulp in a medium bowl. Break the pulp into small pieces with a spoon and combine it with parsley, basil, oregano, garlic, light salt, pepper, parmesan, and bread crumbs. Stir until thoroughly combined.

Spoon the filling into the tomato shells, dividing it evenly among the six shells.

Place in a shallow baking dish, about 2 inches apart.

Bake for 20 to 25 minutes. Serve hot.

SERVING SIZE: 6 Servings, 1 Stuffed Tomato Half Each

PER SERVING: Calories 52   **Fiber:** 1 gram   **Sodium:** 175 mg.

STEWED TOMATOES

 QUICK & EASY

Professional cooks know that stewed tomatoes are one of the few vegetables which appeal to almost everyone. Because this dish is juicy, crafty cooks began adding croutons to absorb the extra fluid. The little chunks of bread added such a pleasant flavor and texture contrast to the acidity of the tomatoes, they fast became an integral part of the recipe.

INGREDIENTS

4 LARGE RIPE TOMATOES, 4 CUPS, PEELED AND CUT UP
1 TEASPOON BUTTER
1 LARGE ONION, CHOPPED
1 CLOVE GARLIC, MINCED
½ LARGE BELL PEPPER, CHOPPED

½ TEASPOON LIGHT SALT
½ TEASPOON BASIL
1 TABLESPOON SUGAR
2 SLICES WHOLE WHEAT BREAD, TOASTED AND THEN CUBED
PARMESAN CHEESE FOR GARNISH (OPTIONAL)

Continued on p. 228.

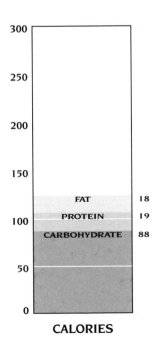

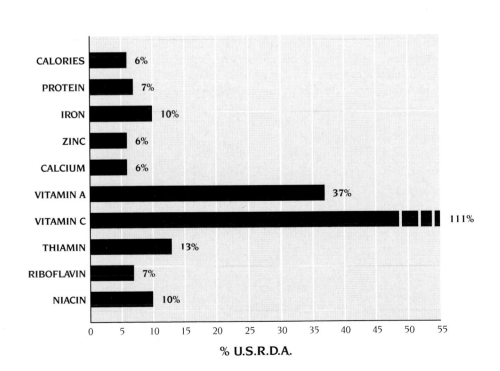

DIRECTIONS

Peel tomatoes and cut in 1-inch chunks or wedges.

Sauté onions and garlic over medium heat in butter in a large nonstick skillet for 12 to 15 minutes. When golden brown, add tomatoes, bell pepper, light salt, basil, and sugar. Mix well.

Simmer, uncovered, for 10 minutes over medium heat to blend flavors and partially reduce liquid.

Add croutons, stir, and serve immediately. Garnish with parmesan, if desired.

SERVING SIZE: 4 Servings, 1 Cup Each

PER SERVING: Calories 125   **Fiber:** 3 grams   **Sodium:** 251 mg.

BASIL CARROTS

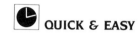 **QUICK & EASY**

A simple recipe—and one of our all-around favorites. On special occasions, substitute whole baby carrots and garnish with sprigs of fresh basil.

INGREDIENTS

5-6 MEDIUM CARROTS (1 LB.)
 2 TEASPOONS BUTTER
 3 TABLESPOONS FRESH BASIL, CHOPPED, OR
1½ TEASPOONS DRIED BASIL

1 TABLESPOON BROWN SUGAR
¼ TEASPOON LEMON RIND, GRATED (OPTIONAL)
 FRESHLY GROUND BLACK PEPPER
 LIGHT SALT TO TASTE

DIRECTIONS

Peel carrots. Slice into ¼-inch rounds.

Using a minimum amount of water, steam or boil sliced carrots for about 20 minutes, or just until tender. Drain or cook off any remaining fluid.

Add butter, basil, brown sugar, and lemon rind, if used.

When butter has melted, toss lightly and season to taste with pepper and light salt.

SERVING SIZE: ¼ Recipe

PER SERVING: Calories 86   **Fiber:** 3 grams   **Sodium:** 80 mg.

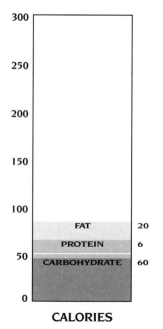

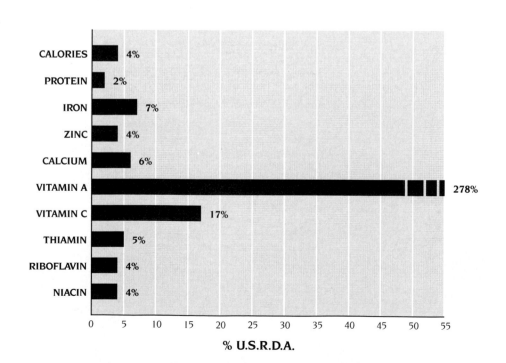

APPLESAUCE GLAZED CARROTS

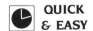 **QUICK & EASY**

INGREDIENTS

4 CUPS CARROTS, SLICED
2 TEASPOONS BUTTER

2 TABLESPOONS BROWN SUGAR
½ CUP UNSWEETENED APPLESAUCE

DIRECTIONS

Preheat oven to 350°.

Boil or steam carrots in a covered saucepan until tender, 15 to 20 minutes.

Combine butter, brown sugar, and applesauce in a small saucepan. Cook over low heat, stirring until the sugar is dissolved.

Turn cooked carrots into a flat baking dish and distribute applesauce mixture over the top.

Bake, uncovered, for 15 minutes or until heated through.

SERVING SIZE: 6 Servings, ⅔ Cup Each

PER SERVING: Calories 65   **Fiber:** 2 grams   **Sodium:** 46 mg.

SUMMER ZUCCHINI SAUTÉ

If you have ever had a vegetable garden—or a neighbor with a vegetable garden—you know that there are certain weeks when you can get your fill of zucchini and tomatoes! This tasty combination takes advantage of the summer bounty and also freezes beautifully.

INGREDIENTS

1 TABLESPOON OLIVE OIL
2 ONIONS, CHOPPED
4 CLOVES GARLIC, MINCED
4 MEDIUM ZUCCHINI, QUARTERED,
   THEN CUT IN ½-INCH SLICES

3 MEDIUM TOMATOES, PEELED AND CUT IN
   1-INCH CUBES
1 TEASPOON LIGHT SEASONED SALT*
1 TEASPOON OREGANO
   DASH BLACK PEPPER

Continued on p. 230.

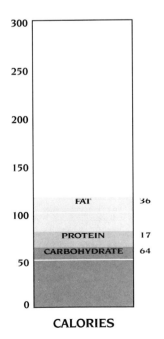

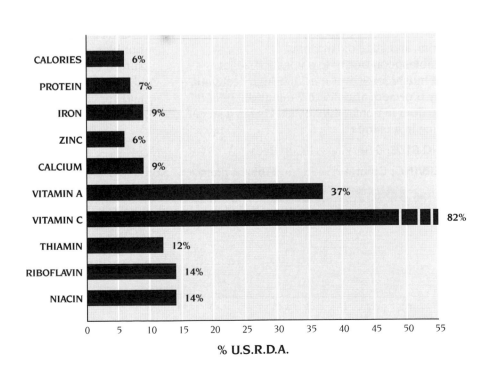

BROCCOLI MUSHROOM STIR-FRY

A harmonious blending of flavors, both subtle and distinct.

INGREDIENTS

1 LARGE ONION, THINLY SLICED
4 CLOVES GARLIC, MINCED
½ LB. MUSHROOMS, 2 CUPS SLICED
1 BUNCH BROCCOLI (1½ LB.)
3 TEASPOONS PEANUT OIL

2 TABLESPOONS SOY SAUCE
1 TABLESPOON SHERRY
2 TEASPOONS SUGAR
1 CAN (8 OZ.) WATER CHESTNUTS, SLICED
(OPTIONAL)

DIRECTIONS

Prepare onion, garlic, and mushrooms as directed above. Cut broccoli into florets; peel and slice the stems into ⅛-inch slices.

Heat 1 teaspoon oil in a nonstick skillet or wok. Stir-fry onion and garlic over high heat, until tender, about 3 to 4 minutes. Remove from skillet.

Heat remaining 2 teaspoons oil. Stir-fry broccoli for 1 minute, then cover and steam for 2 to 3 minutes more.

Combine soy sauce, sherry, and sugar. Add to wok along with mushrooms. Add water chestnuts, if used. Cover and steam 1 minute.

Add cooked onions and garlic. Toss and serve.

SERVING SUGGESTION: For a vegetarian entree, add slices of tofu along with the sauce and mushrooms.

SERVING SIZE: 6 Servings, 1 Cup Each

PER SERVING: Calories 84   **Fiber:** 3 grams   **Sodium:** 306 mg.

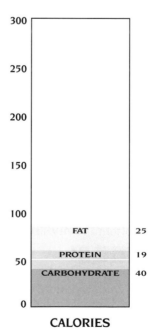

FAT	25
PROTEIN	19
CARBOHYDRATE	40

CALORIES

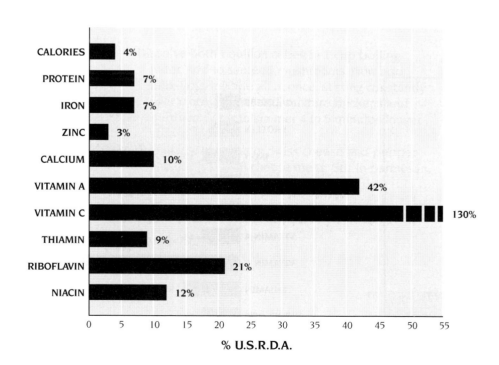

CALORIES 4%
PROTEIN 7%
IRON 7%
ZINC 3%
CALCIUM 10%
VITAMIN A 42%
VITAMIN C 130%
THIAMIN 9%
RIBOFLAVIN 21%
NIACIN 12%

% U.S.R.D.A.

BROCCOLI IN CHEESE CUSTARD

 QUICK & EASY

INGREDIENTS

1 BUNCH BROCCOLI (1½ LB.)
½ CUP SHARP CHEDDAR CHEESE, GRATED
3 EGGS
1½ CUPS NONFAT MILK
1 TEASPOON LIGHT SALT

BLACK PEPPER TO TASTE
¼ TEASPOON NUTMEG
2 TABLESPOONS DEHYDRATED ONION FLAKES (OPTIONAL)

DIRECTIONS

Preheat oven to 350°.

Peel stems of broccoli and cut broccoli into bite-sized pieces. Steam about 15 minutes until tender. Drain well.

Spray an 8-inch by 10-inch baking dish with non-stick cooking spray. Put broccoli into baking dish and sprinkle with cheese.

Beat eggs lightly in a bowl and stir in milk, light salt, pepper, nutmeg, and dehydrated onion, if used.

Pour egg mixture over the broccoli.

Set the baking dish into a large shallow baking pan. Fill the larger pan with hot water to come halfway up sides of baking dish.

Bake, uncovered, for 45 to 60 minutes until custard is set.

SERVING SIZE: 6 Servings, ⅔ Cup Each

PER SERVING: Calories 125   **Fiber:** 2 grams   **Sodium:** 323 mg.

UKOY (PHILIPPINE VEGETABLE FRITTERS)

Ukoy are vegetable fritters sold by street vendors in the Philippine Islands. Shredded squash, bean sprouts, and green onions are encased in an egg batter and fried. The patties stay moist and tasty as the shredded vegetables release steam during cooking. Traditional ukoy hold a large cooked shrimp in the center and are served with a garlic-spiked vinegar dipping sauce.

INGREDIENTS

1 CUP WHOLE WHEAT PASTRY FLOUR
½ TEASPOON LIGHT SALT
½ TEASPOON WHITE PEPPER
1 LARGE EGG
1 CUP WATER
2 CUPS BUTTERNUT SQUASH OR YAMS (10 OZ.) SHREDDED
1 CUP FRESH BEAN SPROUTS

4 GREEN ONIONS, CUT IN FINE JULIENNE STRIPS 2 INCHES LONG
2 TABLESPOONS PEANUT OIL

Filipino Dipping Sauce

½ CUP DISTILLED WHITE VINEGAR
1 OR 2 CLOVES GARLIC, CRUSHED
¼ TEASPOON LIGHT SALT
1 TEASPOON FRESH PARSLEY, FINELY MINCED

DIRECTIONS

Combine all ingredients for dipping sauce. Cover and chill.

Combine flour, light salt, and pepper in a large mixing bowl.

Beat egg well in a small bowl. Add water and beat again.

Add egg and water to flour mixture and beat until blended and most lumps are gone.

Add squash, sprouts, and onions. Stir lightly but thoroughly.

Heat 1 tablespoon peanut oil in a nonstick skillet over medium heat. Spoon half the batter into pan, forming five patties. Do not crowd pan. Flatten patties slightly with spoon. Fry about 3 minutes on each side until golden brown.

Repeat process using the other tablespoon oil and remaining batter.

Drain on paper towels. Serve with dipping sauce.

VARIATION: Shrimp Ukoy: Have 10 large cooked shrimp ready. Position 5 shrimp in heated skillet, spooning batter over each to form 5 patties. Repeat.

SERVING SIZE: 10 Servings, 1 Patty Each

PER SERVING: Calories 101   **Fiber:** 3 grams   **Sodium:** 90 mg.

POTATO CAKES

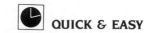 **QUICK & EASY**

So there's a little bowl of leftover mashed potatoes in the refrigerator—not enough to serve the whole family but too much to throw away? Time to make potato cakes! Seasoned with mushrooms, onions, and parsley and strengthened with cracker crumbs and eggs; your dab of potatoes becomes a satisfying side-dish for six or a light entree for three! Serve with a dollop of plain yogurt and a sprig of parsley. This is a nice side dish to accompany fish.

INGREDIENTS

3 TEASPOONS BUTTER
½ LB. MUSHROOMS, 2 CUPS SLICED, OR 1 CAN (8 OZ.), DRAINED
1 SMALL ONION, DICED
1 CUP MASHED POTATOES
2 EGGS (OR 4 EGG WHITES TO REDUCE CHOLESTEROL)

½ CUP WHOLE WHEAT CRACKER CRUMBS
¼ CUP FRESH PARSLEY, CHOPPED
½ TEASPOON LIGHT SALT
BLACK PEPPER TO TASTE
PLAIN YOGURT FOR GARNISH (OPTIONAL)
PARSLEY SPRIGS FOR GARNISH (OPTIONAL)

DIRECTIONS

Using 1 teaspoon butter, sauté onions and mushrooms in a large nonstick skillet over medium heat until golden, about 15 minutes.

Combine mashed potatoes, eggs, cracker crumbs, parsley, light salt and pepper in a medium bowl.

Add the sautéed vegetables to the potato mixture and stir.

In the same skillet, heat 1 teaspoon more butter. Using a large spoon, drop the potato mixture into the hot fat, forming three patties.

Cook over low heat until bottoms are golden brown, 5 to 6 minutes. Turn and brown other side. Repeat for three remaining patties, using the last teaspoon butter.

Garnish and serve.

SERVING SIZE: 6 Servings, 1 Patty Each

PER SERVING: Calories 114   **Fiber:** 3 grams   **Sodium:** 184 mg.

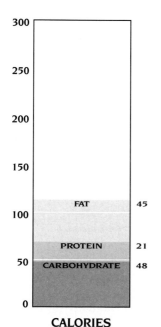

FAT	45
PROTEIN	21
CARBOHYDRATE	48

CALORIES

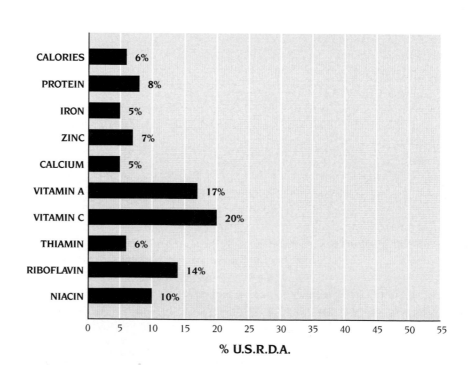

	% U.S.R.D.A.
CALORIES	6%
PROTEIN	8%
IRON	5%
ZINC	7%
CALCIUM	5%
VITAMIN A	17%
VITAMIN C	20%
THIAMIN	6%
RIBOFLAVIN	14%
NIACIN	10%

% U.S.R.D.A.

SWEET POTATO CASSEROLE

INGREDIENTS

- 2 MEDIUM WHITE POTATOES, PEELED AND CUT INTO 1-INCH CHUNKS
- 1 LARGE SWEET POTATO, PEELED AND CUT INTO 1-INCH CHUNKS
- 6 MEDIUM CARROTS, PEELED AND CUT INTO ½-INCH SLICES

- 2 TABLESPOONS BUTTER
- ¼ CUP HONEY
- 1 TEASPOON LEMON RIND
- 2-3 TABLESPOONS LEMON JUICE
  DASH NUTMEG
  LIGHT SALT (OPTIONAL)

DIRECTIONS

Preheat oven to 350°.

Place white potatoes, sweet potatoes, and carrots in a saucepan and add water to cover. Bring to a boil, cover, and cook 15 to 20 minutes until just tender. Reserve 2 tablespoons cooking liquid, then drain thoroughly.

Melt butter in measuring cup or small saucepan. Stir in honey, lemon rind, lemon juice, and nutmeg. Add the 2 tablespoons reserved cooking liquid. Add light salt, if desired.

Place drained vegetables in a 2-quart baking dish. Drizzle sauce over vegetables, turning to distribute evenly.

Bake uncovered for 30 to 35 minutes.

SERVING SIZE: 6 Servings, 1 Cup Each

PER SERVING: Calories 178 **Fiber:** 4 grams **Sodium:** 75 mg.

EGGPLANT CREOLE

INGREDIENTS

- 1 MEDIUM EGGPLANT (1½ LB.), PEELED AND CUBED
- 2 QUARTS WATER
- 2 TEASPOON LIGHT SALT
- 1½ TABLESPOONS BUTTER
- 1 TABLESPOON FLOUR
- 3 LARGE TOMATOES, 2 CUPS CHOPPED

- 1 BELL PEPPER, CHOPPED
- 1 ONION, CHOPPED
- ½ TEASPOON LIGHT SALT
- 1 TABLESPOON FRESH PARSLEY, CHOPPED
- 2 CLOVES GARLIC, MINCED
- ½ CUP DRY WHOLE WHEAT BREAD CRUMBS (2 SLICES BREAD)

DIRECTIONS

Preheat oven to 350°.

Peel eggplant and cut it into ½-inch cubes.

Heat 2 quarts water and 2 teaspoons light salt to boiling in a large saucepan. Add eggplant cubes. Bring back to boiling and cook, uncovered, for 10 minutes. Drain well and turn into a 1½-quart casserole dish.

Melt butter in skillet over low heat and blend in flour. Stir for 30 seconds.

Add tomatoes, bell pepper, onion, light salt, parsley, and garlic. Sauté over medium heat for 10 minutes.

Pour vegetable mixture over eggplant and sprinkle with bread crumbs.

Bake for 30 minutes, uncovered.

SERVING SUGGESTIONS: Serve as a side dish or spoon over a bed of brown rice or whole wheat pasta for a vegetarian entree. If you have a bit left over, it even makes a tasty omelet filling.

SERVING SIZE: 6 Servings, ½ Cup Each

PER SERVING: Calories 106 **Fiber:** 5 grams **Sodium:** 172 mg.

Breads, Muffins, Pancakes & Waffles

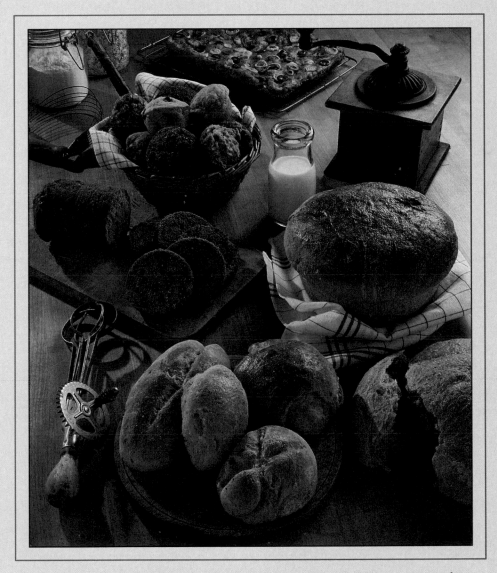

(Clockwise, from top) Foccacia (p. 257), Renee's Oatmeal Bread (p. 249), Apple Cider Bread (p. 250), Potato Chive Bread (p. 251), Molasses Raisin Bread (p. 245), Blueberry Muffins (p. 240), Oatmeal Berry Muffins (p. 239), Blue-Ribbon Bran Muffins (p. 238), Orange Carrot Muffins (p. 241)

ABOUT WHOLE WHEAT FLOUR

Two types of whole wheat flour are used in these recipes, whole wheat flour and whole wheat pastry flour. Both are ground from 100% whole wheat, but the pastry flour is more finely milled and is lower in gluten. Gluten is the wheat protein which develops with kneading and allows the dough to rise. Therefore a higher-protein flour, such as spring hard wheat flour, is best for raised breads while whole wheat pastry flour, ground from soft white wheat, is better for cakes, muffins, and cookies, where a tender crumb is desired. If you can't obtain whole wheat pastry flour through your natural foods store, substitute two parts finely milled regular whole wheat flour plus one part white pastry flour.

Whole grain breads are excellent sources of complex carbohydrate, which is the most desirable energy source for fueling muscle activity. Whole grain breads also provide significant amounts of dietary fiber, protein, B vitamins, and iron. Nutrient profiles are so similar, we've included only representative graphs for muffins, raised breads, quick breads, and pancakes/waffles.

BLUE-RIBBON BRAN MUFFINS QUICK & EASY

This may look like the most basic of muffin recipes. But it's more. We tested at least 30 variations of this recipe to identify the optimal amount of each ingredient. The results? A simple, practically foolproof formula for high-fiber, low-fat baking at its best. (Pictured on p. 237.)

INGREDIENTS

1½ CUPS RAW (UNPROCESSED) BRAN
1¼ CUPS WHOLE WHEAT PASTRY FLOUR
1½ TEASPOON BAKING SODA
¾ TEASPOON LIGHT SALT
2½ TEASPOONS CINNAMON
¼ TEASPOON CLOVES
¼ TEASPOON NUTMEG

½ CUP RAISINS OR CHOPPED PRUNES
⅓ CUP BROWN SUGAR
¼ CUP DARK MOLASSES
3 TABLESPOONS OIL
1 EGG
1 CUP NONFAT MILK

DIRECTIONS

Preheat oven to 400°
Combine bran, flour, baking soda, light salt, cinnamon, cloves, nutmeg, and raisins in a large
    bowl. Mix thoroughly to distribute spices evenly.
Beat brown sugar, molasses, oil, egg, and milk in a small bowl.
Add wet ingredients to dry and stir only until ingredients are moistened. Batter will be thick
    and somewhat lumpy.
Fill 18 nonstick or paper-lined muffin tins about two-thirds full of batter.
Bake for 15 to 18 minutes until toothpick comes out clean.

SERVING SIZE: 18 Servings, 1 Muffin Each

PER SERVING: Calories 94   **Fiber:** 2 grams   **Sodium:** 127 mg.

ANITA'S OATMEAL MUFFINS 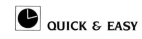 QUICK & EASY

INGREDIENTS

1 CUP WHOLE WHEAT PASTRY FLOUR
¼ CUP SUGAR
1 TABLESPOON BAKING POWDER
1 TEASPOON LIGHT SALT
¾ CUP ROLLED OATS
2 TEASPOONS CINNAMON

½ TEASPOON NUTMEG
¼ TEASPOON CLOVES
1 CUP NONFAT MILK
1 EGG
2 TABLESPOONS OIL

DIRECTIONS

Preheat oven to 400°.

Blend together flour, sugar, baking powder, light salt, oats, cinnamon, nutmeg, and cloves in a medium bowl.

Combine milk, egg, and oil in a separate bowl and add all at once to dry ingredients. Stir just until moistened. Batter will be lumpy.

Spoon into muffin tins which have been lined with cupcake papers or sprayed with nonstick cooking spray.

Bake for 20 to 25 minutes.

VARIATION: Fruited Oatmeal Muffins. Add ½ cup chopped raisins, dates, or nuts to dry ingredients.

Oil-Free Muffins. If muffins will be eaten immediately, oil can be omitted entirely (subtract 20 calories per muffin).

SERVING SIZE: 12 Servings, 1 Muffin Each

PER SERVING: Calories 105 **Fiber:** 1 gram **Sodium:** 163 mg.

OATMEAL BERRY MUFFINS 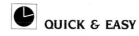 QUICK & EASY

INGREDIENTS

1½ CUPS WHOLE WHEAT PASTRY FLOUR
  1 CUP ROLLED OATS
  ½ CUP PACKED BROWN SUGAR
  2 TEASPOONS BAKING POWDER
  1 TEASPOON BAKING SODA
  1 CUP FRESH OR FROZEN BERRIES, PARTIALLY THAWED (RASPBERRIES, BLUEBERRIES, CRANBERRIES, OR STRAWBERRIES ARE ALL GOOD)
  2 EGGS
  ⅔ CUP BUTTERMILK OR SOUR SKIM MILK*
  2 TABLESPOONS OIL

DIRECTIONS

Preheat oven to 400°.

Mix flour, oats, sugar, baking powder and baking soda in a large bowl. Add berries and gently stir to coat.

Beat eggs with fork in a small bowl. Add buttermilk and oil. Beat until smooth.

Pour into flour mixture and stir just until blended.

Fill 12 large or 18 average muffin cups two-thirds full. Use nonstick muffin tins or spray with nonstick cooking spray. (Using paper liners is not recommended for this recipe because muffins may stick.)

Bake for 15 to 25 minutes until a toothpick inserted in the center comes out clean.

SERVING SIZE: 12 Large or 18 Average Servings, 1 Large Muffin Each

PER SERVING: Calories 156 **Fiber:** 3 grams **Sodium:** 135 mg.

*To sour milk, add 2 teaspoons vinegar or lemon juice to ⅔ cup nonfat milk. Let stand 5 minutes.

BLUEBERRY MUFFINS

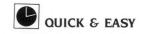 **QUICK & EASY**

Hot, sweet, and aromatic! You can serve these muffins 30 minutes from now— 10 minutes to mix up the batter and 20 minutes to bake. (Pictured on p. 237.)

INGREDIENTS

2 CUPS WHOLE WHEAT PASTRY FLOUR
⅓ CUP SUGAR
1 TABLESPOON BAKING POWDER
½ TEASPOON LIGHT SALT
⅛ TEASPOON CARDAMOM (OPTIONAL)
1 EGG

1 CUP PLUS 2 TABLESPOONS NONFAT MILK
3 TABLESPOONS OIL
1 TEASPOON VANILLA
1 TEASPOON GRATED LEMON RIND (OPTIONAL)
1 CUP FRESH OR FROZEN BLUEBERRIES

DIRECTIONS

Preheat oven to 400°. Spray a 12-muffin tin with nonstick cooking spray.

Thoroughly blend flour, sugar, baking powder, light salt, and cardamom if used in a large bowl.

Beat egg with a fork in a small mixing bowl. Add milk, oil, vanilla, and lemon rind, if used.

Add wet mixture to dry all at once. Stir just until flour is moistened. Batter should be thick and lumpy. Gently stir in blueberries.

Fill prepared muffin tins three-fourths full.

Bake for 20 to 25 minutes until tops are golden brown.

VARIATION: Yogurt Blueberry Muffins. Change the quantities of baking powder and milk, then proceed as above. Use:

2 TEASPOONS BAKING POWDER
¾ TEASPOON SODA

¾ CUP NONFAT PLAIN YOGURT
½ CUP NONFAT MILK

SERVING SIZE: 12 Servings, 1 Muffin Each

PER SERVING: Calories 142   **Fiber:** 2 grams   **Sodium:** 148 mg.

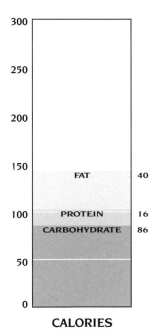

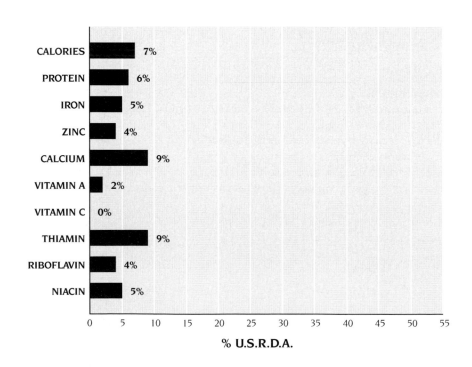

ORANGE CARROT MUFFINS 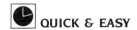 QUICK & EASY

INGREDIENTS

½ CUP NONFAT DRY MILK POWDER
3¼ CUPS WHOLE WHEAT PASTRY FLOUR
3 TEASPOONS BAKING POWDER
½ TEASPOON BAKING SODA
½ TEASPOON LIGHT SALT
1 TEASPOON CINNAMON
¼ TEASPOON NUTMEG
¼ TEASPOON CARDAMOM OR CLOVES
½ TEASPOON ALLSPICE

1 CAN (6 OZ.) FROZEN ORANGE JUICE
  CONCENTRATE
½ CUP HONEY
⅓ CUP OIL
1 TEASPOON ORANGE PEEL, GRATED
½ CUP PLAIN NONFAT YOGURT
1 MEDIUM CARROT, 1 CUP GRATED
4 EGGS
1 TEASPOON VANILLA

DIRECTIONS

Preheat oven to 400°

Combine milk powder, flour, baking powder, baking soda, light salt, and spices in a medium
  bowl. Mix well with pastry blender or wire whisk.

Mix orange juice concentrate, honey, oil, orange peel, yogurt, carrot, eggs, and vanilla in a large
  bowl.

Add dry ingredients to wet, stirring just until combined.

Spoon batter into nonstick muffin tins or use paper liners. Fill cups ⅔ full.

Bake for 15 to 20 minutes until golden.

SERVING SIZE: 24 Servings, 1 Muffin Each

PER SERVING: Calories 143   **Fiber:** 2 grams   **Sodium:** 125 mg.

BANANA WALNUT MUFFINS 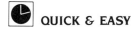 QUICK & EASY

INGREDIENTS

½ CUP WALNUTS
1 CUP WHOLE WHEAT PASTRY FLOUR
1½ CUPS RAW (UNPROCESSED) BRAN
2 TEASPOONS CINNAMON
¼ TEASPOON NUTMEG
¼ TEASPOON CLOVES
½ TEASPOON BAKING POWDER

1½ TEASPOONS BAKING SODA
½ TEASPOON LIGHT SALT
4 RIPE BANANAS (2 CUPS), MASHED
2 EGGS
¼ CUP DARK MOLASSES
½ CUP BUTTERMILK
½ CUP RAISINS

DIRECTIONS

Preheat oven to 375°

Put walnuts, flour, bran, spices, baking powder, baking soda, and light salt in a blender or food
  processor and blend until nuts are ground.

Mash bananas in a large bowl. Add eggs, molasses, and buttermilk. Mix well.

Add dry ingredients to wet, stir just until moistened. Fold in raisins.

Fill nonstick muffin tins, two-thirds full. (Since this batter is sticky, even nonstick muffin cups
  should be sprayed with nonstick cooking spray.)

Bake for 15 to 18 minutes.

SERVING SIZE: 18 Servings, 1 Muffin Each

PER SERVING: Calories 95   **Fiber:** 3 grams   **Sodium:** 98 mg.

OAT BRAN MUFFINS

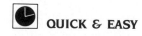 **QUICK & EASY**

INGREDIENTS

2¼ CUPS OAT BRAN CEREAL*
¼ CUP FIRMLY PACKED BROWN SUGAR
1 TABLESPOON BAKING POWDER
½ TEASPOON SALT (OPTIONAL)
¾ CUP NONFAT MILK
½ CUP EGG SUBSTITUTE OR 2 EGGS, BEATEN
¼ CUP HONEY OR MOLASSES
2 TABLESPOONS VEGETABLE OIL
¼ CUP CHOPPED NUTS (OPTIONAL)
¼ CUP RAISINS (OPTIONAL)

DIRECTIONS

Preheat oven to 425°
Combine cereal, brown sugar, baking powder, and salt, if used.
Add milk, egg substitute or eggs, honey, and oil. Mix just until dry ingredients are moistened.
Stir in nuts or raisins, if used.
Grease bottoms only of 12 medium-sized muffin cups or line with paper baking cups.
Fill prepared muffin cups three-fourths full.
Bake for 15 to 17 minutes or until deep golden brown.

PER SERVING: Basic Recipe: Calories 140 **Fiber:** 2 grams **Sodium:** 126 mg.
Variation: Calories 125 **Fiber:** 3 grams **Sodium:** 122 mg.

VARIATION: Applesauce Oat Bran Muffins:
Reduce milk to ½ cup.   Add 1½ cups unsweetened applesauce.
Substitute 2 egg whites for the 2 eggs.   Extend baking time to 25 minutes
Omit honey.

SERVING SIZE: 12 Servings, 1 Muffin Each

*Oat Bran cereal is also available generically. Recipe courtesy of The Quaker Oats Co.

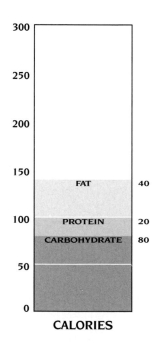

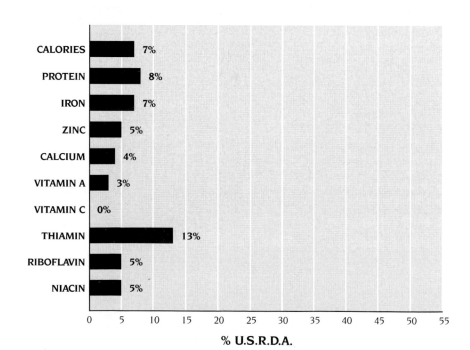

COUNTRY CORNBREAD

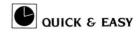 **QUICK & EASY**

INGREDIENTS

- 1 CUP WHOLE GRAIN CORNMEAL
- 1 CUP WHOLE WHEAT PASTRY FLOUR
- 2 TABLESPOONS SUGAR
- 1 TABLESPOON BAKING POWDER
- 1 TEASPOON BAKING SODA
- 1 TEASPOON LIGHT SALT
- 2 EGGS
- 1 CUP NONFAT MILK
- 2 TABLESPOONS CORN OIL

DIRECTIONS

Preheat oven to 400°

Combine corn meal, flour, sugar, baking powder, baking soda, and light salt in a large bowl. Mix well.

Combine eggs, milk, and oil in a small bowl. Mix lightly and pour into dry mixture all at once. Stir only until moistened.

Pour into an 8-inch-square baking dish which has been sprayed with nonstick cooking spray or fill 12 nonstick muffin cups two-thirds full.

Bake bread for 20 to 25 minutes, muffins for 15 minutes.

SERVING SIZE: 12 Servings, 1 Piece or 1 Muffin Each

PER SERVING: Calories 117   **Fiber:** 2 grams   **Sodium:** 283 mg.

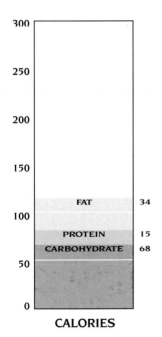

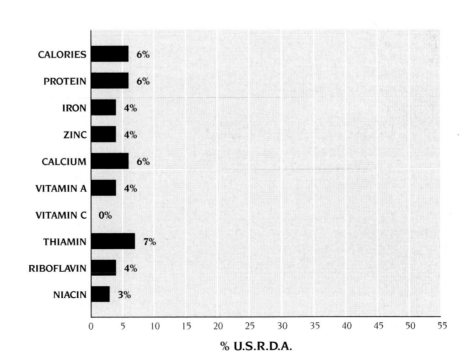

GREEN CHILE CORNBREAD QUICK & EASY

A dense all-corn bread, with added texture and flavor from green chiles and whole-kernel corn—a natural with a bowl of beans or chili.

INGREDIENTS

2¼ CUPS WHOLE GRAIN CORN MEAL
¾ TEASPOON BAKING POWDER
½ TEASPOON BAKING SODA
¼ TEASPOON LIGHT SALT
1½ TABLESPOONS SUGAR

3 EGGS
1½ CUPS BUTTERMILK
¼ CUP GREEN CHILES (2 OZ.), DICED (CANNED OR ROASTED)
1 CUP WHOLE-KERNEL CORN
2 TEASPOONS VEGETABLE OIL

DIRECTIONS

Preheat oven to 350°.
Combine thoroughly corn meal, baking powder, baking soda, light salt, and sugar in a large bowl.
Break up the whole-kernel corn by chopping it a bit or by whirling very briefly in a processor.

Take care not to overprocess, or kernels will lose their texture.
Add eggs, buttermilk, chiles, and corn to dry ingredients. Mix well.
Spread oil in a 9-inch, deep-dish pie pan or an 8-inch square baking dish. Pour batter over oil.
Bake for 30 to 35 minutes or until golden brown.

SERVING SIZE: 12 Servings, 1 Piece Each

PER SERVING: Calories 137   **Fiber:** 4 grams   **Sodium:** 146 mg.

COUNTRY WHOLE WHEAT BISCUITS QUICK & EASY

Biscuits, the most basic of quick breads, are judged by their lightness, flakiness, and buttery flavor. The difference between a prize-winning biscuit and a failure lies in technique. A light hand, a deft wrist, and a midwestern heritage all have been credited as the secrets to success; but—just between us—flakiness begins with layers of butter, and lightness comes from white flour.

Good whole wheat biscuits, like good whole wheat bread, will have a denser texture than white ones. The proportion of white to whole grain flour that you choose will depend on how much of a traditionalist you are about biscuits. Happily, flakiness and butteriness can be achieved with much less fat than is usually called for—and yes, technique does make the difference!

INGREDIENTS

2 CUPS WHOLE WHEAT PASTRY FLOUR OR 1 CUP UNBLEACHED WHITE FLOUR AND 1 CUP WHOLE WHEAT PASTRY FLOUR
1 TEASPOON BAKING SODA
1 TABLESPOON BAKING POWDER
¼ TEASPOON LIGHT SALT

2 TEASPOONS SUGAR
2 TABLESPOONS BUTTER
¾ CUP PLUS 2 TABLESPOONS BUTTERMILK OR 1 CUP NONFAT PLAIN YOGURT
MILK FOR GLAZE (OPTIONAL)

DIRECTIONS

Heat oven to 450°.
In a large bowl combine flour, baking soda, baking powder, light salt, and sugar.
With a pastry blender or two knives, cut in butter until butter bits are the size of split peas.
Add buttermilk or yogurt and stir quickly with a fork just until dough clings together. Dough should be stiff but sticky. If it's too dry, add milk, 1 tablespoon at a time, until dough is sticky.

With floured hands knead dough 10 to 15 times on a lightly floured surface. Then roll dough out to a ½-inch thickness.
Cut dough with a biscuit cutter or the rim of a glass dipped in flour. Place biscuits on an ungreased baking sheet. Brush tops with milk to glaze, if desired.
Bake for 10 to 12 minutes.

SERVING SIZE: 12 Servings, 1 Biscuit Each

PER SERVING: Calories 97   **Fiber:** 2 grams   **Sodium:** 238 mg.

MOLASSES RAISIN BREAD 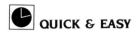 QUICK & EASY

A dark, rich, full-flavored quick bread—reminiscent of steamed Boston brown bread—it's ideal with baked beans, but also very nice for breakfast. Try it toasted with a mild low-fat cheese and crisp apple slices. (Pictured on p. 237.)

INGREDIENTS

¾ TEASPOON BAKING SODA
2 TABLESPOONS HOT WATER
⅔ CUP DARK MOLASSES (NOT BLACKSTRAP)
1 EGG
1 CUP NONFAT MILK

3 CUPS WHOLE WHEAT PASTRY FLOUR,
   2 TABLESPOONS RESERVED
2 TEASPOONS BAKING POWDER
1 TEASPOON LIGHT SALT
1 CUP RAISINS

DIRECTIONS

Preheat oven to 325°.

Dissolve baking soda in 2 tablespoons hot water in large bowl.

Add molasses and egg. Stir well.

Add milk slowly, stirring constantly.

Mix flour (save out 2 tablespoons to dust raisins), baking powder, and light salt in a small bowl.

Add dry ingredients to wet ingredients. Stir well.

Dredge raisins in 2 tablespoons reserved flour. Add raisins to mix.

Pour into 9-inch by 5-inch by 3-inch loaf pan which has been sprayed with nonstick cooking spray. The pan will be almost full. For an interesting presentation, bake the batter in 2 greased 24-oz. cans, as shown in the photograph.

Bake for 1 hour until a knife inserted in the center comes out clean.

SERVING SIZE: 16 Servings, 1 Slice Each

PER SERVING: Calories 140   **Fiber:** 3 grams   **Sodium:** 176 mg.

LEMONY BANANA LOAF 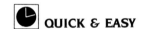 QUICK & EASY

More a cake than a bread, it's rich and delicately fruity. The fresh aroma of lemon lends distinction to the sweetness of bananas. Densely textured and easy to slice, this is a lovely tea loaf.

INGREDIENTS

1 TABLESPOON LEMON PEEL, GRATED
4 MEDIUM RIPE BANANAS, 2 CUPS MASHED
½ CUP HONEY
4 EGG WHITES
¼ CUP VEGETABLE OIL
1½ TEASPOONS VANILLA

¼ CUP WALNUTS
1⅔ CUPS WHOLE WHEAT PASTRY FLOUR
⅓ CUP RAW (UNPROCESSED) BRAN
1 TEASPOON BAKING SODA
½ TEASPOON LIGHT SALT
¼ TEASPOON NUTMEG

DIRECTIONS

Preheat oven to 375°.

Grate lemon peel.

Blend bananas, honey, egg whites, oil, and vanilla with lemon peel in food processor or blender, until smooth.

Add walnuts and blend for just a few seconds until nuts are finely chopped.

Combine flour, bran, baking soda, light salt, and nutmeg in large mixing bowl.

Add wet ingredients to dry, stirring just until moistened.

Turn batter into a 9-inch by 5-inch by 3-inch loaf pan sprayed with nonstick cooking spray.

Bake for 45 to 50 minutes or until a toothpick inserted in the center comes out clean.

SERVING SIZE: 16 Servings, 1 Slice Each

PER SERVING: Calories 145   **Fiber:** 2 grams   **Sodium:** 99 mg.

Breads-Muffins-Pancakes-Waffles

SHREDDED VEGETABLE BREAD

QUICK & EASY

This moist, spicy loaf bakes up nicely when made with any vegetable or fruit that will shred. Carrots, zucchini, yellow squash, apples, yams, and pears all work well.

INGREDIENTS

2 CUPS WHOLE WHEAT PASTRY FLOUR
2 TEASPOONS BAKING POWDER
½ TEASPOON BAKING SODA
½ TEASPOON LIGHT SALT
2 TEASPOONS CINNAMON

⅔ CUP FRUIT JUICE OR BUTTERMILK
3 EGGS
¼ CUP PEANUT OIL
½ CUP SUGAR
3 CUPS CARROTS OR VEGETABLES OR FRUIT, SHREDDED

DIRECTIONS

Preheat oven to 350°.

Mix flour, baking powder, baking soda, light salt, and cinnamon in a large bowl.

Combine juice or buttermilk, eggs, oil, and sugar in a medium bowl or blender.

Add wet to dry ingredients. Stir just until moistened. Fold in shredded vegetables.

Pour into a 9-inch by 5-inch by 3-inch loaf pan which has been sprayed with nonstick cooking spray. Bake for 55 to 65 minutes until knife inserted in center comes out clean.

SERVING SIZE: 16 Servings, 1 Slice Each

PER SERVING: Calories 130 **Fiber:** 2 grams **Sodium:** 134 mg.

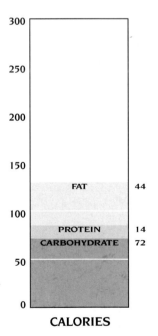

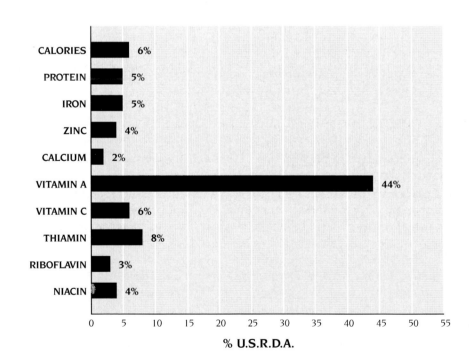

KAREN MINER'S BREAD

As owner of Grass Roots Natural Foods in South Lake Tahoe, California, Karen Miner developed a wide variety of irresistible recipes. Fast food addicts and health nuts alike would crowd into the small, homey bakery to buy bread, cookies, muffins, and pies. Karen was kind enough to share with us one of her most popular bread recipes and her secrets to successful whole grain bread baking. Karen recommends the use of high-protein, whole wheat spring flour because the rising qualities and tenderness of this flour are superior. She also varies this bread by adding "goodies" to the recipe.

INGREDIENTS

2 CUPS HOT WATER (105° TO 115°)
¼ CUP HONEY
1½ TABLESPOONS ACTIVE DRY YEAST

½ TABLESPOON LIGHT SALT
3 TABLESPOONS OIL
5½-6½ CUPS WHOLE WHEAT FLOUR

DIRECTIONS

Put hot water, honey, and yeast in a large bowl. Stir and let sit a few minutes until mixture starts to bubble.

Mix in light salt, oil, and 3 cups flour. This thin batter is called the sponge and should be beaten thoroughly (150 strokes) until it begins to look slightly stringy. This develops the gluten that will hold the bread up once it rises. At this point, stirring will become very difficult, and you can begin working in the final 2½-3½ cups of flour by hand. Add the last cups of flour in ½-cup increments, working in each addition before adding more. You will know to stop adding flour when it no longer works easily into dough.

When dough is smooth and not sticky, place it in a greased bowl, cover with a damp towel, and put in a warm place (80° to 105°)—near the stove or on a sunny window sill—to rise until it doubles in size, about 1 hour.

When dough is doubled in size, place it on a lightly floured surface and knead for 10 minutes until it is smooth, elastic, and not sticky.

Preheat oven to 350°.

Spray two loaf pans (9-inch by 5-inch by 3-inch) with nonstick cooking spray. Divide kneaded dough in half and shape into two smooth loaves. Place loaves in pans. Cover and let rise again in a warm place for 15 to 25 minutes until dough has risen to tops of loaf pans.

Bake at 350° for 45 minutes to 1 hour until golden brown and hollow-sounding when you "thump" them. Remove from pans and let cool for about an hour.

VARIATIONS: Add up to ½ cup of any mixture of nuts and seeds—favorites are pumpkin, sunflower, sesame, alfalfa, poppy, and flax.

Add ¼-½ cup of cracked or whole grains such as a nine-grain cereal, millet, or cracked wheat for a wonderful crunchiness.

Replace a portion of the whole wheat flour with a variety of flours (rye, buckwheat, soy, sunflower meal, or bran). To do this, subtract an equal amount of whole wheat flour. Don't replace more than one-fourth of the total flour volume or the bread won't rise. You can compensate for the addition of extra-heavy items by adding ¼-½ cup gluten flour. This adds height and lightness to any bread.

Substitute molasses, rice syrup, raisin syrup, maple syrup, or any combination of sweeteners for a taste treat.

After the loaves are shaped, dip tops of bread in water and then dip into sesame or poppy seeds.

Karen's favorite bread uses molasses for a sweetener, ½ cup bran, and is rolled in sesame seeds.

SERVING SIZE: 32 Servings, 1 Slice Each

PER SERVING: Calories 96   **Fiber:** 2 grams   **Sodium:** 53 mg.

SESAME MILLET BREAD

Hearty, rich and crunchy, this bread is slightly higher in calories than plain whole wheat bread because of the sesame seeds—but these nutritious seeds give the bread a nutty flavor that can't be matched.

INGREDIENTS

3 CUPS WARM WATER (105° TO 115°)
2 PACKAGES ACTIVE DRY YEAST
½ CUP HONEY
1 CUP NONFAT DRY MILK POWDER
    OR 3.2 OZ. ENVELOPE INSTANT
4 TEASPOONS LIGHT SALT

2 CUPS UNBLEACHED WHITE FLOUR
6 CUPS WHOLE WHEAT FLOUR, DIVIDED
1 CUP SESAME SEEDS, GROUND IN BLENDER OR
    PROCESSOR, OR 1 CUP SESAME MEAL
2 CUPS MILLET, CRACKED IN BLENDER
    OR PROCESSOR

DIRECTIONS

Dissolve yeast in warm water in a large bowl.

Add honey, dry milk, and light salt. Stir.

Stir in 2 cups white and 2 cups whole wheat flour to form a thick batter. Beat 150 strokes.

Cover bowl with a damp cloth, let rise in a warm place (80° to 105°) for 1 hour.

Stir in ground sesame seeds, cracked millet, and 2 more cups whole wheat flour. Stir in additional flour in small increments just until dough pulls away from the sides of the bowl.

Knead dough on a floured board for 10 to 15 minutes until smooth, using more flour, as needed, to keep dough from sticking to the board.

Shape dough into a ball; place in a greased bowl, turning dough to grease top. Cover and let rise again in a warm place for 50 minutes or until doubled in bulk.

Punch down. Let rise again until doubled—about 40 minutes.

Preheat oven to 350°.

Shape dough into three loaves and place in greased 9-inch by 5-inch by 3-inch loaf pans.

Let rise 20 to 40 minutes until dough reaches tops of pans.

Bake at 350° for 40 to 45 minutes.

SERVING SIZE: 48 Servings, 1 Slice Each

PER SERVING: Calories 113   **Fiber:** 3 grams   **Sodium:** 103 mg.

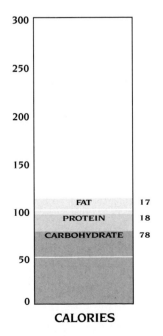

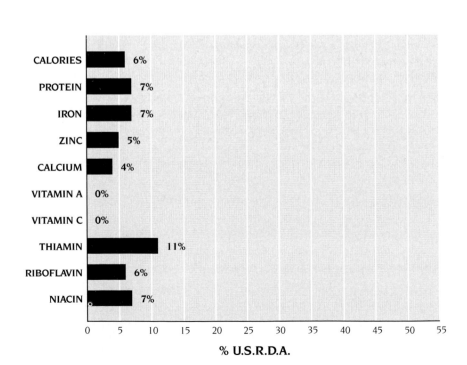

RENEE'S OATMEAL BREAD

Renee Fisher's oatmeal bread is so delicious that she is asked to bake her secret recipe every time the church has a dinner, the office has a party, or the club has a bake sale. The day she found herself agreeing to bake 48 loaves for yet another worthy cause she wondered if some secrets are really worth keeping. As it turned out, her dilemma was solved shortly thereafter. She was asked to do a baking demonstration on TV—so she decided to let *everyone* in on the secret! Thanks, Renee. (Pictured on p. 237.)

INGREDIENTS

4 CUPS WATER
2 CUPS QUICK-COOKING OATMEAL
6 TABLESPOONS HONEY
2 TABLESPOONS LIGHT SALT
1 CUP LUKEWARM WATER (105° TO 115°)

2 PACKAGES ACTIVE DRY YEAST
8 CUPS WHOLE WHEAT FLOUR, DIVIDED
3 CUPS WHITE FLOUR
2 TABLESPOONS BUTTER

DIRECTIONS

Bring 4 cups of water to a boil in a medium saucepan. Add oatmeal and cook for 1 minute, stirring constantly.

Turn into a very large bowl. Add honey and light salt. Mix and allow to cool to lukewarm.

Dissolve yeast in 1 cup lukewarm water. Add to oatmeal mixture with 4 cups of the whole wheat flour. Beat vigorously for 100 strokes.

Cover bowl with a damp towel, set in a warm place (80° to 105°) and let rise for about 50 minutes until light and spongy.

Gradually beat in the remaining 4 cups of whole wheat flour to form a dough that is stiff enough to handle.

Turn dough out onto kneading surface covered with white flour. Knead in enough of the 3 cups of white flour to form a dough that is smooth and elastic.

Use 1 tablespoon butter to grease a large bowl and the other tablespoon to grease 3 loaf pans (9-inch by 5-inch by 3-inch).

Shape dough into a ball; place in greased bowl, turning dough to grease top. Cover again with a damp towel and set in a warm place to rise for about an hour until doubled in size.

Punch down. Divide into three equal parts. Form each part into a loaf by stretching it into a 6-inch by 12-inch oval and then rolling into a 6-inch loaf. Place loaves in prepared pans.

Cover pans and let rise again for 30 to 45 minutes until doubled in size and almost to tops of loaf pans.

Preheat oven to 400°.

Bake loaves for 15 minutes at 400°. Reduce heat to 350° and bake 30 to 40 minutes longer until loaves are well browned and sound hollow when tapped.

Remove from pans and cool on wire racks.

SERVING SIZE: 48 Servings, 1 Slice Each

PER SERVING: Calories 113 **Fiber:** 2 grams **Sodium:** 144 mg.

Graph on p. 250

Renee's Oatmeal Bread (p. 249)

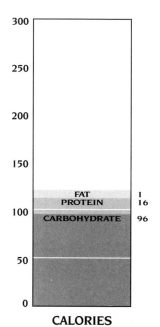

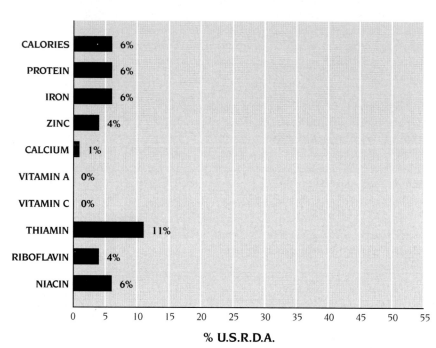

APPLE CIDER BREAD

This recipe is a gift from Waldie Evans, one of the world's first and finest natural food cooks. Waldie makes her own apple cider and lets it begin fermenting by leaving it at room temperature for 48 hours. This sparkling cider is the secret ingredient that earned Waldie a blue ribbon for this recipe at the El Dorado County Fair. If you don't have a cider press, don't worry—this bread turns out beautifully with bottled juice, as well. (Pictured on p. 237.)

INGREDIENTS

3 CUPS SPARKLING APPLE JUICE OR CIDER
2 PACKAGES OR 2 TABLESPOONS DRY YEAST
1 EGG

1½ TEASPOONS LIGHT SALT
1 TABLESPOON OIL
4-4½ CUPS WHOLE WHEAT FLOUR

DIRECTIONS

Make "sponge" by combining cider, yeast, egg, light salt, oil, and 1 cup flour in a large bowl. Beat 150 strokes to blend. Let stand 20 minutes in a warm place until light and foamy.

Stir down sponge, add 2 more cups flour, beating with a wooden spoon or electric mixer until soft dough is formed.

Turn onto floured surface; knead lightly, adding flour as needed (1 to 1½ cups) to prevent sticking. Continue kneading dough until it is smooth and elastic, 5 to 10 minutes.

Shape dough into a ball; place in a greased bowl, turning to oil top. Cover with a damp cloth and

let rise in a warm place (80° to 105°) until dough has doubled in size, 30 to 60 minutes.

Cut dough ball in half and knead each half lightly with oiled hands. Form two loaves and place in two greased 9-inch by 5-inch by 3-inch loaf pans.

Preheat oven to 350°.

Let rise until dough reaches top of pan, 20 to 30 minutes.

Bake for 30 minutes or until light golden brown. Cool on wire racks.

VARIATION: Substitute ½ cup gluten flour for ½ cup of whole wheat flour in the sponge. The added gluten will make a dough that's easier to handle.

SERVING SIZE: 32 Servings, 1 Slice Each

PER SERVING: Calories 69   **Fiber:** 2 grams   **Sodium:** 54 mg.

POTATO CHIVE BREAD

INGREDIENTS

½ LB. POTATOES, 1¾ CUPS PEELED AND CUBED
2 CUPS NONFAT MILK
3 TABLESPOONS BUTTER
¼ CUP SUGAR
1 TABLESPOON LIGHT SALT

1 PACKAGE ACTIVE DRY YEAST
4 CUPS WHOLE WHEAT PASTRY FLOUR
1 CUP UNBLEACHED WHITE FLOUR
⅓ CUP SNIPPED CHIVES OR THINLY SLICED GREEN ONION TOPS

DIRECTIONS

Boil potatoes in water to cover until tender, 20 to 25 minutes. Drain well, place in a large mixing bowl, and mash.

Combine milk, 2 tablespoons butter, sugar, and light salt in a small heavy saucepan. Heat to just below boiling. Pour over potatoes in the mixing bowl and beat until smooth. Cool to 105° to 115°, or until mixture feels warm to the fingertips, but not hot.

Sprinkle yeast over mixture, then stir in. Add 2 cups whole wheat flour. With electric mixer or wooden spoon, beat dough for 4 to 5 minutes. Stir in remaining 2 cups whole wheat flour to make a soft dough.

Sprinkle kneading surface with some of the white flour. Turn out dough and knead until smooth and elastic, about 10 to 12 minutes. Work in more of the white flour as needed.

Use 1 teaspoon of the remaining butter to grease the bread bowl. Shape dough into a ball and place in the greased bowl, turning to coat the entire surface. Cover bowl with towel. Let dough rise in a warm place (80° to 105°) until it doubles in bulk, about 1½ hours.

Return dough to kneading surface, sprinkle with chives or green onions, punch down, and knead until smooth, about 1 to 2 minutes.

Replace in bowl, cover with towel, and let rise again until doubled, about 1 hour.

Use remaining 2 teaspoons butter to grease two loaf pans (9-inch by 5-inch by 3-inch) or 2 round (1½ quart) casserole dishes. Divide dough in half, shape into two loaves, place in prepared pans.

Cover pans with towel, let dough rise until it reaches the tops of the loaf pans, or doubles in size, about 45 minutes.

Preheat oven to 375°. Bake loaves for 30 to 35 minutes until they are golden brown and sound hollow when tapped. Cool on wire racks.

VARIATION: Individual Potato Loaves. Omit chives. Divide dough into six portions. Shape into potato-like miniloaves. Place on a buttered cookie sheet. Cover with towel. Let rise until doubled. Bake for 25 to 30 minutes at 375°.

SERVING SIZE: 32 Servings, 1 Slice Each

PER SERVING: Calories 91   **Fiber:** 2 grams   **Sodium:** 124 mg.

CLEAR CONSCIENCE WAFFLES 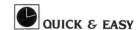 QUICK & EASY

INGREDIENTS

2¼ CUPS WHOLE WHEAT PASTRY FLOUR
4 TEASPOONS BAKING POWDER
½ TEASPOON LIGHT SALT
2 EGG WHITES
1 EGG YOLK
2¼ CUPS NONFAT MILK
1 TABLESPOON OIL

DIRECTIONS

In a medium bowl, mix flour, baking powder, and light salt until thoroughly combined.

In small bowl or blender, beat egg whites, yolk, milk, and oil.

Add wet ingredients to dry. Stir just until mixed. Batter will be lumpy.

Spoon onto waffle iron. Use a nonstick waffle iron or spray with nonstick cooking spray.

SERVING SUGGESTIONS: Serve waffles with pureed fresh fruits or thawed frozen fruits. Low fat yogurt or cinnamon-sugar make good toppings, too.

SERVING SIZE: 6 Servings, 1 Large or 4 Small Waffles Each

PER SERVING: Calories 220 **Fiber:** 4 grams **Sodium:** 350 mg.

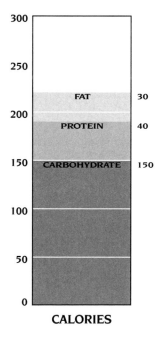

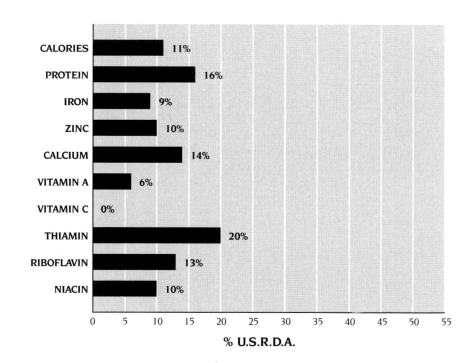

FRENCH TOAST FOR TWO 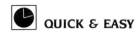 QUICK & EASY

INGREDIENTS

2 EGGS*
½ CUP NONFAT MILK
⅛ TEASPOON LIGHT SALT
½ TEASPOON VANILLA

PINCH CARDAMOM OR NUTMEG
4 SLICES WHOLE WHEAT BREAD
2 TEASPOONS BUTTER

DIRECTIONS

Combine eggs, milk, light salt, vanilla, and spices in a blender or small bowl. Beat well.

Pour half the mixture into a large, flat baking dish. Lay bread in dish and pour remaining mixture over top.

Allow to sit 5 to 10 minutes until egg mixture is completely absorbed by bread.

Melt butter in a large nonstick skillet. Add bread and cook over medium heat for about 5 minutes per side until golden brown and puffy.

SERVING SUGGESTIONS: Top with fresh fruit and vanilla yogurt or ricotta cheese mixed with honey. Maple syrup and butter are great, too, for children, athletes, and any others who aren't worried about calories.

SERVING SIZE: 2 Servings, 2 Slices Each

PER SERVING: Calories 250   **Fiber:** 3 grams   **Sodium:** 444 mg.

*If you are concerned about cholesterol, simply substitute 3 egg whites for the 2 whole eggs.

ORANGE WHOLE WHEAT PANCAKES QUICK & EASY

Dollar pancakes—plump, round, and golden. Try them with smooth Orange-Yogurt Topping.

INGREDIENTS

2 CUPS WHOLE WHEAT PASTRY FLOUR
½ TEASPOON BAKING SODA
½ TEASPOON LIGHT SALT
1½ CUPS ORANGE JUICE
2 EGGS
2 TABLESPOONS MELTED BUTTER OR OIL

Orange Yogurt Topping*

1 CUP NONFAT PLAIN YOGURT
2 TABLESPOONS FROZEN ORANGE JUICE CONCENTRATE, THAWED
½ TEASPOON VANILLA
SWEETENER (OPTIONAL)

DIRECTIONS

Sift flour, baking soda, and light salt together in a measuring cup or bowl.

Blend orange juice, eggs, and 1 tablespoon melted butter or oil in a large bowl.

Add dry ingredients. Beat just until blended.

Heat remaining butter or oil, 1 teaspoonful at a time, in a large nonstick skillet.

Drop thick batter by rounded tablespoonfuls to make "dollar" pancakes.

Fry over medium heat until bubbles burst and bottoms are golden brown, about 2 to 3 minutes.

Flip pancakes and brown other side. Makes about 24 dollar pancakes.

To make Orange Yogurt Topping: Mix yogurt with orange juice concentrate and vanilla. Taste and sweeten, if desired.

SERVING SIZE: 6 Servings, 4 Pancakes Each

PER SERVING: Calories 208   **Fiber:** 4 grams   **Sodium:** 222 mg.

*Not calculated into recipe totals.

OATMEAL RAISIN PANCAKES

The first step of this recipe takes place the night before, so plan ahead.

INGREDIENTS

2 CUPS ROLLED OATS
2 CUPS LOWFAT BUTTERMILK
2 EGGS, LIGHTLY BEATEN
½ CUP RAISINS
⅛ TEASPOON ALMOND EXTRACT (OPTIONAL)
½ CUP WHOLE WHEAT PASTRY FLOUR

2 TABLESPOONS BROWN SUGAR OR HONEY
1 TEASPOON BAKING POWDER
1 TEASPOON BAKING SODA
½ TEASPOON CINNAMON
¼ TEASPOON LIGHT SALT
1-2 TEASPOONS BUTTER FOR FRYING

DIRECTIONS

In a large bowl combine oats and buttermilk. Cover and refrigerate until the next day.

Add lightly beaten eggs, raisins, and almond extract, if used.

In another bowl, stir together flour, brown sugar, baking powder, baking soda, cinnamon, and light salt. (If honey is used, add it to the wet ingredients).

Add dry ingredients to wet and stir just until moistened. Batter will be thick. (If slightly thinner batter is desired, thin with 1-2 tablespoons non-fat milk or water.)

Preheat a nonstick skillet or griddle over medium-low heat. Grease lightly, using ½-1 teaspoon butter per skillet.

Spoon batter by ¼ cupfuls into skillet. Spread with spoon to make 3- to 4-inch circles.

Cook until tops bubble and edges appear dry, about 2 to 3 minutes. Turn and cook other side until brown.

SERVING SIZE: 6 Servings, 4 Pancakes Each

PER SERVING: Calories 269 **Fiber:** 4 grams **Sodium:** 368 mg.

CORN CAKES

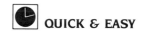 QUICK & EASY

A delicious change of pace, these pancakes are wonderful on a cold winter morning or for a light, cozy fireside supper.

INGREDIENTS

1 CUP WHOLE WHEAT PASTRY FLOUR
½ TEASPOON BAKING POWDER
½ TEASPOON BAKING SODA
¼ TEASPOON LIGHT SALT
1 TABLESPOON SUGAR
1 LARGE EGG

1 CUP BUTTERMILK
¼ CUP NONFAT MILK
1 TABLESPOON BUTTER, MELTED
1 CUP FROZEN WHOLE-KERNEL CORN, THAWED, OR
  1 CUP CANNED CORN, DRAINED

DIRECTIONS

Mix flour, baking powder, baking soda, light salt, and sugar in a medium bowl.

Beat egg until foamy in large bowl. Add buttermilk, milk, and butter. Beat to blend.

Add flour mixture and stir just until moistened. (If a thinner batter is desired, add small amount nonfat milk or water.)

Fold in corn.

Drop batter by scant one-fourth cupfuls onto a medium-hot, nonstick griddle or nonstick skillet. Bake until bottoms are brown and bubbles break on top, about 3 minutes. Turn and bake until done.

SERVING SIZE: 4 Servings, 3 Corn Cakes Each

PER SERVING: Calories 223 **Fiber:** 5 grams **Sodium:** 333 mg.

ZUCCHINI PANCAKES

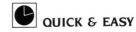 **QUICK & EASY**

INGREDIENTS

3 SMALL ZUCCHINI, 3 CUPS COARSELY GRATED
1 EGG, LIGHTLY BEATEN
2 TABLESPOONS NONFAT MILK
½ CUP WHOLE WHEAT PASTRY FLOUR

1 TEASPOON BAKING POWDER
PINCH NUTMEG
LIGHT SALT AND FRESHLY GROUND PEPPER TO TASTE
2 TEASPOONS BUTTER

DIRECTIONS

Combine all ingredients except butter in a medium bowl.

Melt 1 teaspoon butter in a large nonstick skillet or griddle over medium heat. Using half the mixture, drop by rounded teaspoonfuls into hot fat to form six 3-inch pancakes. Flatten batter slightly, if needed.

Turn heat to low. Brown 3 to 4 minutes per side to allow zucchini to cook. Repeat with remaining fat and batter.

SERVING SIZE: 4 Servings, 3 Pancakes Each

PER SERVING: Calories 103 **Fiber:** 4 grams **Sodium:** 148 mg.

LAZY DUMPLINGS

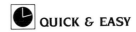 **QUICK & EASY**

The original recipe for lazy dumplings comes from an old Polish cookbook and calls for shaping the soft dough into a rope on a floured board, then cutting off chunks and sliding them into the boiling water. This procedure may have been considered a shortcut at the turn of the century, but by today's flash-fix standards, it didn't merit a "lazy" rating. Luckily, a bit of experimentation proved that we could eliminate the rope step entirely without losing the soft doughy texture and mild cheesy flavor which made these dumplings a childhood favorite.

INGREDIENTS

3 QUARTS WATER
3 LARGE EGGS
1½ CUPS LOW-FAT COTTAGE CHEESE

½ TEASPOON LIGHT SALT
2 CUPS WHOLE WHEAT PASTRY FLOUR

DIRECTIONS

Bring about 3 quarts of water to a rolling boil in a large kettle.

In a blender or food processor, blend eggs, cottage cheese, and light salt until smooth.

Pour mixture into a medium bowl. Add flour and stir just until combined.

Drop dough by teaspoonfuls into the boiling water, about a dozen at a time.

Dumplings will begin floating to the top after they simmer for 1 to 2 minutes and will puff up to about twice their original size.

After about 5 minutes of simmering, when they are all afloat and look light and fluffy, remove from water with a slotted spoon.

Keep dumplings warm while cooking the others.

SERVING SUGGESTION: Traditionally, these high-protein dumplings were served as a Lenten (meatless) entree, with vegetables and a buttered bread-crumb topping. The children always liked them best with just sugar or honey, but they are also delightful topped with parmesan cheese or sprinkled with toasted wheat germ or smothered with applesauce and yogurt, or . . . you get the idea.

SERVING SIZE: 6 Servings, 6 Dumplings Each

PER SERVING: Calories 223 **Fiber:** 4 grams **Sodium:** 351 mg.

POTATO PANCAKES

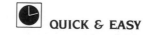 **QUICK & EASY**

... childhood memories of potato pancakes—distinctively flavorful, golden brown cakes, served fresh and hot with applesauce and a dollop of sour cream. They were wonderful, but a rare treat—a special Sunday breakfast or perhaps an early Lenten supper. Making potato pancakes for the whole family was an ordeal. You had to be in the mood to peel, then hand-grate a dozen or so potatoes and an onion or two. (For those of you who have never grated a raw onion, it's a knuckle-scraping, eye-watering experience, at best.) However, with a food processor or a blender, you can treat your family to fresh potato pancakes in less than 30 minutes with nary a nicked knuckle to show for it! Substitute nonfat yogurt for the sour cream and use unsweetened applesauce for the ultimately streamlined version of this very traditional dish.

INGREDIENTS

4 MEDIUM POTATOES (1 LB.)
½ SMALL ONION
2 EGGS
3 TABLESPOONS FLOUR

½ TEASPOON LIGHT SALT
⅛ TEASPOON BLACK PEPPER
4 TEASPOONS BUTTER, FOR FRYING

DIRECTIONS

Scrub or peel potatoes. Peel onion. Cut into 1-inch chunks.

In food processor: Use basic mix-chop blade, process potato and onion until chopped to pea-sized chunks. Add eggs, flour, light salt, and pepper. Process until all ingredients are well combined and potatoes and onions are coarsely ground.

In blender: Place eggs in blender container, add potato and onion chunks. Sprinkle with flour, light salt, and pepper. Blend at low speed just until potatoes are uniformly grated, but not liquified.

Heat 2 teaspoons butter in a large nonstick skillet. Drop half the batter by rounded tablespoonfuls into the hot fat.

Cook over medium-low heat until golden brown, about 3 to 4 minutes on each side. Repeat with other half of batter and serve immediately. Makes about 20-24 dollar-sized cakes.

SERVING SIZE: 4 Servings, 5 to 6 Pancakes Each

PER SERVING: Calories 177   **Fiber:** 2 grams   **Sodium:** 212 mg.

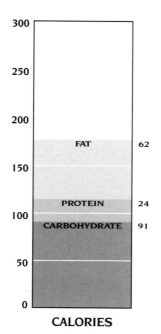

FAT	62
PROTEIN	24
CARBOHYDRATE	91

CALORIES

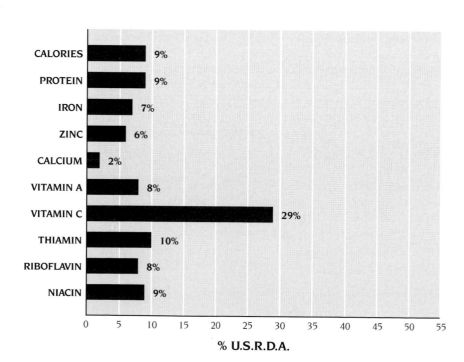

	% U.S.R.D.A.
CALORIES	9%
PROTEIN	9%
IRON	7%
ZINC	6%
CALCIUM	2%
VITAMIN A	8%
VITAMIN C	29%
THIAMIN	10%
RIBOFLAVIN	8%
NIACIN	9%

% U.S.R.D.A.

BANANA FRENCH TOAST

A spectacular breakfast entree, suitable for Sunday brunch at its show-stopping best. Each recipe can be made independently of the others. The toppings are good on pancakes or waffles.

INGREDIENTS

Banana Toast

2 EGGS
2 SMALL RIPE BANANAS
1 TEASPOON CINNAMON
½ TEASPOON VANILLA
4 SLICES WHOLE GRAIN BREAD
½ TABLESPOON BUTTER OR OIL
  ORANGE SLICES, CHOPPED PEANUTS, OR
  CINNAMON FOR GARNISH (OPTIONAL)

Orange Rum Topping

¼ CUP ORANGE JUICE
2 TABLESPOONS RUM
2 SMALL BANANAS

Yogurt Sauce

½ CUP NONFAT YOGURT
1 TEASPOON PEANUT BUTTER
½ TEASPOON VANILLA
  SWEETENER TO TASTE

DIRECTIONS

Preheat oven to 400°.

Prepare French toast batter in a blender or mixing bowl by beating together eggs, bananas, cinnamon, and vanilla.

Lay bread slices in a flat dish, pour batter over bread, and soak while preparing Orange Rum Topping.

To make Orange Rum Topping: Combine orange juice and rum in a measuring cup. Peel bananas and cut in half lengthwise. Lay flat in a small baking dish and pour orange juice and rum over the top. Bake for 10 minutes. Turn oven to broil and brown bananas for 30 seconds. Set aside.

Melt butter in a 10-inch nonstick skillet. Add bread slices and spoon any unabsorbed batter over top.

Brown over a low flame for 8 minutes per side.

While toast and bananas are cooking, prepare Yogurt Sauce by blending yogurt, peanut butter, vanilla, and sweetener in a small bowl.

To serve, warm plates and slice fresh oranges for garnish. On each plate, place 1 slice banana toast and top with half a baked banana. Drizzle with orange rum sauce from the baked bananas and top with a dollop of Yogurt Sauce. Sprinkle with cinnamon or peanuts and garnish with orange slices.

SERVING SIZE: 4 Servings, 1 Slice Each with Toppings

PER SERVING: Calories 244 **Fiber:** 3 grams **Sodium:** 180 mg.

FOCCACIA 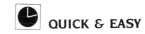 **QUICK & EASY**

"Foccacia" is Italian for "freshly baked bread dough topped with aromatic seasonings." It's something between a light pizza and a fancy garlic bread. Cut it in little squares for hors d'ouvres or in large, satisfying pieces when you just want something delicious. (Pictured on p. 237.)

INGREDIENTS

1 LOAF (1 LB.) FROZEN WHOLE WHEAT BREAD
  DOUGH, THAWED
3 TEASPOONS OLIVE OIL
1 TABLESPOON POLENTA (COARSELY GROUND
  CORN MEAL)

Toppings
Onion

¼ CUP SPAGHETTI SAUCE
½ MEDIUM ONION, THINLY SLICED
2 CLOVES GARLIC, MINCED
1 TABLESPOON FRESH SAGE, CHOPPED, OR 1
  TEASPOON DRIED SAGE LEAF

Continued

PINEAPPLE CHEESE PIE

Cool, smooth and creamy, this pie makes a delightful finish to any meal. We like to dress it up with sliced kiwifruit to serve after a spicy Szechuan dinner. Be sure to plan ahead; this dessert requires an 8-hour head start for proper chilling and is really best made a day ahead.

INGREDIENTS

5 GRAHAM CRACKERS (5-INCH BY 2½-INCH), CRUSHED
¼ CUP ALMONDS, GROUND TO A PASTE, OR 2 TABLESPOONS BUTTER
1 TABLESPOON PLAIN NONFAT YOGURT
¼ CUP WATER
3 TABLESPOONS SUGAR
1 ENVELOPE UNFLAVORED GELATIN
1 CUP UNSWEETENED PINEAPPLE JUICE

3 CUPS LOW-FAT COTTAGE CHEESE
3 TABLESPOONS SUGAR
¼ TEASPOON ORANGE PEEL, GRATED
1 CAN (8½ OZ.) JUICE-PACKED CRUSHED PINEAPPLE
2 TEASPOONS CORNSTARCH
1 TABLESPOON WATER
⅛ TEASPOON ORANGE PEEL, GRATED

DIRECTIONS

Combine graham cracker crumbs, ground almonds or butter, and yogurt. Mix well and press into bottom of an 8-inch springform pan or pie plate sprayed with nonstick cooking spray. Chill.

In blender, combine water, sugar, and gelatin. Let stand for 5 minutes to soften gelatin. Bring pineapple juice to a boil and add it to gelatin. Blend for 30 seconds and let cool to room temperature.

Add cottage cheese and sugar to blender in several additions, blending briefly after each.

Add grated orange peel.

Pour mixture into chilled crust. Refrigerate until firm—several hours or overnight.

About 2 hours before serving, make topping: Bring juice-packed pineapple, cornstarch, and water to a boil, stirring. Cook 1 minute. Add grated orange peel and let cool for 15 minutes. Spread over cheese pie. Chill at least 1 hour more and serve.

SERVING SIZE: 1/12 Recipe

PER SERVING: Calories 131 **Fiber:** 2 grams **Sodium:** 270 mg.

POSSIBLE PUMPKIN PIE

A magical pie that bakes its own crust! It takes 6 minutes to assemble, provides 83% of your daily vitamin A in a single serving and tastes absolutely delicious!

INGREDIENTS

1 CAN (12 OZ.) NONFAT EVAPORATED MILK
2 CUPS COOKED PUMPKIN OR 1 CAN (1 LB.)
2 EGGS
¾ CUP SUGAR
2 TEASPOONS VANILLA
½ CUP WHOLE WHEAT PASTRY FLOUR

¾ TEASPOON BAKING POWDER
¼ TEASPOON LIGHT SALT
2 TABLESPOONS MELTED BUTTER OR OIL
1 TEASPOON CINNAMON
½ TEASPOON GINGER
¼ TEASPOON CLOVES

DIRECTIONS

Heat oven to 350°.

Lightly butter a 9-inch deep-dish pie plate or spray with nonstick cooking spray.

Combine all ingredients in a mixing bowl, blender, or food processor. Blend until smooth (1 minute in blender or processor, 2 minutes with hand mixer).

Pour into prepared pie plate. Bake for 50 to 55 minutes until a knife inserted in the center comes out clean.

SERVING SIZE: 1/8 Recipe

PER SERVING: Calories 202 **Fiber:** 2 grams **Sodium:** 184 mg.

CARROT CAKE

We tried many low-calorie adaptations of carrot cake without success. When we were about to give up, Eve's mother took over, diligently baking a new version each day until she came up with a cake so moist, sweet, and richly flavored, it does not even require an icing! Her secret? Retaining most of the traditional ingredients! Her rationale? If dessert does not taste like dessert, why bother? We agree wholeheartedly; in fact, we even added a ricotta cheese filling! But do not despair, our cake is still just 183 calories per serving, while that classic recipe with cream cheese frosting provides 540 calories for the same size slice!

INGREDIENTS

2¼ CUPS WHOLE WHEAT PASTRY FLOUR
1½ TEASPOONS BAKING POWDER
 1 TEASPOON BAKING SODA
 1 TEASPOON CINNAMON
½ TEASPOON NUTMEG
½ TEASPOON ALLSPICE
¼ TEASPOON CLOVES
¼ TEASPOON LIGHT SALT
 2 LARGE CARROTS, 2 CUPS SHREDDED
 1 CUP WATER
½ CUP GOLDEN RAISINS, CHOPPED

½ CUP HONEY
 2 TABLESPOONS VEGETABLE OIL
½ CUP WALNUTS, FINELY CHOPPED
 2 TABLESPOONS BROWN SUGAR
 1 CAN (8 OZ.) JUICE-PACKED CRUSHED PINEAPPLE (DO NOT DRAIN)
 2 TEASPOONS VANILLA
 2 TEASPOONS FRESH GINGER, THINLY SLICED, THEN GRATED IN FOOD PROCESSOR (TO AVOID "STRINGS")
 POWDERED SUGAR FOR TOPPING

Filling

 1 CUP LOW-FAT RICOTTA CHEESE
1½ TABLESPOONS SUGAR
½ TEASPOON VANILLA

DIRECTIONS

Preheat oven to 350°.

Combine all the listed ingredients in the order given, first blending dry ingredients well, then adding wet ingredients and stirring just until moistened.

Divide the batter between two 9-inch layer cake pans sprayed with nonstick cooking spray or use a 9-inch by 13-inch sheet cake pan.

Bake for about 25 minutes or until knife inserted in center comes out clean.

Cool cakes on rack, then remove from pans.

Combine ricotta cheese, sugar, and vanilla to make cake filling.

Place bottom layer on a serving plate upside down. Spread top only (not sides) with ricotta filling. Place top layer over filling, right side up, sprinkle lightly with powdered sugar, and serve.

SERVING SUGGESTION: For a truly elegant presentation, create a lace pattern, as pictured on p. 261. Just before serving, place a paper doily on top of *cooled* Carrot Cake. Put about ¼ cup powdered sugar in a sieve or flour sifter. Sift sugar over doily. Very carefully remove paper doily leaving the sugar lace pattern.

VARIATION: Napolean Cream is also an excellent filling for this cake (p. 271).

SERVING SIZE: 1⁄16 Recipe

PER SERVING: Calories 183   **Fiber:** 3 grams   **Sodium:** 116 mg.

WALNUT ANGEL CAKE

Light and elegant with an intriguing flavor—our slimmed-down version of an award-winning recipe. (Pictured on p. 261.)

INGREDIENTS

1 CUP WHOLE WHEAT PASTRY FLOUR
1½ CUPS POWDERED SUGAR
½ CUP WALNUTS OR ALMONDS, GROUND OR FINELY CHOPPED
1½ TEASPOONS CINNAMON
12 EGG WHITES (1½ CUPS)

1½ TEASPOONS CREAM OF TARTAR
¼ TEASPOON LIGHT SALT
¾ CUP GRANULATED SUGAR
2 TEASPOONS VANILLA EXTRACT
¼ TEASPOON ALMOND EXTRACT

DIRECTIONS

Preheat oven to 375°.

Combine pastry flour, powdered sugar, ground nuts, and cinnamon in a medium bowl.

Beat egg whites in a large bowl with cream of tartar and light salt until foamy. Gradually beat in all granulated sugar, 2 tablespoons at a time. Continue beating until meringue holds stiff peaks.

Gently fold in vanilla and almond extracts.

Sprinkle dry ingredients over meringue and fold in gently, just until sugar mixture disappears.

Pour into an ungreased angel cake pan. Gently cut through batter five or six times.

Bake for 35 to 40 minutes until a toothpick inserted in the center comes out clean.

Remove from oven and immediately invert by placing a funnel on the counter and inverting cake so air can circulate under it.

When completely cooled, run a spatula around edges of the pan to loosen cake. Turn out onto a cake plate and sprinkle lightly with powdered sugar or drizzle with a thin glaze.

SERVING SIZE: 1/16 Recipe

PER SERVING: Calories 185 **Fiber:** 1 gram **Sodium:** 53 mg.

APPLESAUCE LOAF CAKE

INGREDIENTS

⅓ CUP SUGAR
1 TEASPOON BAKING POWDER
1 TEASPOON BAKING SODA
1 TEASPOON CINNAMON
1 TEASPOON NUTMEG
½ TEASPOON CLOVES

1½ CUPS WHOLE WHEAT PASTRY FLOUR
½ TEASPOON LIGHT SALT
½ CUP RAISINS, CHOPPED
1 TABLESPOON VEGETABLE OIL
2 CUPS UNSWEETENED APPLESAUCE

DIRECTIONS

Preheat oven to 350°.

Mix sugar, baking powder, baking soda, spices, flour, and light salt in a medium bowl.

Add raisins and mix again.

Add oil and applesauce. Stir just until mixed.

Turn batter into a 9-inch by 5-inch loaf pan that has been sprayed with nonstick cooking spray.

Bake for 45 minutes to 1 hour or until a toothpick inserted in the center comes out clean.

SERVING SIZE: 1 Large Slice, ⅛ Recipe

PER SERVING: Calories 169 **Fiber:** 4 grams **Sodium:** 229 mg.

RICOTTA CHEESECAKE

A solid, firmly textured cheesecake with a ruby crown of cherries and an almond-studded crust. (Pictured on p. 261.)

INGREDIENTS

Graham Cracker Crust

- ¾ CUP GRAHAM CRACKER CRUMBS (8, 2-INCH SQUARES)
- ⅓ CUP ALMONDS, FINELY CHOPPED
- ⅓ CUP SUGAR
- 2 TABLESPOONS BUTTER

Filling

- RIND OF 1 LEMON, GRATED
- 4 TABLESPOONS LEMON JUICE
- 1 LB. LOW-FAT (PART-SKIM) RICOTTA CHEESE
- 3 EGGS

Filling (continued)

- ½ CUP NONFAT YOGURT
- ⅓ CUP SUGAR
- ½ TEASPOON LIGHT SALT
- 1½ TEASPOONS VANILLA EXTRACT
- ½ TEASPOON ALMOND EXTRACT

Topping

- 1 CAN (1 LB.) SOUR CHERRIES, PITTED
- 6 TABLESPOONS SUGAR
- 2 TABLESPOONS CORNSTARCH
- ¼ TEASPOON ALMOND EXTRACT

DIRECTIONS

Preheat oven to 350°.

Thoroughly combine graham cracker crumbs, chopped almonds, sugar, and butter. Press into the bottom of a buttered 8-inch springform pan.

Blend all filling ingredients in food processor or blender for 5 minutes until very smooth.

Pour over crumb crust and bake for 1 hour. Remove from oven. (Center will not look done, but will solidify as cake cools.) Cool to room temperature.

Drain all liquid from cherries into a 2-cup measure. Add water to make 1½ cups.

In a medium saucepan, combine sugar and cornstarch. Gradually add cherry liquid, stirring to dissolve cornstarch.

Heat, stirring constantly, until mixture thickens and becomes clear.

Remove from heat; add almond extract and cherries. Stir gently to combine.

Cover and allow mixture to cool to room temperature.

Spread topping on cooled cheesecake. Chill.

VARIATION: Spiked Cherry Cheesecake. Add a shot of kirsch or brandy to topping along with the cherries.

SERVING SIZE: 1/12 Recipe

PER SERVING: Calories 233 **Fiber:** 2 grams **Sodium:** 170 mg.

OLD-FASHIONED RICE PUDDING

A dessert Grandmother made, rice pudding is as nourishing and comforting now as it was then.

INGREDIENTS

- 3 CUPS NONFAT MILK
- 3 EGGS
- ½ CUP SUGAR
- 2 TEASPOONS VANILLA
- ½ TEASPOON CINNAMON
- 2 CUPS COOKED BROWN RICE
- ½ CUP RAISINS
- NUTMEG

Continued

DIRECTIONS

Cook rice if necessary.

Preheat oven to 350°.

Scald milk by heating to just below boiling.

Beat eggs in a medium bowl. Add sugar, vanilla, and cinnamon. Continue beating until frothy.

Slowly add scalded milk, beating continuously.

When blended, stir in cooked rice and raisins.

Turn mixture into a 2-quart baking dish or into eight custard cups. Sprinkle with nutmeg.

Put baking dish or custard cups into a large, shallow pan on the oven rack. Pour very hot water into the large pan to come to within ½-inch of the top of the baking dish or custard cups.

Bake for 45 to 55 minutes until a knife inserted 1 inch from the edge comes out clean.

Remove from water to cool.

SERVING SIZE: 8 Servings, ⅔ Cup Each

PER SERVING: Calories 193 **Fiber:** 2 grams **Sodium:** 142 mg.

LOIS GORDON'S BREAD PUDDING

Carla and her brother Geff grew up in a century-old Victorian farmhouse in the grape country near Lodi, California. When the kitchen bread box filled up with leftover odds and ends of bread, they knew it wouldn't be long until Mom made bread pudding. And now, this homey dessert is also a favorite of Carla's daughter Kristin and her cousins, Matthew and Daniel.

INGREDIENTS

2 CUPS NONFAT MILK

2 TABLESPOONS BUTTER

2 CUPS CUBED WHOLE WHEAT BREAD (ABOUT 5 SLICES)

½ CUP SUGAR

1 TEASPOON CINNAMON

1 TEASPOON NUTMEG

DASH CLOVES

DASH LIGHT SALT

1 TEASPOON VANILLA

1 CUP RAISINS

Lemon Sauce

1 TABLESPOON CORNSTARCH

¼ CUP HONEY

1 TEASPOON GRATED LEMON RIND

1 CUP WATER

¼ CUP LEMON JUICE

1 TABLESPOON BUTTER

DIRECTIONS

Preheat oven to 350°.

Heat, but do not boil milk. Remove from heat. Add butter to hot milk, stirring to melt.

In a small bowl, mix sugar, cinnamon, nutmeg, cloves, and light salt, if desired.

Spray an 8-inch square baking dish with nonstick cooking spray. Place bread cubes in dish. Sprinkle with sugar and spice mixture. Pour hot milk and butter over the bread and let stand until cooled.

Add vanilla and raisins. Stir gently to mix.

Bake, uncovered, for 1 hour until top is brown and mixture is set.

Meanwhile, make sauce by mixing cornstarch, honey, lemon rind, and water in a small saucepan. Bring to boiling over medium heat. Boil, stirring constantly, for 5 minutes. Remove from heat and blend in lemon juice and butter. If sauce is too tart, a small amount of additional honey may be stirred in.

Serve sauce over pudding. It's good either warm or cold.

SERVING SIZE: 8 Servings, ½ Cup Each

PER SERVING: Calories 233 **Fiber:** 2 grams **Sodium:** 157 mg.

BANANA CREAM PUDDING

This oldie but goodie is smooth, sweet, delicious—and so nutritious you'll feel good about serving it to the ones you love.

INGREDIENTS

⅔ CUP SUGAR
¼ CUP CORNSTARCH
½ TEASPOON LIGHT SALT
3 CUPS NONFAT MILK
4 EGG YOLKS
4 TEASPOONS VANILLA
3 MEDIUM BANANAS, QUARTERED OR HALVED LENGTHWISE, THEN SLICED

DIRECTIONS

Stir together sugar, cornstarch, and light salt in a medium saucepan.
Blend milk and egg yolks. Gradually pour into sugar mixture, stirring to dissolve lumps.
Cook over medium heat, stirring constantly, until pudding thickens and begins to boil.
Remove from heat and stir in vanilla. Cover pan to prevent skin from forming. Cool to room temperature.
Stir sliced bananas into cooled pudding. Spoon into six small bowls. Cover and chill.

VARIATION: Banana Cream Pie. Slice bananas into a 9-inch prebaked pie shell. Pour cooled pudding over bananas. Chill.

SERVING SIZE: 6 Servings, ¾ Cup Each

PER SERVING: Calories 257 **Fiber:** 1 gram **Sodium:** 165 mg.

CORN PUDDING

A simple, satisfying dessert that's not too sweet.

INGREDIENTS

½ CUP SUGAR
3 TABLESPOONS CORNSTARCH
2 EGGS
1 CAN (1 LB.) CREAM-STYLE CORN
1 CAN (12 OZ.) EVAPORATED NONFAT MILK

DIRECTIONS

Preheat oven to 350°.
In a medium bowl, mix sugar and cornstarch.
Add eggs, corn, and milk. Mix well.
Pour into a 1½-quart baking dish which has been sprayed with nonstick cooking spray.
Bake for 1 hour or until the center is firm.
Serve warm or cold.

SERVING SIZE: 8 Servings, ½ Cup Each

PER SERVING: Calories 172 **Fiber:** 3 grams **Sodium:** 223 mg.

VALERIE'S CHOCOLATE MOUSSE

Valerie Parker, co-author of *Lowfat Lifestyle*, was kind enough to let us use her prize recipe. She prepares this chocolate mousse when she gives cooking demonstrations and tells us, "This recipe convinces even nonbelievers that low-fat eating can be fabulous!"

INGREDIENTS

- 1 TABLESPOON INSTANT COFFEE
- 1 TABLESPOON BOILING WATER
- 4 OZ. SEMISWEET CHOCOLATE
- 2 EGGS PLUS 2 EGG WHITES
- 4 TABLESPOONS SUGAR
- 2 TABLESPOONS BRANDY

DIRECTIONS

Dissolve coffee in boiling water in a small saucepan. Add chocolate and melt slowly over very low heat. Let cool.

Separate eggs and beat the 4 egg whites until stiff. Set aside.

In a separate bowl but with the same beaters, beat the 2 yolks until thick. Add sugar and beat until well dissolved.

Pour cooled chocolate-coffee mixture and brandy into egg yolks and stir until well mixed. Fold this mixture carefully into the beaten egg whites.

Fill six small dessert dishes and chill for 4 hours before serving.

SERVING SIZE: 6 Servings, ½ Cup Each

PER SERVING: Calories 175 **Fiber:** 0 **Sodium:** 37 mg.

PUMPKIN PIE CUSTARD

Pumpkin pie flavor without a calorie-laden crust! This sweet indulgence assembles in minutes and provides 4 days worth of vitamin A in a single serving!

INGREDIENTS

- 1 CAN (12 OZ.) EVAPORATED SKIM MILK
- 2 EGGS
- 1 CAN (1 LB.) PUMPKIN
- ¾ CUP SUGAR
- 1 TEASPOON CINNAMON
- ¼ TEASPOON CLOVES
- ½ TEASPOON GINGER
- ½ TEASPOON LIGHT SALT

DIRECTIONS

Preheat oven to 375°.

Select a deep-dish pie pan, a 10-inch quiche pan, or eight individual custard dishes. Spray with nonstick cooking spray.

In a blender, processor, or mixer bowl, blend all ingredients well.

Pour custard into prepared pan or dishes. Place in a large, flat baking pan. Pour hot water into the large pan to come to within ½ inch of the top of the custard dishes.

Place in oven and bake at 375° for about 1 hour for a large custard or 40 minutes for individual dishes. Custard is done when a knife inserted in the center comes out clean.

SERVING SIZE: 8 Servings, ½ Cup Each

PER SERVING: Calories 142 **Fiber:** 1 gram **Sodium:** 141 mg.

NAPOLEAN CREAM

A very thick custard sauce, this can be used as a cake filling or served with fruit for dessert.

INGREDIENTS

1 CUP NONFAT MILK
1 EGG
2 TABLESPOONS SUGAR

2 TABLESPOONS WHITE FLOUR
½ TEASPOON VANILLA EXTRACT

DIRECTIONS

Heat milk to scalding (just to the point that it begins to foam, but not boil) in a medium-sized, heavy saucepan.

Beat egg until frothy in a blender or small mixing bowl. Add sugar and continue beating until smooth and cream colored.

With blender or mixer running on low speed, slowly pour hot milk into egg mixture. Add flour. Beat just long enough to combine. Return mixture to saucepan.

Over medium heat, bring mixture to a boil stirring constantly. Boil 1 minute and stir until thickened. Remove from heat and stir in vanilla.

Turn mixture into a small bowl. Lay plastic wrap over surface of custard to prevent a skin from forming. Chill. Makes 1 cup.

SERVING SIZE: 4 Servings, ¼ Cup Each

PER SERVING: Calories 72 **Fiber:** 0 **Sodium:** 47 mg.

PIÑA COLADA WHIP

A thick, rich, flavorful pudding—almost a mousse—Piña Colada Whip is an elegant finale for any meal, especially when served in crystal stemware. (Pictured on p. 261.)

INGREDIENTS

1 ENVELOPE UNFLAVORED GELATIN
3 TABLESPOONS COLD WATER
1 CAN (20 OZ.) JUICE-PACKED CRUSHED PINEAPPLE
1 EGG
2½ TABLESPOONS SUGAR

1½ TEASPOONS RUM EXTRACT
½ TEASPOON VANILLA EXTRACT
1⅓ CUP LOW-FAT (PART SKIM) RICOTTA CHEESE
2 TEASPOONS SHREDDED COCONUT FOR GARNISH (OPTIONAL)
SLICED KIWIFRUIT GARNISH (OPTIONAL)

DIRECTIONS

Put gelatin in blender or food processor and add cold water. Let stand 2 minutes to soften.

Drain pineapple juice into a measuring cup. Add water to make 1 cup. In a saucepan or microwave, bring juice to a boil, then pour over softened gelatin in blender. Process for 30 seconds to dissolve.

Add egg; blend 30 seconds more.

Add sugar, rum extract, and vanilla. Blend again for 30 seconds.

Add about half of the pineapple and all of the ricotta. Blend until smooth, about 3 minutes. Pour mixture into a bowl and stir in remaining pineapple. Do not blend.

Ladle into eight individual dessert dishes or one 8-inch soufflé dish. Chill at least 2 hours. Just before serving, garnish with shredded coconut or sliced fresh kiwifruit.

SERVING SIZE: 8 Servings, ½ Cup Each

PER SERVING: Calories 132 **Fiber:** 1 gram **Sodium:** 61 mg.

FRUIT GELATIN MOUSSE

This versatile mousse can be used as a tangy salad or refreshing dessert. Simply vary the gelatin flavors, yogurts, and fruits.

INGREDIENTS

1 PACKAGE (0.6 OZ.) SUGAR-FREE FRUIT-FLAVORED GELATIN (8-SERVING SIZE)
2 CUPS BOILING WATER
1 CONTAINER (8 OZ.) PLAIN OR FRUIT-FLAVORED NONFAT YOGURT
1 CAN (15 OZ.) JUICE-PACKED CRUSHED PINEAPPLE
¾ CUP COLD WATER

DIRECTIONS

Pour gelatin into a medium bowl and add 2 cups boiling water per package directions, stirring to dissolve.

Put hot mixture in blender or food processor. Add yogurt and whirl until frothy and well mixed.

Add pineapple with its juice; blend briefly just to mix.

Return mixture to a bowl and add cold water. (If a molded mousse is desired, omit cold water.) Stir.

Chill several hours until set. Mousse can be chilled in its mixing bowl or individual serving dishes.

VARIATIONS: Strawberry Banana Mousse. Use strawberry-flavored gelatin, 2 cups boiling water, and plain yogurt, as above. Substitute 2 large ripe bananas for the pineapple and juice. Blend till smooth, omit cold water. Fold in 2 cups fresh or frozen sliced strawberries. Chill in parfait glasses. (6 Servings; 90 calories, 104 mg. sodium each.)

Lemon Creme. Use lemon-flavored gelatin, 2 cups boiling water, and vanilla-flavored yogurt. (To keep calories to a minimum, use nonfat plain yogurt, as above, plus ½ teaspoon vanilla and sweetener to taste.) Substitute 1½ cups cold nonfat milk for canned pineapple. Omit cold water. Chill in a 1-quart mold. (6 servings; 48 calories, 136 mg. sodium each.)

Lemon-Raspberry Bombe. Make lemon creme, as above. Fold in 3 cups fresh or frozen raspberries. Chill in a fancy 6-cup mold. (6 servings; 79 calories, 136 mg. sodium each.)

SERVING SIZE: 6 Servings, 1 Cup Each

PER SERVING: Calories 76 **Fiber:** 1 gram **Sodium:** 104 mg.

OATMEAL RAISIN COOKIES

Eliminating fat and sugar completely transforms a cookie recipe into a recipe for soggy crackers. These cookies are a happy compromise—with just enough sugar and butter to keep the cookie quality and plenty of whole grain nutrition to rationalize the calories. When this recipe was tested by Carla's 10-year-old daughter, Kristin, she used chocolate chips because, as Kristin puts it, "Raisins are just plain yucky!"

INGREDIENTS

3 CUPS ROLLED OATS
1 CUP WHOLE WHEAT PASTRY FLOUR
1 TEASPOON LIGHT SALT
1 TEASPOON BAKING SODA
1-2 TEASPOONS CINNAMON (OPTIONAL)
½ CUP RAISINS, CHOCOLATE CHIPS, CAROB CHIPS, NUTS, OR DATES

¼ CUP BUTTER, MELTED
1 CUP BROWN SUGAR, PACKED
2 EGGS
½ CUP PLAIN NONFAT YOGURT
1 TEASPOON VANILLA

DIRECTIONS

Preheat oven to 350°.

Combine oats, flour, baking soda, light salt, cinnamon, if desired, and raisins (or other choice).

Beat butter, brown sugar, eggs, yogurt, and vanilla in a large bowl until creamy.

Add dry ingredients and mix well.

Spray cookie sheet with nonstick cooking spray. Drop by rounded teaspoonfuls onto cookie sheet and bake for 12 to 15 minutes.

SERVING SIZE: Makes 4 Dozen Cookies

PER COOKIE: Calories 65 **Fiber:** 1 gram **Sodium:** 41 mg.

GIANT GINGER COOKIES

INGREDIENTS

2 CUPS WHOLE WHEAT PASTRY FLOUR
1½ TEASPOONS BAKING SODA
1 TEASPOON GROUND CLOVES
½ TEASPOON LIGHT SALT
2 OZ. FRESH GINGER ROOT (ABOUT A 4-INCH PIECE), 3-4 TABLESPOONS PROCESSED

¼ CUP BUTTER
1 CUP SUGAR
1 EGG
2 TABLESPOONS DARK CORN SYRUP
2 TABLESPOONS SUGAR
½ TEASPOON GROUND CINNAMON

DIRECTIONS

Combine flour, baking soda, cloves, and light salt in a large bowl.

Peel ginger root, slice thinly, and grate in food processor or spice grinder. (You should have 3 to 4 tablespoons ground ginger root.)

Cream butter with sugar and egg until light and fluffy. Beat in corn syrup, then grated ginger.

Add wet ingredients to dry. Stir to combine thoroughly. Turn dough out of bowl onto a sheet of plastic wrap or waxed paper. Wrap tightly and refrigerate until easy to handle (2 hours, up to a week).

When ready to bake, preheat oven to 350°.

Spray two large cookie sheets with nonstick cooking spray.

Cut dough ball in half. Divide each half into eight equal pieces.

Roll each piece into a 2-inch ball.

Combine sugar and cinnamon in a small bowl. Roll cookies in this mixture, then place them 3 inches apart on prepared cookie sheets.

Bake one sheet at a time for 15 to 18 minutes until very lightly browned.

Cool on wire racks.

SERVING SIZE: 16 Cookies—4-inch diameter—1 Cookie Each

PER SERVING: Calories 139 **Fiber:** 2 grams **Sodium:** 150 mg.

STRAWBERRY RHUBARB SAUCE

Strawberries and rhubarb combine beautifully in this rose-pink compote. It's wonderful over ice-milk or stirred into vanilla yogurt.

INGREDIENTS

¼ CUP SUGAR
¾ CUP HOT WATER
2 CUPS FRESH STRAWBERRIES, RINSED, TRIMMED, AND HALVED
½ LB. FRESH RHUBARB, ABOUT 2 CUPS RINSED, TRIMMED, AND CUT INTO 1-INCH PIECES
4 SPRIGS FRESH MINT FOR GARNISH (OPTIONAL)

Continued on p. 274.

DIRECTIONS

Stir sugar and water together in a 1½ quart shallow
  baking dish until sugar is partially dissolved.
  Add strawberries and rhubarb. Stir to combine.
Place in cold oven. Turn to 350°.
Bake until rhubarb is tender, 25 to 30 minutes.
  Baste once or twice during baking, but do not
  stir. Set dish on wire rack to cool. Refrigerate to
  chill slightly before serving, if desired.
Spoon into serving dishes. Garnish each with a
  mint sprig, if desired.

SERVING SIZE: 4 Servings, ½ Cup Each

PER SERVING: Calories 88   **Fiber:** 3 grams   **Sodium:** 1 mg.

MICROWAVE DIRECTIONS

Pour sugar and water into a 3-quart glass dish. Stir
  to dissolve sugar partially.
Add rhubarb and strawberries. Stir gently.
Cover and microwave on high until rhubarb is ten-
  der, about 8 minutes. Let stand 2 minutes.
Remove cover and move to a wire rack to cool.
Refrigerate to chill slightly before serving, if
  desired.

BAKED APPLES AND PEARS

Cinnamon and lemon peel add a special zest to these baked apples and pears. They've always
been a favorite at the Bailey Fitness Seminars.

INGREDIENTS

   4 LARGE APPLES (ROME BEAUTIES ARE BEST)*
   4 LARGE PEARS
   4 TABLESPOONS SUGAR
      PEEL OF 1 LARGE LEMON, SLIVERED
   1 TEASPOON CINNAMON
   ½ CUP WATER

DIRECTIONS

Preheat oven to 350°.
Remove yellow outer peel from lemon with potato peeler, then cut into thin slivers.
Core apples and pears. Arrange in a large shallow baking dish, so each fruit is upright.
Mix sugar, lemon peel, and cinnamon.
Fill hollowed out fruit with this mixture. Pour water around fruit into bottom of dish.
Bake, uncovered, for 30 minutes (or omit water and microwave on high 12 to 15 minutes
  in a covered baking dish).
Spoon sauce from pan over fruit before serving.

SERVING SIZE: 8 Servings, 1 Apple or 1 Pear Each

PER SERVING: Calories 152   **Fiber:** 5 grams   **Sodium:** 2 mg.

*Any apple can be used, but Rome beauties are nice
because their skins don't split during baking.

MERINGUE KISSES (BEZY)

From the French *bese*, to kiss. These light, airy, delicate, and formal meringue kisses are incredibly low in calories. They're so sweet they taste deceptively fattening, yet they're nothing more than whipped egg white with a pinch of sugar. (Pictured on p. 261.)

INGREDIENTS

2 EGG WHITES (AT ROOM TEMPERATURE)
¼ TEASPOON CREAM OF TARTAR
¼ TEASPOON LEMON EXTRACT
½ CUP SUPERFINE SUGAR (OR GRANULATED SUGAR, WHIRLED IN BLENDER OR PROCESSOR UNTIL FINELY GROUND)
    OTHER FLAVORING INGREDIENTS, AS DESIRED (SEE VARIATIONS)

DIRECTIONS

Preheat oven to 225°.

Line a large baking sheet with aluminum foil or paper (waxed, brown, or parchment all work well).

Beat egg whites and cream of tartar in a small, deep bowl with an electric mixer at high speed until foamy.

Add lemon extract.

Add sugar, about 2 tablespoons at a time, beating constantly until sugar is dissolved and whites are glossy and stand in stiff peaks. (To test meringue, rub a little between your fingers to feel if the sugar has dissolved.)

Gently fold in variation ingredients as desired. Food coloring may be added.

Drop by rounded teaspoonfuls or pipe through a pastry tube onto lined baking sheet.

Bake for about 1 hour until firm. Turn oven off. Let kisses stand in oven with the door closed until cool, dry, and crisp (at least 1 additional hour.)

Store in a tightly sealed container. If they become soggy, you can refresh them by placing in a preheated oven at 200° for 15 minutes.

VARIATIONS*

Coconut Almond: ¼ teaspoon almond extract and 1 tablespoon shredded coconut.

Almond: 2 tablespoons ground almonds and ½ teaspoon almond extract.

Citrus: ¼ teaspoon lemon extract and ½ teaspoon grated orange peel.

Chocolate: ¼ cup unsweetened cocoa powder and 1 teaspoon vanilla.

Chocolate Mint: ¼ cup unsweetened cocoa powder and ¼ teaspoon mint extract.

Mint: ¼ teaspoon mint extract and a drop of green food coloring.

SERVING SIZE: 36 Kisses, 1 Kiss Each

PER SERVING: Calories 12   **Fiber:** 0   **Sodium:** 3 mg.

*Any flavoring or very finely chopped dried fruit or nuts can be added successfully in small quantities. Take care though not to add wet ingredients or the whole mountain of meringue turns into a little puddle at the bottom of the bowl.

INDEX